**TOM VENUTO** is a fat-loss expert, health and fitness writer, and steroid-free bodybuilder with more than 25 years of experience. Tom holds a degree in exercise science and is a member of the American College of Sports Medicine (ACSM), the International Society of Sports Nutrition (ISSN), the National Strength and Conditioning Association (NSCA), and the International Association for the Study of Obesity (IASO). Tom was praised by O magazine as being 'honest' about what it really takes to lose weight, and Greatist.com named Tom one of the 100 most influential people in fitness. Visit Tom's website at www.BurnTheFatFeedTheMuscle.com.

# BURN THE FAT

# FEED THE MUSCLE

**The Secrets of the Leanest People in the World**

# TOM VENUTO

**V**ermilion
LONDON

First published in 2013 by Vermilion, an imprint of Ebury Publishing
A Random House Group company

First published in the USA by The Crown Publishing Group,
a division of Random House, Inc., in 2013

The Random House Group Limited Reg. No. 954009

Addresses for companies within the Random House Group can be found at
www.randomhouse.co.uk

Penguin Random House is committed to a sustainable future for
our business, our readers and our planet. This book is made from
Forest Stewardship Council® certified paper.

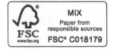

Printed and bound in Great Britain by Clays Ltd, Elcograf S.p.A.

ISBN 9780091954925

To buy books by your favourite authors and register for offers visit
www.randomhouse.co.uk

# CONTENTS

## ACTIVATE: CARDIO TRAINING (The 3rd Element) 229

## NEW BODY: WEIGHT TRAINING (The 4th Element) 253

## THE NEXT LEVEL: ADVANCED STRATEGIES 286

## APPENDIX: EXTRA TOOLS

## ACKNOWLEDGEMENTS 329

## ONLINE RESOURCES 330

# My Story: From Fat Boy to Fat-Loss Expert

I wasn't always a best-selling author, personal trainer, and fat-loss expert, getting written up in *Men's Fitness* and *O, The Oprah Magazine*. I certainly wasn't winning bodybuilding contests or doing photo shoots. All that came much later. At first, I simply had to be honest with myself. I was getting chubby. I was never obese, but I do know what it feels like to hate my body and be paralysed with self-consciousness.

When I was a 14-year-old freshman in high school, that's when it hit me: I had a roll of fat around my waist and what I thought was the worst affliction a warm-blooded male teenager could have – "man boobs." I dreaded taking my shirt off for swimming class, and when we played basketball in the gym, I prayed I'd be called to play for "shirts," not "skins," so nobody would see my "moobs" and ab flab jiggling up and down the court.

That same year, I watched a movie called *Conan the Barbarian*, starring Arnold Schwarzenegger. The moment I saw Arnold on the big screen, my whole world stopped. I stared, frozen in awe. I had seen cartoons and superhero characters with that kind of body, but I couldn't believe a real human being could look like that: He had gladiator pecs with slabs of muscle inches thick, shoulders like cannonballs, the V-shaped back tapering down to the tiny waistline, chiselled six-pack abs, and the arms – they were the most mind-blowing of all – huge, sinewy and rock hard, with biceps like mountain peaks. It was the most awesome physique I'd ever seen. That was the moment I knew I wanted muscles.

The next day at the newsstand, I picked up a magazine that had a cover photo of Arnold as Conan, slathered in warpaint, gripping a sword, biceps bulging. I thumbed through the pages and was blown away a second time. The magazine was filled with pictures of dozens of men who looked a lot like Arnold, and women who looked like "warrior goddesses" straight out of the fantasy novels. None of the bodies in that *Muscle and Fitness* magazine seemed to have an ounce of fat on them.

When I saw an ad for Arnold's book *Arnold: The Education of a Bodybuilder*, I bought it on the spot and devoured it in a day. It was part autobiography, part training manual, and I started doing the workouts from the back of the book. The first programme consisted of body weight, or what Arnold called "freehand" exercises. I did it for a month but got bored very quickly. He emphasized that these were not sissy exercises, and anyone who has tried a body weight pull-up the first time knows it's true. But I wanted to do what Arnold did – pump iron – so I moved on to the "real workouts" – the ones with barbells and dumbbells in chapter 17.

From the first workout, I was hooked. If you wanted to stop me from training, you'd have had to pry the barbell out of my cold, dead hands. I kept after it. By my senior year in high school I didn't look anything like Arnold, but I had put on about 25 pounds (11 kg) of muscle. I was stronger and I did look a lot better. But I didn't have it right yet. I had been building up the muscle, but the whole burning-fat part eluded me.

After four years of lifting weights, my abs were still hidden underneath my belly fat. I still couldn't take my shirt off in public without feeling self-conscious. Maybe you can relate to this feeling. You've worked hard for a long time, maybe years, but still feel trapped inside a body that's not doing what you want, no matter what you try. You think your frustration just can't get any worse. Well, mine did.

It happened when I went to college … and discovered beer. Combined with late-night pizza, cheese fries, and burgers, plus hungover Sunday morning binges on syrup-smothered pancakes, I quickly gained the classic "freshman 15" (for me, it was more like 20). I was now 45 pounds (20 kg) heavier than I was when I started high school, so I was no pipsqueak, but believe me, it wasn't all muscle. I was what you'd call "bulked up." My college roommates even had a nickname for me: "Bob's Big Boy," after the fast food restaurant's chubby mascot. Sometimes they just called me "Fat Boy."

I took the taunting quietly and laughed along with them, but deep down I was humiliated because I was a die-hard bodybuilding fan and self-proclaimed "muscle guy," but I had a beer belly to go with my biceps. What made matters worse was that I'd declared my major in exercise science. I was in college, planning for a career in fitness after graduation, but my behaviour and physical condition were incongruent with my goals. I felt like a hypocrite.

I knew at that point I had to do something. Fortunately, I never stopped lifting weights. Even with one foot in the college party lifestyle, I still kept the other in the gym. My friends at the gym always supported me and told me exactly what to do: Enter a bodybuilding contest for motivation. Why not? I had already built the foundation of muscle underneath the fat. I'd thought about competing before and prattled on about doing it all the time. But up until then I was all talk and no walk. The only title I had won was "Mr. Procrastinator."

Something had to give, or I would be the laughing stock of my gym as well as the clients I would soon be training. It wasn't until my gym buddies challenged me to stop talking and commit to training for a contest that everything started to change.

I finally got serious about figuring out what these guys were doing right. They certainly were doing something to get lean and ripped that I wasn't doing.

I read everything I could get my hands on about competition prep and picked the brain of every bodybuilder I met. My training partners and gym friends who had already competed taught me their unique "bodybuilder's diet" that they used to strip off all the fat, right down to the six-pack abs – just like the models in the magazines. I paid attention, I listened, and I took action.

I started working out and eating in a certain way, and it quickly became clear that I was onto something. "Contest training" was by far the most effective programme I had ever followed. My body was changing faster than ever and the belly fat seemed to melt away by the day.

I came to some realizations about my past mistakes. First, I knew I'd been missing a major piece of the puzzle. It's not enough to work out; you have to get the nutrition right. That's the most important element. The cliché "You can't out-train a bad diet" is absolutely true. When I added the proper nutrition on top of the right training, the magic started happening. Second, I realized the importance of having a goal and an emotional reason why you absolutely must achieve that goal.

This combination of nutrition and training with a motivating goal worked so well that I not only got second place in my first competition, I did better every time I stepped onstage. I won my weight class in my second competition and I won the overall title in my third. I captured the Pennsylvania, New Jersey, and New York state championships and then went on to regional competition, winning the mid-Atlantic states and my weight class at the Natural Eastern Classic. I went as far as runner-up at the Natural Mr. America and Natural North America. All of these competitions were drug tested and I reached contest condition 100 per cent drug-free.

Beer belly? Gone. Moobs? Nowhere in sight. I traded the six-packs of beer for six-pack abs. I was not only ripped for the first time in my life (finally!), my abs were on the front page of the sports section in our small-town newspaper! It wasn't long before I was in the magazines.

Maybe you've seen that old Charles Atlas ad where the skinny kid gets sand kicked in his face by a muscle-bound bully, then gets in shape and beats up the bully? That's kind of how it felt. It felt like redemption. It was like getting to tell the world, "Hey, remember that kid from gym class with the man boobs? Well, take a look at this!" I'm not saying any of this was easy. I'm saying it was worth it.

I'm also not telling you this story to brag or hold myself up as some kind of "poster boy." Quite the opposite. For years I've been an under-the-radar kind of coach and athlete, who doesn't care much about being in the limelight. I get more satisfaction from making fitness stars out of my clients and readers. There are literally thousands of my client's stories that are more inspiring than mine ... stories from ordinary men and women who have no interest in entering a bodybuilding contest, yet use this same "bodybuilder science" to achieve their own personal goals, with massive success.

I've always loved seeing other people succeed, so immediately after graduating, armed with a degree, two certifications, and eight years of experience training myself, I dived headfirst into my career training others. I worked with hundreds of men and women one-on-one in the gym. Even though I was a trainer, not a nutritionist, my appreciation for the nutrition element in the fat-loss equation continued to grow when I saw how two clients followed the same workout but one got better results than the other. None of them were slackers. My clients trained their butts off. The difference was what they did when they left the gym. Some of them controlled what they ate and drank and some of them didn't.

When I realized that my clients' diets were making or breaking the results of our workouts, I knew I had to give them guidance about what to eat. Left to their own devices, who knows what they would have done? They might have followed one of those weird weight-loss gimmicks they saw in the tabloids or on TV. They might have resorted to diet pills. Or they might have done it right, all week long, only to undo it in one weekend binge. The first thing that popped into my mind was "Why don't I show them how I do it?" I was working in mainstream health clubs, so very few of my clients were bodybuilders. But I figured if I could go from a "fat boy" chugging six-packs of beer to a bodybuilder with six-pack abs, why wouldn't the same system work for my clients?

Put simply, if you want to learn how to get really lean, who better to learn from than the leanest people in the world? So I decided to share the secrets. I wrote down my fat-burning formula and gave it to my clients. It worked like magic! For all of them! Men and women. From soccer moms to stockbrokers. From twenty-somethings to retirees.

As I kept teaching my method to my personal-training clients, I also launched a coaching programme for people who wanted more intensive nutrition guidance, combined with the accountability of a personal motivation coach. After 600 clients completed my 12-week coaching programme, I had it down to a science. I realized that as long as the nutrition was customized for each individual, it would work for almost anyone to achieve any goal, whether that was burning the last few pounds of stubborn fat or overcoming serious obesity, from just "firming up" to "ripping up," from brides shaping up for weddings to guys chiselling down for the beach.

By this point, I had amassed an incredible amount of real-world data from all kinds of people. I had also developed a food and nutrition manual to give to all my training clients. One day when I was printing out the manual for a client consultation, it occurred to me that if I added a few more pieces of vital information, I would have my entire coaching system transferred into book form. I went to work, and with some late nights and a lot of strong coffee, in a few months I held the first-ever copy of *Burn the Fat, Feed the Muscle*.

It was 2003. It had taken me nearly 14 years of trial, error, research, and experimentation to put the system together. I had already used it to help hundreds of clients transform their bodies, one person at a time. I had also written a mission statement for myself:

**I will coach and inspire as many people as possible to strengthen and transform their bodies and reach all their health and fitness goals, the natural way.**

To be true to my mission, I had to ask myself, "How can I help more people?" It didn't take long to find an answer. A colleague told me that getting a publisher was "almost impossible" when you're an unknown personal trainer. So he self-published his books and made them available on the Internet for instant downloads. I said, "Wait a minute. You mean I don't have to print these or haul them to the post office? And people can download this in any country? And my readers don't have to wait – they get the books instantly? And I can do it all myself?"

He said, "Yes."

I said, "Say no more." I became an Internet publisher too. I put up a new website, started an e-mail newsletter, and made *Burn the Fat, Feed the Muscle* available as an e-book.

Back then, most people didn't even know what e-books were. They said no one would pay for a download; information on the Internet is free. They laughed at me. But, like the critics who told me I'd never make it as a bodybuilder without taking steroids, I ignored them and did it anyway.

The original *Burn the Fat, Feed the Muscle* became an online sensation. It debuted at number one on the fitness e-book charts and stayed there for five years straight, a record that still stands to this day. The book reached customers in 154 countries and built a huge online community. It pioneered the entire fitness e-book industry, which exploded in the next decade. Many other successful authors followed. People went from calling me a fool to calling me the father of fitness e-books.

I could have stopped there and retired or kept chugging along quietly online, but my mission statement, tacked onto my office bulletin board, kept staring me in the face every day. Again I asked, "How can I help more people?" At this point, I was no longer an unknown. Millions of people had visited my website and a quarter of a million were subscribed to my newsletter. Now agents and publishers were knocking on my door. When the offer came to put *Burn the Fat, Feed the Muscle* into a print edition, I had my answer.

This brand-new edition is revised and improved. If the original had any kinks, they've been straightened out. If parts fell out of date, they've been updated. If anything was overcomplicated, it's been simplified. This book contains new material and new workout plans never before published. The flagship training programme is called The New Body 28 (TNB-28). The original TNB was beta tested and fine-tuned for three years by my inner-circle members. The schedule fits a busy lifestyle so well, and the results were so astonishing, it became the most popular and talked-about workout I ever created.

TNB-28 is the latest evolution of the plan. The new workout has been perfected and is now available to you in chapters 16 and 17 of this book, with extra tools and exercise guides available for free on the website at www.BurnTheFatFeedTheMuscle.com.

Although *Burn the Fat, Feed the Muscle* retains every effective core principle of the original, it has been reengineered so that even more people can now easily make the *Burn the Fat* eating principles a part of their lifestyles. In the past, the bodybuilding style of eating was acknowledged as the most powerful and effective system in the world for burning fat and building muscle. But it was also known for being strict, even dogmatic. Not any more. This is the next generation of fat-burning and muscle-building nutrition.

The new *Burn the Fat, Feed the Muscle* is structured and flexible at the same time. You can customize it to fit your schedule, your tastes, and your lifestyle. You can customize your mealtimes, number of meals, type of foods, and even the amount of carbs. No foods are off-limits; you can eat anything you want, if you follow a few reasonable guidelines you'll learn in the nutrition part of the book.

There are four elements to the plan – nutrition, cardio training, weight training, and mental training – and all four of them can be customized and fine-tuned week by week to help you reach your goals. Whether you want to burn 10 pounds (4.5 kg), 20 pounds (9 kg), or 100 pounds (45 kg), whether you want to build muscle or just look "toned," this programme is for you. It's not about becoming a bodybuilder, it's about using the "bodybuilder's secrets" to reach your own personal goals. It's about developing the leanest you, the fittest you, the best you.

Almost everyone is missing at least one piece of the puzzle, and that's what holds them back. If you've never put all four elements together before, then do it with all you've got for the next 28 days. You'll be in the best shape of your life and you'll be on the road to even bigger – and permanent – changes as you make this plan a part of your long-term lifestyle.

When you look back at the origins of this programme, you could say that *Burn the Fat, Feed the Muscle* was 30 years in the making and 20 years in the perfecting. You have in your hands one of the most tested and proven fat-burning systems ever created. It's the original bible of fat loss for hundreds of thousands of people worldwide. I hope this brand-new edition of a fat-loss classic becomes your health and fitness bible as well.

# PART I

# PHILOSOPHY

# CHAPTER 1

# Fat-Burning Secrets of the Leanest People in the World

"If you want to know about fat loss or muscle building, ask top level body-builders. These guys know it. In other words, quit buying fat loss devices off of late night TV ads, quit buying 'fat loss' stuff that grandma tried when her cribbage partner mentioned it, and quit trying fad diets. Instead, listen to the best of the best."

– Dan John, strength coach and author of
*Never Let Go: A Philosophy of Lifting, Living and Learning*

Life is short, time is precious, and you are busy. You don't have hours to waste and you want results as quickly as possible. So what's the fastest way to burn fat and get in great shape? Simple: Model yourself after an expert. Any time you attempt something new, there's a learning curve, but if you have the right coach, you can bypass years of trial, error, and frustration. The big question is, with all the noise in the diet and fitness world today, how do you choose your mentors? Who should you listen to? What sources can you trust?

Let me suggest the same strategy to you that I've put to use for my personal training and coaching clients for years: If you want to shed fat and build lean muscle, learn from the leanest, best-built people in the world – bodybuilders. Why? Again, it's simple: Bodybuilders and other physique athletes (figure, fitness, fitness model, and bikini competitors) are the world's greatest experts in the art and science of body transformation.

Athletes in physique sports do things differently from – sometimes the exact opposite of – everyone else. Here's just a taste of what this programme will reveal about their methods.

1. **Physique athletes don't diet – not in the conventional sense.** Diets don't work; you'll find out why in the next chapter. In fact, bodybuilders are well-known for

how much food they eat. It doesn't seem possible that you can "eat more and burn more," but on this plan, you really can.

2.  **Physique athletes are masters at stripping off the last 10 to 15 pounds (4.5 to 7 kg) of stubborn fat.** Most people get stuck on those final pounds, but this method can strip off *all* the fat – all the way to six-pack abs. You may not want to get so lean that people say, "Wow, you are ripped!" But if you do, this is how it's done.

3.  **Physique athletes don't lose muscle.** What good is it to lose weight if half of it is lean body mass? If you want to lose 20 pounds (9 kg) as fast as possible, we could saw off one of your legs. That sounds ridiculous, but it's exactly what most people are doing with crazy starvation diets: burning off their own muscle. Follow this plan and you won't just lose weight, you'll burn fat, keep muscle, and completely transform your body.

4.  **Physique athletes know how to break plateaus.** By tracking body composition (instead of only body weight), charting progress, and using a performance feedback loop system, you can break any plateau. You'll know when you're stuck and what to do to get "unstuck."

5.  **Physique athletes (and fitness models) have to show up in shape on a specific date.** If you use their system, you can "dial it in" whenever you want to get in peak shape – for a vacation, a reunion, a wedding, a whole summer, a body transformation contest, or even your own photo shoot. You can get as lean as you want, *when you want*. You'll be in complete control of the timing and speed of your results.

I could go on and on about the unique tactics that bodybuilders use: nutrient timing, carb cycling, modified low-carb diets, protein optimization, hydration strategies, macronutrient tweaks that no one else talks about – not to mention the unique training style designed to make you stronger and healthier and look great naked at the same time. But we'll get to these topics soon enough.

For now, it's sufficient to know that *Burn the Fat, Feed the Muscle* is a health and fitness philosophy that has been quietly tested and proven in the bodybuilding and physique world for decades. These are the secrets of the leanest people in the world. Until now the only place you could get this kind of information is if you were one of my personal clients, if you are a member of my inner circle, or you had your own coach who was privy to the physique athlete style of nutrition and training. Now I can be your coach through this book.

It's important to know that this book was written by a bodybuilder, but it's not just for bodybuilders. Think of using this programme as simply "stealing" some of their secrets to help you achieve your own personal goals. I do work with physique competitors, and the advanced acceleration strategies in the final chapters of this book can be used to go all the way to competition-stage or photo-shoot shape. But this book is for any man or woman who wants to shed fat, get lean, and transform their body without losing muscle and without starvation, drugs, or diet gimmicks.

Most people don't want to be bodybuilders. But let me bounce an idea off you. *Burn the Fat, Feed the Muscle* is not about dieting your body down as much as it's about building your body up. When you follow this programme, you'll build strength, health, energy, discipline, and self-confidence, not to mention lean muscle. I always believed that anyone who lifts weights and feeds their body nutritiously could call themselves a "bodybuilder."

So after you start the programme, why not try that and say, "I am a bodybuilder." Or say something similar that resonates with you more, like "I am a body sculptor," "I am a strength athlete," or "I am a fitness athlete." You may not look or feel like one yet, but when you affirm it, you'll get there faster. It's miraculous how the words you use to describe yourself can shape your identity, change your self-image, and, in turn, change your behaviour. You'll learn more about the psychology of affirmations in chapter 6. It really is amazing!

## WHY THIS IS THE MOST UNIQUE AND EFFECTIVE FAT-LOSS AND BODY-TRANSFORMATION PROGRAMME IN THE WORLD

Before you dive into the programme, I want to give you a quick overview of the *Burn the Fat, Feed the Muscle* principles. I'll explain the ten most important ways this programme is unique, and why I believe this is the most powerful fat-loss and body-transformation system ever developed. This will give you the big picture, and I hope it gets you even more excited about the journey you're about to begin.

### 1. *Burn the Fat, Feed the Muscle* is not a weight-loss programme, it's a fat-loss programme.

Weight loss and fat loss are not the same thing. The scale can be misleading if it's the only way you measure your progress, because the scale doesn't tell you the difference between fat weight and muscle weight. For example, a woman could weigh 110 pounds (7 st 12 lb/50 kg) but have 33 per cent body fat. That's what you call a "skinny fat person." On the other hand, a well-trained female athlete could weigh

150 pounds (10 st 10 lb/68 kg) and be very lean, with 16 per cent body fat. That's what you call "solid muscle."

What matters most is your ratio of muscle to fat – your body composition. With this distinction in mind, losing weight should not be your only goal. Your main focus should be burning the fat and keeping the muscle. As long as your body is mostly muscle, then you shouldn't worry so much about your total body weight. *Burn the Fat, Feed the Muscle* will teach you how to measure your body fat and use body composition to track your progress. You'll learn how to get results as fast as possible, but you'll also be reminded that there's a world of difference between rapid weight loss and permanent fat loss.

### 2. *Burn the Fat, Feed the Muscle* is not a diet, it's a nutrition programme.

Crash diets are tempting because they can produce quick weight loss, at least in the beginning. The problem is, when you cut calories too much, or banish entire food groups, you may not get enough vitamins, minerals, essential fatty acids, or fibre. Reduce your carbohydrates too much, and your energy level takes a nosedive. If you fall short on protein, you could lose lean body mass, which slows your metabolism and makes you softer and weaker. You might weigh less and fit into a smaller size, but your body still looks flabby.

Even if you grit your teeth and willpower your way through an extreme diet for a few months, the consequences outweigh the benefits. Deprivation diets make you lethargic, hungry, and miserable. You can't stay on them forever, so the weight loss rarely lasts. As you read this book, you'll discover that if you eat the right foods, you can actually eat more and nourish your body with all the nutrients it needs. You'll not only burn fat faster and keep it off, you'll also get healthier and feel more energized at the same time.

### 3. *Burn the Fat, Feed the Muscle* is not about nutrition or training; it's about both.

You'll lose weight on any diet with a calorie deficit, but when you add training, you'll burn more fat without slowing down your metabolism or losing muscle. Putting training and nutrition together is the difference between transforming your body and simply losing weight. Research has also proven that exercise is critical for long-term weight maintenance. You might take the fat off with dieting alone, but you'll have a hard time keeping it off.

When you make training a part of your lifestyle, you can eat more and still have the caloric deficit you need to burn fat. And when your training includes lifting weights, not just cardio, more of what you eat is partitioned into muscle. Don't starve the fat with diets: *Burn the fat* with training and *feed the muscle* with nutrition.

## 4. *Burn the Fat, Feed the Muscle* is not only about looking better but also about becoming healthier.

The nutrition and training guidelines I give for transforming your body are the same simple lifestyle changes I recommend for good health. If you want to look like a fitness model, get ripped, or peak for a photo shoot, a stricter and more sophisticated plan may be necessary. I explain how to ramp up your training and tighten up your nutrition to accelerate fat loss in the last part of the book. But after a special peaking event is over, you return to the same balanced lifestyle plan.

There's nothing wrong with training harder and using stricter diets to pursue extreme leanness at times. And there's nothing wrong with setting purely cosmetic ("vanity") goals. But there's more to *Burn the Fat, Feed the Muscle* than getting super lean. You're going to be setting a lot of goals in this programme. To keep yourself in balance, make sure you set goals for looking great and getting healthier. This means following sensible nutrition and training practices, as well as avoiding drugs or potentially harmful diet pills. It means 100 per cent natural!

## 5. *Burn the Fat, Feed the Muscle* is a lifestyle, not a quick fix.

The word "diet" comes from the Latin *diaeta*, meaning "way of life." Today, however, I think the word "diet" carries too much negative baggage to use so loosely. The way I define it, a diet is any temporary change in your eating behaviour to try to lose weight. When you say you're going on a diet, you're implying that at some point you're going off it.

*Burn the Fat, Feed the Muscle* is not something you go on and off; it's a lifestyle. The only way you'll get lean and stay lean is to choose new behaviours, develop new habits, and maintain them for life. You'll need a calorie deficit during your fat-loss phase, but the rest of your nutrition will be similar all year round, regardless of whether your goal is burning, building, or maintaining.

This programme is not a quick fix. But you will get results quickly. If you've never used a programme like this before – one that covers all bases – and if you diligently put into action all four elements of the plan at the same time, you will see incredible results in the first 28 days. You will lose pure fat, not just weight, you will transform your body shape, and you will already have new habits established that will keep you lean for life.

## 6. *Burn the Fat, Feed the Muscle* is based on science and experience, not one or the other.

Most scientists live by the credo "Prove all things." That's good advice for the rest of us, too, especially when we're evaluating claims that seem too good to be true. Science and critical thinking are important tools for helping us design our fitness programmes, sort through information overload, and avoid being taken by charlatans and con artists.

However, being so scientific and sceptical that you trust studies over your own experience can be hazardous to your progress. That's why this book is based on both science *and* real-world results. We should never deny or ignore the results of well-performed research. We should never dismiss the results of our own experience, either, when results are the one thing that counts the most. At some point in your journey, you have to start experimenting, measuring progress, and drawing conclusions based on your own results.

Some of the nutrition and training methods used by bodybuilders are controversial, and throughout this book I'll be sure to point that out wherever that's the case. Research results may be conflicting or there's not much evidence either way. But if you wait for enough studies to validate every nutrition and training technique that has already been proven effective out in the trenches, you could be waiting a long time. When it comes to body transformation, physique athletes are often ahead of the science, and the results they've achieved prove it.

## 7. *Burn the Fat, Feed the Muscle* is simple, but it's not easy.

Burning fat is simple, but that doesn't mean it's easy. "Simple" means uncomplicated. "Easy" implies little or no effort. Losing weight is a simple matter of achieving a calorie deficit. There's nothing complicated about that. But balancing energy in and energy out in a modern, sedentary, temptation-filled environment is easier said than done.

Fat loss isn't always easy. Most diet experts won't admit it, because "effortless and overnight" is marketable. "Hard work" scares people away. But hard work is the only way anyone accomplishes great things. Everything worth having in life has a price attached to it. Legendary American football Green Bay Packers coach Vince Lombardi put it best when he said, "The dictionary is the only place success comes before work. Hard work is the price we must all pay for success."

### 8. *Burn the Fat, Feed the Muscle* pursues the truth, not the fads.

I launched my first website in 1999. Since then I've shared my hard work and no-gimmicks philosophy with millions of visitors. To this day, my Burn the Fat websites and social communities are still growing. That kind of longevity not only requires results, it also requires honesty. I make my living from the health-and-fitness business, but I will go broke and starve to death before I "sell out" or compromise my values. Believe me, I've had no shortage of opportunity. Let me tell you a quick story.

Years ago, the editor of a major fitness magazine contacted me with a proposition. He was so impressed with my online articles that he wanted to hire me. He offered me $1,000 (£630) to interview some of the top supplement gurus, including the CEO of one of the largest nutrition companies in the world. My assignment was to write a two-page article about the latest developments with a popular but controversial product. A thousand bucks is temptingly good pay for one short article, but then he threw in the catch: Because of his magazine's relationship with the supplement company, he told me I couldn't write anything bad about the product. In fact, I had to put a "positive spin" on it. I turned it down. It went against everything I believed in about truth and objectivity.

By selectively quoting research, magazines can promote a new diet pill or exercise fad every month and make it look like a breakthrough every time. By putting product information into articles, the claims sound more legitimate, and the advertisements feed off the articles. That makes magazines – online or in print – the perfect vehicles for selling supplements. Publishers see it as the ultimate business model. I see it as a conflict of interest. That's why, years ago, I made a public pledge that I would never go into the supplement business or use my books or websites to sell them.

As you read *Burn the Fat, Feed the Muscle*, you can rest assured that there's no hidden agenda. I'm not here to sell you magic weight-loss potions or the latest training trend; I'm here to sell you on getting strong, healthy, and fit.

### 9. *Burn the Fat, Feed the Muscle* is about real food, not supplements.

It's tempting to think that all you need to solve a body fat problem is a fat-burning pill or diet drink. The supplement companies certainly want you to believe that. The truth is that training and good nutrition from whole foods are all you'll ever need. Protein shakes and meal replacement products are sometimes helpful, but they have no magical fat-reducing properties. They're essentially just powdered food.

The majority of so-called fat-burning products available over-the-counter are worthless and have no scientific evidence validating their use. Pills that rely on stimulants, thermogenics, or appetite suppressants might help a little, but they aren't as effective as many advertisements claim, and there are potential dangers if they're abused.

Most people want overnight health cures and fat-loss miracles. But those are fantasies. If there really were a magic pill that burned off fat without work, there wouldn't be millions of overweight people in the world today. If you want to see a real miracle, try training hard and eating real food consistently for a few months. The sooner you accept this reality, the sooner you'll be the proud owner of a lean body.

### 10. *Burn the Fat, Feed the Muscle* is custom-tailored, not one-size-fits-all.

Some nutrition laws are universal: They apply to everyone. But after you've mastered the fundamentals, you'll need to customize your plan to fit your goals and your body type. No two people are exactly alike. Each person has a metabolism, digestive system, hormonal profile, sugar tolerance, and body structure as unique as their fingerprint. That's why one-size-fits-all diet or exercise plans almost always fail.

*Burn the Fat, Feed the Muscle* identifies all these differences and accommodates them. You'll also have enough flexibility to adjust your nutrition and training to fit your schedule and satisfy your personal tastes. Customizing your programme enables you to do the very best you can with what Mother Nature gave you.

### PUTTING IT ALL TOGETHER

*Burn the Fat, Feed the Muscle* is an amazingly thorough and detailed programme. It covers all four elements of the fat-burning equation:

LEARN: Mental training
EAT: Nutrition
ACTIVATE: Cardio training
NEW BODY: Weight training

It's a simple formula, but don't underestimate its power. Almost everyone is missing at least one of these crucial elements, and many are missing two or even three. Only when all four are in place will you fully maximize your potential.

This book was designed to be the definitive guide to body transformation. Thousands of readers already call this their "fat-loss bible" and come back to it over and over again as a reference manual. The information came from thousands of academic and real-world sources. I've updated this book based on the latest research, but the core concepts are principle-based, so they'll never go out of date. Popular trends always change, but fundamentals never do.

Some of this information may be new or surprising to you, depending on your current level of knowledge. Most of it, however, is so simple and straightforward, you'll wonder why it didn't "click" for you sooner. What's different about *Burn the Fat, Feed the Muscle* is the way all the isolated bits and pieces you may have heard before are pulled together into a single comprehensive and organized system.

Throughout the rest of the book, I'll take you through all the nutrition and training principles you need to know to get the results you want. I'll show you what to do and give you just enough science so you know why you're doing it. You'll get all the essentials first. We'll finish with advanced strategies to break plateaus and accelerate your results. You'll be able to customize everything to match your goals, suit your tastes, and fit your lifestyle.

At first, it may seem like a lot to take in, but it all comes together in the end, and the payoff is extraordinary. By the time you reach the final chapters, you'll experience a sort of "nutritional enlightenment." But you can't reach that state of knowledge and understanding without first passing through the initial learning curve. My goal is to shorten that curve for you, inspire you, and help you reach your goals as fast as possible.

If you want to get started quickly, you can. Chapter 14 contains the *Burn the Fat, Feed the Muscle* eating plan, sample meal plans, and food lists, making that an excellent "nutrition quick-start guide." Chapters 15, 16, and 17 contain the workout, including the 28-day training plan. Jump in!

It's especially important, however, that you begin with the first element: mental training. If you've ever sabotaged yourself or fallen off the fitness wagon before, the reason always comes back to lack of focus and an untrained mind. Do the goal-setting exercises in chapter 6 before going on to the other three elements. Hundreds if not thousands of readers have told me over the years that what they learned in that chapter about mental training made a bigger difference in their results than anything they'd ever read in a diet or fitness book before.

## NOW GET STARTED!

As you read, remember that knowledge unused is worthless; only knowledge applied is power, so begin using what you learn immediately. Don't obsess over getting the whole programme perfect from day one. As you learn new tips on each page, put them to use. Start today! Start with your very next meal! I like the way the late, great

American motivational speaker Jim Rohn said it: "Don't let your learning lead to knowledge, let your learning lead to action."

One more thing: You don't have to do this alone. Support is a major key to motivation and long-term success. You can connect with me and hundreds of thousands of *Burn the Fat* fans on our social media sites including www.facebook.com/burnthefat and twitter.com/tomvenuto. You can get the free tools and resources that go with this book at www.BurnTheFatFeedTheMuscle.com. And if you want to join thousands of fellow "burners" at our private, members-only support community, visit the *Burn the Fat* Inner Circle at www.BurnTheFatInnerCircle.com.

# CHAPTER 2

# Why Diets Fail and Why This Plan Won't

"Dieting is not effective in controlling weight. You can get a temporary weight loss with a diet, but each scheme ultimately gives way to weight gain, and subsequent losses become increasingly difficult. Worst of all, you get progressively fatter on less food. Dieting actually makes you fatter!"

– Dr. Lawrence E. Lamb, author of *The Weighting Game:*
*The Truth About Weight Control*

## WHY DIETS NEVER WORK

In the first part of this chapter, you'll learn why most people struggle to lose weight and keep it off long term. You'll also realize why most diets are fundamentally flawed and doomed to fail before they're even started. All it takes is a basic understanding of metabolism, hormones, and your body's remarkable protective mechanism known as the "starvation response." In the second part, you'll discover six strategies that guarantee you'll burn off fat forever without starving yourself or giving up your favourite foods. All of these strategies are built right into the foundations of the programme. By following the training and eating plans from this book, you'll automatically be using every one of these strategies and setting yourself up to succeed.

By our definition, a diet is the temporary and unsustainable restriction of food or calories. Most popular weight-loss diets call for very low calories: 800 to 1,200 per day or less for women and 1,500 to 1,800 per day or less for men is not uncommon. When you cut calories to these extremes, you *will* lose weight, at least for a little while. However, there are two major problems with this approach.

The first is that restrictive low-calorie diets are almost impossible to follow for long, so the weight loss almost never lasts. According to research by the American National Weight Control Registry, 95 per cent of people who lose weight on conventional diet programmes eventually regain it. The second problem is that most people neglect proper training while dieting, so much of the weight they lose is lean body mass, not fat. Best-case scenario: A dieter somehow keeps the weight off, but they end up a smaller version of their old self; they haven't reshaped their body nor become any stronger, healthier, or fitter.

If your only interest is *weight* loss and you don't care where the weight comes from, how long it stays off, or whether you harm yourself in the process, then you could say, "All diets work." If your goal is to shed *fat* permanently and safely without losing muscle, it's truer to say, "Diets never work."

There are more diet programmes today than ever, yet there's more obesity than ever. According to the American National Institutes of Health, more than 133 million people in the United States are overweight; that's 64 per cent of the adult population. The Centers for Disease Control and Prevention says that the number of clinically obese people increased in the United States from one in eight in 1991 to nearly one in five in 1999. Today, 63 million, or one in three adults, are clinically obese (at least 30 per cent over their ideal weight), which means they're at risk for over 30 health problems associated with excess body fat.

You see diet ads everywhere proclaiming that the Holy Grail of weight loss has been found, but the statistics don't lie: The way most people are dieting for weight loss doesn't work – and there are scientific reasons why.

## WHY THE CALORIE MATHS DOESN'T ADD UP

The law of energy balance says that if you eat fewer calories than you burn, you will lose weight. There are 3,500 calories in a pound of stored body fat. If you cut 1,000 calories per day from your daily maintenance level, it adds up to a 7,000-calorie deficit in one week and – on paper – should produce weight loss of 2 pounds (0.9 kg) every week. Simple maths, right? Not exactly.

When you introduce a calorie deficit at the start of a diet, you'll lose weight, but it doesn't take long before weight loss slows and sometimes stops completely. Why does this happen? With a 1,000-calorie deficit below your initial daily maintenance level, why don't you lose 50 pounds (23 kg) in 25 weeks or 100 pounds (45 kg) in 50 weeks? The answer is simple: The maths equation changes!

The number of calories you burn initially may not be the same six months or a year later. In other words, energy balance is dynamic. A calorie deficit is a moving target. When you lose body weight, you need fewer calories to support your smaller body. When you drop your calories, you also tend to drop your activity levels, sometimes unconsciously. But most people fail to adjust their calorie intake to match their lower energy needs.

In addition, most people don't train properly to maintain muscle (or they don't work out at all). Instead, they try to starve the fat. That only makes it worse, because your body has a complex and redundant series of defence mechanisms to protect you from starvation and maintain a stable weight.

## UNDERSTANDING THE STARVATION RESPONSE

If our ancient ancestors wanted to eat, they had to forage for food, grow it, or kill it (which required a lot of physical activity, something modern humans don't get). Ancient humans may not have even known when their next meal was coming. During the lean times, they may have eaten substantial meals only after successful hunts. Scientists theorize that adaptive mechanisms, collectively known as the "starvation response," developed to ensure survival of the species.

You can survive a long time without food. You may have heard stories about people lost in the wilderness for weeks with no food, or confined in a prisoner-of-war camp for years with little food. There are case studies of lean individuals on hunger strikes surviving up to two months without food and obese individuals surviving 200 days or longer without eating. Two things make it possible to survive so long under starvation and semi-starvation conditions:

1. Your body can easily and efficiently store energy as fat when food is plentiful, as insurance against future shortages.
2. Your body can decrease energy expenditure and increase food-seeking behaviours when body-fat stores are running low and food is scarce.

## YOUR BODY CAN'T TELL THE DIFFERENCE BETWEEN DIETING AND STARVATION

During long periods of starvation, your body slowly feeds off itself for energy, burning through fat stores, then muscle and eventually vital organs. If you continued to burn calories at your normal rate while your food intake fell far below normal, you would quickly exhaust your reserves of stored energy and die soon after your food supply was cut off. Your body's starvation response keeps you alive longer.

This type of adaptation was a blessing to our ancestors during times of famine. But in modern, affluent societies today, this same life-preserving mechanism can work against you when you're trying to lose fat. When your body senses calorie deprivation, your survival responses kick in, even though a diet is not a life-or-death situation. Your body tells itself, "It looks like this is all the food you're getting for a while, so you'd better stop burning so many calories, start conserving your energy, and increase the drive for finding food."

Whether a real famine or a low-calorie diet, your body can't tell the difference. Either way, if the calorie shortage is severe and prolonged, there are consequences, and they're hardwired into your genes. The only way to avoid them is to avoid severe calorie shortages!

## THE TOP TEN REASONS TO AVOID EXTREME LOW-CALORIE DIETS

The negative side effects of very low-calorie dieting can be physiological or psychological in nature – usually both. They include increases in hunger and food-seeking behaviour, drops in energy or activity level, loss of lean body mass, decreases in metabolic rate, and problems with hormones. If you're not aware of them, these forces conspire to get you burning less, eating more, and relapsing when the diet is over.

### 1. Diets increase hunger and cravings.

The first thing you notice during a calorie shortage is the hunger. You should expect a little hunger when you're in a calorie deficit, but with extreme diets you become ravenous. It's almost impossible to stay on a diet when you're battling voracious hunger and all you can think about is food. More than a dozen hormones influence how hungry or full you feel. The urge to eat can also be psychological or environmental. You tend to want what you can't have, so if your diet is too low in calories or it sets too many rules about what you can't eat, the feeling of deprivation triggers cravings and binges. It's worse when you're surrounded by temptations and eating cues all day long.

### 2. Diets slow down your metabolic rate.

Your basal metabolic rate is the number of calories you burn at rest every day. When you lose a lot of weight, you burn fewer calories simply because you have a smaller body. But calorie restriction causes your metabolic rate to decrease even more than a drop in body weight would predict. This is known as "adaptive thermogenesis" and it's one of the reasons why progress slows over time and why it's harder for most people to lose those last stubborn 10 to 15 pounds (4.5 to 7 kg).

### 3. Diets may increase the risk of muscle loss.

When your body is being starved, it looks for ways to conserve energy. Since muscle burns calories and muscle is extra weight you have to lug around, getting rid of it is an easy way for your body to burn less. Lean people who already have low body fat are more likely to lose muscle than overweight people, but it can happen to anyone. Dieting without resistance training can cause 30 per cent to 50 per cent of your weight loss to come from lean tissue. The risk of muscle loss is higher if your protein intake is too low. Even when you're lifting weights and eating enough protein, if your diet is too severe, some of the lost weight can still come from muscle.

### 4. Diets decrease non-exercise activity thermogenesis.

Non-exercise activity thermogenesis, also known as NEAT, is the scientific name for all your physical activity throughout the day, excluding formal exercise. This includes all the calories you burn from casual walking, shopping, gardening, housework, standing, pacing, and even little things like chewing, changing posture, and fidgeting. Obviously, most of those activities don't burn many calories individually, but over time the total burn from NEAT can really add up. Studies by Dr. James A. Levine at the Mayo Clinic found that when you cut calories, your NEAT level drops. Many people already know that low-calorie diets make them lethargic. If they make it to the gym at all, they work out with less gusto. Unless you consciously counter this tendency by keeping yourself active, your weight loss will slow down automatically as you keep dieting.

### 5. Diets decrease your energy and work capacity.

Some people do better than others when training under less-than-ideal conditions. But as a general rule, low-calorie diets are not conducive to good workouts or an active lifestyle. One of the first signs of undernutrition is loss of energy and the ability to sustain intense training. Without enough fuel coming in, you'll fatigue faster, your strength will suffer, your performance will plummet, and your results will be compromised. To maximize your fat burning and build your best body, you must be able to train hard. If you're hardly eating, you can hardly train.

### 6. Diets decrease thyroid hormones.

Low-calorie diets can have a major impact on hormone levels. Since thyroid levels help regulate your metabolic rate, maintaining thyroid function is important for successful fat loss as well as overall health. Endocrinologists have measured reductions in triiodothyronine (T3) and thyroxine (T4) levels as quickly as one week after starting a very low-calorie diet, even before there is a decrease in body weight. As the severity and duration of the diet increases, the risk of negative effects increases. You need that calorie deficit to burn fat, but cutting calories too far – especially when you slash the carbohydrates too low – can wreak havoc with the very hormones you need working at peak efficiency.

### 7. Diets decrease the hormone leptin.

Leptin is a hormone produced primarily in your fat cells that also plays a major role in regulating metabolism and body weight. When you're well fed and your body fat levels are stable, leptin sends a signal to your brain saying, "Everything is okay in the food supply and fat storage department." If food intake or body fat stores go down, your leptin levels drop. When leptin is low, it signals your brain that body fat reserves are declining and starvation is impending. This is why leptin is often called the "anti-starvation hormone," and it may be the hormone that triggers the entire cascade of starvation responses, from increased hunger to reduced metabolism.

### 8. Diets increase the stress hormone cortisol.

Cortisol is a catabolic (muscle-wasting) hormone produced by your adrenal glands in response to various types of physical and mental stress, including dieting. Research has shown that cortisol is inversely related to calorie levels. What about those pills that claim to suppress high cortisol levels and help burn fat? Don't bother. Even if they help reduce high cortisol, a pill is only a plaster. If starvation dieting and other stressors are causing a hormonal imbalance, you need to address those issues rather than trying to treat the symptoms.

### 9. Diets decrease testosterone.

Testosterone also takes a hit when you cut calories too much. This makes perfect sense from an evolutionary point of view because if you can't even feed yourself, you're in no condition to bear and feed offspring, are you? In a study from the *Journal of Applied Physiology*, army rangers who were fed only 1,000 calories a day under conditions of stress, sustained workload, and inadequate sleep experienced a drop in testosterone that approached castration levels. (Make note: Sleep deprivation, stress, and a low-calorie diet are a really bad combination.) Most research says that a conservative calorie cut of 20 per cent below maintenance level won't affect testosterone. As the calorie cuts get more aggressive and your body gets leaner and leaner, low testosterone becomes more of a concern.

### 10. Diets increase the chance of weight regain.

Almost everyone loses weight at the beginning, but later on, when the weight loss slows down and the hunger pangs intensify, most people give up. Even worse, they end their diet with a binge. That's bad news, because dieting can prime your body to regain weight more easily and leave you fatter than when you started. Eventually, you get sucked in by the newest fad diet, and the yo-yo diet cycle starts all over again. This up-and-down pattern of weight loss and regain is known as weight cycling, and many people suffer through this for years or even their entire lifetime. Not only is it unhealthy, but with each cycle your metabolism becomes less efficient and you may actually get fatter more easily while eating less food than before.

## WHY DIETING CAN ACTUALLY MAKE YOU FATTER

You can now see the great irony in the weight-loss world today: Dieting can actually make you fatter in the long term. Because most of the best-selling popular diets today promote very low calories and ignore proper training, they're actually causing the very problem they claim to cure.

Let's see how these biological and psychological responses to extreme diets affect real-world results. Chris is a typical dieter with a goal of losing 20 pounds (9 kg).

BEFORE THE DIET
**200 pounds (14 st 4 lb/91 kg) body weight**
**36 pounds (16 kg) (18 per cent) body fat**
**164 pounds (74 kg) lean body mass**

Like most people, Chris was told that the best way to lose body fat is to slash calories, so he went on a 1,500-calorie-per-day diet (which is semi-starvation for an active man of his size). In the first week he lost 5 pounds (2.3 kg) and was very happy, even though he suspected a pound or two was water weight. The second week he lost 4 pounds (1.8 kg). In weeks three through six he lost 3 pounds (1.4 kg) per week for a grand total of 21 pounds (10 kg).

Chris now weighs 179 pounds (12 st 11 lb/81 kg) and he lost weight steadily without hitting a plateau (although the weight loss did slow down). Judging by the scale alone, he's reached his goal. If we look at the numbers more closely, however, we find that he hasn't been so successful after all.

AFTER THE DIET
**179 pounds (12 st 11 lb/81 kg) body weight**
**26.5 pounds (12 kg) (14.8 per cent) body fat**
**152.5 pounds (69 kg) lean body mass**
**21 pounds (10 kg) weight loss**
**9.5 pounds (4.3 kg) fat loss**
**11.5 pounds (5 kg) lean body mass loss**

By rating his results in terms of body composition instead of scale weight, it becomes clear how Chris has failed. Fifty-five per cent of his weight loss came from lean body mass. The drop in lean body mass decreased his metabolism, so he is now burning fewer calories each day than when he started. This has set him up for a relapse.

Even if he doesn't give in to hunger and binge, but simply goes back to the way he used to eat, his body no longer burns calories as efficiently as before. Therefore, the number of calories that used to maintain his weight now makes him gain weight. As the weeks pass, the weight slowly creeps back on until he finally regains all the fat he lost.

SIX WEEKS AFTER THE DIET ENDS
**200 pounds (14 st 4 lb/91 kg) body weight**
**41.1 pounds (19 kg) (20.5 per cent) body fat**
**158.9 pounds (72 kg) lean body mass**

Chris now weighs the same as when he started, with one difference: He has less muscle, more fat, and a slower metabolic rate than when he began. He has "damaged" his metabolism and it will now be harder to lose weight than before.

The same thing happens to women. The difference is that women have naturally higher body fat levels, lower total body mass, lower calorie needs, and different hormonal concerns. It's not a stretch to say that fat loss is harder for women than men, and women are more susceptible to metabolic damage than men.

## SIX STRATEGIES TO BURN THE FAT FOREVER, WITHOUT DIETING OR DEPRIVING YOURSELF

The odds of you losing fat permanently with traditional low-calorie diets are stacked against you biologically, psychologically, and environmentally. It sounds grim, but the good news is you can bypass these problems if you avoid the typical diet mentality. Instead, do what bodybuilders and fitness models do. Let me introduce you to six no-diet strategies you can use to burn the fat and keep it off for good. These are the secrets of the leanest people in the world. Even if you've used starvation diets in the past and you're afraid you've caused damage from previous dieting mistakes, don't worry. These same guidelines will help you bring your metabolism back up to speed.

### 1. Think "habit" not "diet."

You can't achieve permanent fat loss by going on and off diets, especially if you're always hopping from one diet trend to the next. You achieve permanent results by adopting new habits that you can maintain for the rest of your life. These habits must include the way you eat, the way you think, and the way you move.

Good habits aren't easy to form, but once they're established, they're just as hard to break as the bad ones. American motivational writer Orison Swett Marden put it this way: "The beginning of a habit is like an invisible thread, but every time we repeat the act we strengthen the strand, add to it another filament, until it becomes a great cable and binds us irrevocably."

Nature abhors a vacuum. If you simply remove a bad habit, it leaves a void begging to be filled by another one. An old proverb says that a negative habit can most easily be driven out by a positive habit, just as a nail can be driven out by another nail. The best way to get rid of undesirable habits such as drinking fizzy drinks, spending hours on the sofa watching TV, and thinking like a pessimist is by replacing them with new ones, rather than trying to overcome them with willpower. Throughout this book, you'll hear many ideas for "out with the old and in with the new."

Initially, there's a period where starting the new habit will feel uncomfortable. Be patient: Everything is difficult in the beginning. Accept the challenge! For a new behaviour to become entrenched in your nervous system, it could take months. However, the roots of nutrition and exercise habits can be formed in less than 28 days. That's why it's so important to give 100 per cent effort and commitment in the beginning while you build up momentum. After those four weeks, you'll be leaner and on your way to making your new habits as effortless and natural as brushing your teeth or taking a shower.

## 2. Maintain your muscle.

Billionaire investor Warren Buffett is well-known for saying that rule number one in making money is never lose money. It's the same with making a body transformation. A simple strategy for permanent fat loss is never lose muscle. Muscle is your fat-burning secret weapon. Muscle is your metabolic furnace. The more muscle you have, the more calories you burn at rest as well as during exercise. Obviously, weight training is a huge factor when it comes to keeping your muscle while you're shedding the fat, so when you get to the chapter on training, read it carefully and take it seriously. On the nutrition side, the biggest keys to maintaining muscle include getting enough protein and being conservative with calorie cuts.

## 3. Cut calories conservatively.

You must have a calorie deficit to burn body fat, but most people cut calories much too fast. Your body can't be forced to lose fat more quickly than nature intended; you must coax it. The smartest, safest, and healthiest approach for permanent fat loss is to start with a small deficit, add exercise, then continue to cut calories if necessary as your weekly results dictate. Do it slowly and progressively in stages, not all at once.

In chapter 7, I'll show you the exact formulas to calculate your personal calorie requirements to maintain your weight, burn fat, and build muscle. If you don't like crunching numbers, I'll also show you the quick start shortcuts as well. Here's what you need to know now – and this should be music to your ears: If you eat the right foods and do the type of training I recommend, you'll be able to eat a lot more than you think and the fat will still melt away. Welcome to *Burn the Fat, Feed the Muscle*, good-bye to starvation diets.

## 4. Burn the fat, don't starve the fat.

There's more than one way to create a calorie deficit. You can decrease your calorie intake from food or increase the calories you burn from training and other activity. Unless you're physically unable to exercise, a combination of both is ideal. Using exercise to maintain muscle and expand your calorie deficit has huge advantages over dieting alone.

Most people are too focused on cutting calories and removing foods while training little or not at all. With the right kind of training, you build muscle, increase your strength, reshape your body and boost your metabolism. Plus you can eat more and still keep losing fat. As paradoxical as it might sound, the fastest way to transform your body is to *eat more and burn more*. You eat more to provide energy, nutrients, and building material. You burn more to stoke metabolism, build muscle, gain strength, and improve fitness.

Why deprive yourself by eating less when you can eat more and fire up your metabolic furnace? All you need to do is add the right kind of training on top of a sensible nutrition programme. Compared to dieting alone, the results you get from combining cardio, weight training, and nutritious eating to achieve a specific goal are nothing short of miraculous.

Here are some reasons why training (weight training and cardio training combined) is superior to dieting for losing body fat:

| Training (burn more) | Dieting (eat less) |
|---|---|
| Raises your metabolic rate | Slows down your metabolic rate |
| Creates a caloric deficit without triggering the starvation response | Triggers the starvation response |
| Provides countless health benefits | May be harmful to your health |
| Builds and maintains lean body mass | Promotes loss of lean body mass |
| Increases fat-burning hormones | Decreases fat-burning hormones |

### 5. Use the calorie "cycling" method (don't stay in a deficit too long).

You probably know at least one person who always seems to be on a diet. While these "professional dieters" may lose some weight in the beginning, they never seem to reach their long-term goals. They're always hitting plateaus and struggling to avoid regaining the weight they lost. God bless them – they never give up! Unfortunately, that's part of the problem. Each time they plateau or see the scale start creeping up again, they either panic and cut calories more, or they try all over again with the latest crash "diet of the month."

When your fat loss slows down or you hit a fat-loss plateau the first time, dropping calories is usually the right decision. But if your calories are already low and you've been dieting for a long time, cutting calories more can dig you into a deeper metabolic rut. It seems counterintuitive, but sometimes the best thing you can do to "reset" a sluggish metabolism is to eat more before going back to the caloric deficit again.

Inserting occasional higher-calorie days between lower-calorie days is a simple technique that gives you a nice physical and psychological break from days or weeks of continuous deficit. After months of lower-calorie eating, a full week or two of higher-calorie (maintenance level) eating optimizes your hormones and re-stokes your metabolic fire.

This method of raising your calories periodically instead of staying low all the time is known as the "cycling" or "zigzagging" method. The bigger your calorie deficit has been, the longer you've been in it, and the lower your body fat becomes, the more important it is to take these diet breaks or "re-feeding" days. This plan will teach you how to know when your body needs this extra surge of calories to keep burning fat.

### 6. Lose weight at the right rate for you.

Most people sell themselves short and greatly underestimate the calibre of physique they can develop over time. I've seen people go from obesity to the fitness stage in one year; no one even recognized them with their new bodies. In the short term, however, most people are impatient and expect too much weight loss too fast, so it's important to set weekly goals thoughtfully.

Setting lots of short-term goals is crucial. But if you set them so high that they're physiologically impossible to achieve in the time frame you've chosen, and your results fall short of your expectations, you end up disappointed. Even if you set weekly weight-loss goals too high and actually do reach them, it doesn't always mean victory. Recall Chris the dieter, who lost 21 pounds (10 kg) in six weeks but half the weight was lean body mass, and he regained every pound of fat and more.

People with high body fat levels can usually drop fat faster without as many negative side effects. People who are already lean need to lose more slowly, or the risks – especially muscle loss – are greater. Women lose more slowly as well, especially short or small-framed women, because they have lower metabolisms to start with. "Slow burners" should celebrate every pound of progress, be patient, and keep in mind that old fable of the tortoise and the hare.

The best way to burn fat and keep it off for good, *without losing muscle,* and without making your life miserable, is to lose weight at the right rate for you. Many fitness experts recommend 2 pounds (0.9 kg) per week. That's a sensible general guideline, but it could be too fast for a petite female and too slow for a big man. Dropping 1 per cent of total body weight each week is a safe and realistic goal that's customized for each individual. That would be only 1.5 pounds (0.7 kg) per week for someone at 150 pounds (10 st 10 lb/68 kg) and 3 pounds (1.4 kg) per week for someone at 300 pounds (21 st 6 lb/136 kg).

Your mileage may vary. Most important of all: You will track your progress as you make this journey. You'll learn to measure your body fat and lean body mass. You'll always be on target if you give your body the nutrition it needs because the weight you lose will be pure body fat.

## PUT THESE STRATEGIES TO WORK
## AND YOU'LL NEVER DIET AGAIN

You'll learn more about how to implement these no-diet nutrition strategies in the upcoming chapters, and of course you'll find the ultimate lean-muscle training programme in chapter 17. The best part is everything can be custom tailored for your goals, your metabolism, your schedule, your lifestyle, and your body type. It's all about you, and in the next chapter you'll find out just how important that is.

# CHAPTER 3

# Understanding Your Body Type and Customizing Your Plan

"Some people are born with the propensity to become fatter than others. There are naturally skinny ectomorphs and naturally fatter endormorphs. Some individuals are given more fat cells by heredity, some fewer. But the set point is affected by environment and behaviour as well as heredity. You can vary your set point considerably depending on what and how you eat, as well as what kind and how much exercise you do."

– Neal Spruce, author, speaker, bodybuilder

## THE GENETIC BELL CURVE

There are seven billion people on our planet today and no two are exactly the same. Just as individuals are born with various hair, eye, and skin colours, each person also inherits different physical and metabolic traits that influence how easily they can build muscle and shed fat. One of the greatest secrets of body transformation is to "know thyself" and customize your training, nutrition, and lifestyle to suit your body type instead of blindly following someone else. Understanding the uniqueness of your body also helps you set expectations as well as keeps you motivated when the going gets tough.

Dr. Michael Colgan, author of *Optimum Sports Nutrition: Your Competitive Edge* once said, "As a part of biochemical individuality, people differ widely in their inherited tendencies to accumulate fat." Many people who struggle to lose weight would certainly agree. In physique and strength sports, genetically gifted people seem to simply touch the weights and their muscles get bigger and stronger.

When I was a beginner in bodybuilding, seeing other people get results more easily than I did was always frustrating. I was eating *perfectly* while pushing, working, struggling, and straining with every bit of energy I could muster for every ounce of muscle I could gain. Then some "genetic freaks" would come along and pass right by me without breaking a sweat. To add insult to injury, it seemed like they were breaking every training and nutrition rule in the book. When some of them took steroids on top of their hereditary gifts, their muscle growth exploded! I learned quickly that a genetic superior on drugs is not a good role model.

The law of averages dictates that the distribution of body types is statistically predictable based on percentiles. This phenomenon, known as the genetic bell curve, is similar to the distribution of grades among students. Sixty per cent of students will receive passing grades (Bs, Cs, and Ds), 20 per cent will fail, and 20 per cent will get As.

With regard to body type, most people (about 60 per cent of the population by my estimate) are genetically average. If you fall into this middle category, you'll respond favourably and predictably to any sensible plan. All it takes is a following a well-designed training programme and covering all the nutritional bases, including calories, protein, carbs, fats, fibre, vitamins, minerals, and water.

The 20 per cent of the population on the right side of the curve represents those genetically above average. This lucky group sheds fat quickly and easily, even if their nutrition and training aren't perfect. They have more leeway and can get away with fewer workouts and more cheat days. On the extreme right edge of the curve, you have the outliers who appear to eat chocolate and doughnuts all day long, hardly work out, yet have six-pack abs. These are the genetically gifted – or the genetic freaks, as I endearingly call them.The remaining 20 per cent, on the left side of the curve, are the genetically below average. These people have a more difficult time shedding fat and need to work harder than others. Getting results may require a stricter nutrition programme, more disciplined training, and a lot more patience. The farther to the left side of the genetic bell curve you are, the more challenging it is to get lean and muscular.

You can't deny that it's easier for some people to burn fat and build muscle than it is for others. Nor *should* you. The best approach is "realistic optimism." Not everyone has the genetic raw material to become a Mr. Universe, a fitness model, an Olympic sprinter, or an elite marathon runner. However, *everyone can improve their fitness and physique above and beyond where it is today.* Your goal should be to achieve your personal best while avoiding comparisons to others who have different genetics than you. The information in this chapter will help you do it.

First we'll look at genetic variability and what "good genetics" really means. You'll then learn about the three basic body types and how to identify which one you are. You'll also get action strategies to customize your plan to suit your type. We'll wrap up with some advice on mind-set, because when it comes to how genetics affect your health and your body, your attitude can make you or break you.

# THE TEN MAJOR GENETIC VARIABLES THAT AFFECT FAT LOSS, MUSCLE GROWTH, STRENGTH, AND ATHLETIC ABILITY

A good place to start is to answer the basic question: Why is burning fat and building muscle easier for some than for others? There are ten major genetic variables that affect your ability to burn fat, build muscle, increase strength, and reach high levels of athletic achievement. Studying these variables will help you understand how nutrition and training can affect you differently than other people.

## 1. Basal metabolic rate

Your basal metabolic rate (BMR) is the amount of energy you burn at rest every day just to maintain normal body functions such as breathing, circulation, digestion, and so on. The average male has a BMR of about 1,900 calories and the average female 1,400 calories. (You will use the formulas in chapter 7 to calculate your customized BMR numbers). Naturally, BMR can vary a lot based on body size and lean mass. But BMR can also vary between people who weigh the same because of differences in thyroid, organ mass, and other genetic factors. Some people are like cars that idle fast: They burn more fuel even while sitting still. When these people are highly active – and they usually are – they're like calorie-burning machines.

## 2. Number of fat cells

Some people are born with more fat cells than others, and women have more fat cells than men. Obviously, the person with more sites for fat storage has a disadvantage. A healthy, normal weight adult has between 25 billion to 30 billion fat cells. A typical overweight adult has about 75 billion fat cells, but with severe obesity, that number can be as high as 250 billion to 500 billion! Fat cells can increase in both size and number. They can multiply during rapid weight gain, which is another reason to keep your calories in check and your weight under control. Fat cell number cannot be decreased except through liposuction, and that can be expensive, painful, and risky. (It's also nothing more than cosmetic surgery, not a permanent solution, because new fat cells can be formed so easily). The good news is, with the right nutrition and training, even someone with a large number of fat cells can shrink them all and get dramatically leaner.

### 3. Number of muscle fibres

Like fat cells, you were born with a predetermined number of muscle fibres. Muscle fibres can get larger, in a process called hypertrophy, or they can get smaller, or atrophy. Unlike fat cells, muscle cells can't multiply in number. Hyperplasia, the process of splitting existing muscle fibres into new fibres, has been hypothesized but never proven in humans. This means that if you were born with a large number of muscle fibres, you have a greater potential to grow muscle than someone with fewer fibres.

### 4. Muscle fibre type

There are also different types of muscle fibre. Some are suited to endurance work (slow-twitch fibres) while others are suited for strength, power, and explosive work (fast-twitch fibres). The differences in each person's ratio of muscle fibres may explain why some people make better endurance athletes while others gravitate to strength or power sports.

### 5. Muscle insertions

The muscles insert onto the same bones in all humans; however, the exact point of insertion varies. Even a tiny difference in insertion points can create large increases in mechanical advantage. This partly explains why certain people are naturally stronger than others: They have better leverage because of their muscle insertion points.

### 6. Limb length

Some people are born with long legs and long arms, others with short legs and short arms. Limb length can affect your body's shape and symmetry. It can also influence your strength, athletic prowess, and ability to gain muscle. Long limbs mean long levers, which can create a mechanical disadvantage when performing certain exercises. Some people are born with fantastic leverage and that's why they become naturally strong.

### 7. Joint size

Joint size affects the way your body is shaped, but being "big-boned" has nothing to do with body fat or your ability to burn it. You can measure joint circumference with a tape measure. A simple test is to wrap your hand around your opposite wrist. If your thumb and middle finger overlap, you are small jointed (usually 6- to 7-inch/15- to 18-cm wrists); if your thumb and middle finger touch, you are medium jointed (usually 7- to 8-inch/18- to 20-cm wrists); if your thumb and middle finger do not touch, you are large jointed (usually 8 inches/20 cm or more in wrist circumference). In general, women lean toward the smaller-jointed side.

### 8. Digestive differences

The structure and function of each person's digestive system varies dramatically. The width of the oesophagus can vary at least fourfold and this can affect the amount of food swallowed. Human stomachs also vary in size: some can hold six to eight times as much as others. Secretion of digestive enzymes and gastric fluids can vary. Some people have more efficient digestion and absorb and utilize nutrients better. Hormones that affect how full or hungry you feel are also produced in the gastrointestinal tract, and hormonal response can differ from one person to the next.

### 9. Food allergies and sensitivities

Some people are born with the tendency toward food allergies or sensitivities. Two common examples are lactose intolerance (an inability to properly digest dairy products) and gluten intolerance (an allergy to the protein found in wheat and certain other grains). Through years of trial and error, most people instinctively favour certain foods while shying away from others. Some people become vegetarians, while others are carnivores simply because of the way each food or diet makes them feel. Other people ignore their body's signals and suffer the consequences, from mild gastrointestinal disturbances to more serious health problems.

### 10. Carbohydrate tolerance

Some people's bodies don't handle carbohydrates very well. Carb-intolerant individuals often suffer from blood-sugar- and insulin-related metabolic disorders and may have problems with appetite regulation. Their condition gets worse if they eat large doses of sugar or other concentrated carbohydrates. This explains why one person can stay lean, healthy, and energetic on a meal plan high in rice, potatoes, whole grains, and other high-carb foods, while another gains fat and suffers from mood swings, low energy, and health problems eating the same thing.

## THE TRUTH ABOUT GENETICS AND YOUR POTENTIAL

Judging by the list of traits that can't be changed, you might think the only surefire road to athletic success or a super-lean body is to choose the right parents. The great news is that fat loss and fitness are not determined by genetics alone. The way your body looks today is the result of genetics, behaviour, and environment all put together. The truth is the factors you can't control are small potatoes compared to the ones you can.

Dedication, discipline, and hard work can take you so far, it can appear as if you've shattered your genetic "limits." The reality is that most people never come close to fulfilling their full potential. A belief in limitations stops many from even exploring it. How much potential do you have? You'll never know unless you get busy and find out.

If you're below average on the genetic bell curve, you'll have to accept that getting lean or muscular might be more challenging or take longer for you than others. So ignore what the others are doing, especially the genetic freaks, because anything works for them. Instead, accept the challenge of lifelong personal improvement. Regardless of your genetics, you can transform yourself as long as you follow the right plan and customize it for your body type.

## HOW TO IDENTIFY YOUR BODY TYPE:
## THE SOMATOTYPE SYSTEM

In the 1930s and 1940s, American psychologist William Herbert Sheldon became engrossed in the study of human body types. Sheldon's main objective was to discover how variations in human physiques were related to personality types or temperaments. Part of his research included studying more than 4,000 photographs, from which he pioneered a system for identifying body types known as somatotyping.

Sheldon's system said that you can discern a person's body type by visual inspection (the photoscopic method). You simply compare how you look to a list of body-type characteristics. The modern body-typing method we use goes beyond external structure alone, and considers body fat, lean mass, metabolic traits, behavioural tendencies, and a person's tendency toward weight and body composition change.

There are three basic body types:

- *Endomorphs* are the large, fatter types. They have a soft roundness and often have difficulty losing body fat.
- *Mesomorphs* are mostly muscular types. They are lean, hard, and naturally athletic, and gain muscle with ease.

- *Ectomorphs* are the lean, skinny types. They are thin and bony, with fast metabolisms and extremely low body fat.

Pure body types are rare; a combination is more common. For example, someone who gains muscle easily but also has a tendency to gain fat along with the muscle is an endomorphic mesomorph (endo-meso). This body type is typical of American football linemen, heavyweight wrestlers, and powerlifters; they have lots of muscle, but it's often covered with a layer of fat. The ectomorphic mesomorph (ecto-meso) is the person who is lean and linear, with moderate amounts of muscle. Basketball players are often ecto-meso body types (think Michael Jordan).

Keep in mind that the somatotype system gives only general guidelines, and the lines between body types are somewhat subjective. What's most important is knowing your *predominant* type and understanding how to use that knowledge in a practical way.

To help classify yourself, the next step is to take a closer look at the body type characteristics. We'll also go through a list of action strategies to help you customize your nutrition, training, and lifestyle plan to get the best results for your body type.

## ENDOMORPHIC CHARACTERISTICS AND TENDENCIES

Endomorphs are the naturally round, fatter types. Endomorphs have a tendency for weight gain and slower weight loss. They often struggle with cycles of weight loss and regain throughout their lives. Santa Claus is the archetypal endomorph. Endomorphs typically:

- have naturally high levels of body fat (often overweight)
- are usually big-boned, large jointed
- have short, tapering arms and legs
- have soft, round body contours (round or apple-shaped body)
- have a wide waist and hips (waist dominates over chest)
- describe themselves as having a "slow metabolism"
- have a moderate or poor carb tolerance
- respond better to higher protein and low or moderate carbs
- tend to partition excess calories into fat (can't get away with overeating)
- have difficulty losing weight (it requires more effort)
- tend to gain fat easily when exercise is stopped
- tend to lose fat slowly, even on a reduced-calorie diet
- respond best to longer, more frequent cardio sessions

- find it challenging to keep fat off after it is lost
- fall asleep easily and sleep deeply
- tend to be sluggish and tired, and lack energy
- have low activity and NEAT levels.

## Endomorphic Training, Nutrition, and Lifestyle Strategies

When it comes to fat loss, a well-planned, strategic approach is more important for the endomorph than any other body type. Their bodies are very unforgiving, so they require stricter compliance to their meal plans and more careful tracking of daily calorie and macronutrient goals. Many endomorphs respond well to reducing carbs. The endomorph strategy calls for high levels of activity, including an active lifestyle, weight training, and cardio. Endomorphs must be disciplined and consistent in everything they do.

### REDUCE CARBOHYDRATES

Endomorphs often have varying degrees of carb intolerance, so high-carb, low-fat diets are usually not ideal. The endomorph nutrition strategy leans toward more protein, healthy fats, and fibrous carbs, with natural starches and whole grains eaten in moderation. Carbs may be included successfully if they are cycled and used strategically around training times. You'll learn more about nutrient timing and carb cycling strategies in upcoming chapters.

### KEEP CHEAT MEALS TO A MINIMUM

Everyone can include their favourite indulgence foods in their meal plans if they do it sensibly. However, endomorphs have unforgiving bodies, so they have to do it more cautiously. They cannot eat whatever they want whenever they want or indulge in free-for-all cheat days and expect to get away with it. Plan cheat meals in advance, and make sure they fit into your daily calorie and macronutrient limits. Most endomorphs do best with a fairly strict 90 per cent compliance rule. That means limiting junk foods to 10 per cent or less of weekly calories, or allowing no more than two cheat meals per week.

### INCREASE CARDIO DURATION OR INTENSITY

A simple way to burn more fat is with longer or harder cardio workouts. Twenty to thirty minutes is a good starting point, but to maximize fat loss, most endomorphs get better results building up to 40 to 45 minutes. In some cases, up to 60 minutes per day may be ideal. This could also be split into more than one session. Once you've reached your goal, you can return to shorter workouts for maintenance. For time efficiency, a great strategy is to increase the intensity of the cardio you're already doing and burn more calories in the same amount of time. Either way, endomorphs should focus on burning more.

### INCREASE TRAINING FREQUENCY

Endomorphs must stay in motion to keep their metabolism revved up. Think of your metabolic rate as a spinning top. You twist the top and it starts spinning at maximum velocity, but soon after you let go, the top is already slowing down. Eventually it starts to wobble. You have to spin it again before it loses its momentum and topples over. By spinning it more frequently, the average rpms stay higher and the top never slows to a wobble.

Every bout of intense training "spins" your metabolic rate, but this exercise-induced boost doesn't last long. Building more muscle with weight training can create a long-term increase in metabolism, but the only way to keep your metabolism "spinning" is with frequent and consistent exercise. Cardio and resistance training combined give you the best results.

### USE METABOLISM-STIMULATING RESISTANCE EXERCISES

Resistance training is essential. By choosing large muscle full-body and lower-body exercises, you not only build lean mass and strength, you also increase metabolism, burn more calories, and stimulate hormones that improve body composition. Squats, dead lifts, lunges, pull-ups, rows, presses, and other compound exercises are your best choices. Exercises like yoga, Pilates, and tai chi have some great benefits, including flexibility and stress reduction, but for the endomorph they're not the ideal way to maximize fat loss. If you enjoy these activities, do them to supplement – not replace – your weight training.

### ADOPT A MORE ACTIVE LIFESTYLE

The natural endomorph's disposition is to take it easy and relax. Endomorphs like to kick back in an easy chair for the weekend, while their ectomorphic or mesomorphic counterparts might "relax" with a 100-mile bike ride or a hike through the mountains. The best strategy for the endomorph is to get some kind of activity daily. Get out of your chair at regular intervals throughout the day. Walk everywhere. Take up some sports or recreational activities in addition to your regular workouts in the gym.

### AVOID OVERSLEEPING

Sleep is important for recovery and overall health, but endomorphs should become early risers and avoid excessive sleeping. Endomorphs often have the urge to hit the snooze button. Resisting this habit and getting up early to review your goals and train is one of the best strategies to get a positive start on the day.

### WATCH LESS TV

Any pastimes or hobbies that glue your rear end to a sofa or easy chair are not ideal for an endomorph, especially if you spend 40 hours or more behind a desk each week. Replace as much TV time as possible with physical recreation or exercise – unless your workout machine is parked in front of the TV and you're on it.

### ALWAYS BE ON THE LOOKOUT FOR SOMETHING TO MOTIVATE AND INSPIRE YOU

Endomorphs sometimes lack motivation, especially if results are slow. The solution is to be on constant lookout for anything to inspire you. Read biographies, watch sports or the Olympics, get a training partner, read motivational books, listen to inspiring audio programmes, hire a trainer, get a coach, rewrite your goals every day, go watch a bodybuilding or fitness contest, or even enter a body transformation contest yourself. Do whatever it takes to stay mentally pumped!

### BE CONSISTENT

Except for occasional planned layoffs and vacations, the endomorph can't relax his efforts or it will take a long time to achieve big goals. Endomorphs must be very consistent and disciplined in eating and training habits 7 days a week, 52 weeks a year. Spurts of starting and stopping never work for the endomorph. Get your momentum going and keep it going.

### BE PATIENT

Endomorphs often lose fat more slowly than the other body types. However, endomorphs can reach their body composition goals just like everyone else. It simply may take a little longer. Patience is a virtue that all endomorphs must cultivate.

### MAKE A LIFELONG COMMITMENT TO EXERCISE

Exercise is one of the most important factors in successful weight-loss maintenance and it's more important for the endomorph than anyone else. The endomorph tendency is to gain fat when sedentary and regain fat when exercise is stopped. Every time you stop working out for an extended period, body fat will start to creep back on. Burning fat is one thing. Keeping it off is another. It takes a lifetime commitment to stay lean.

## ECTOMORPHIC CHARACTERISTICS AND TENDENCIES

Ectomorphs are naturally lean, skinny types. Ectomorphs have a tendency to lose weight easily and have a hard time gaining muscle. They rarely have trouble with excess body fat during their entire lives. The 1960s model Twiggy was the quintessential ectomorph. Ectomorphs typically:

- have long limbs and are linear
- have small joints and are small-boned
- have a small waist and narrow shoulders
- have angular, projecting bones
- are naturally lean; they lose fat very easily
- consider themselves "hard gainers"
- have low strength levels prior to starting a training programme
- have a fast metabolism and burn up everything they eat
- have good carbohydrate tolerance
- have a high energy level
- tend to be overactive and restless
- sometimes suffer from insomnia
- have high levels of NEAT
- sometimes find it hard to maintain weight
- find it extremely hard to gain weight
- respond best to low-volume, brief, infrequent, heavy weight training.

### Ectomorphic Training, Nutrition, and Lifestyle Strategies

The common complaint of the ectomorph is: "I've always been too skinny. No matter what I eat, I can never gain weight." Many ectomorphs start weight training to fill out their bony frames. Although ectomorphs rarely develop the muscle size of mesomorphs, with hard work and persistence most of them can build impressive physiques with the advantage of staying lean without much effort. However, if they quit training or allow their calories to drop too low for too long, they'll eventually slide back toward the level of thinness to which their bodies are naturally inclined.

Most *Burn the Fat, Feed the Muscle* readers are not pure ectomorphs, because this is a fat-loss-focused book and ectomorphs are naturally lean. There are some exceptions, such as the combination ecto-endo body type with skinny legs, skinny arms, and a large belly. An ectomorph can successfully use many of *Burn the Fat, Feed the Muscle*'s strategies, but the average ecto is more likely to use them for muscle gain than fat loss. Eating more and doing less cardio is the common prescription.

The following guidelines will help maximize results for the ectomorphic body type.

## SLOW DOWN AND REDUCE STRESS

Because ectomorphs are thin, hyperactive people with fast metabolisms, the first and most obvious solution is less activity. Like an engine idling too fast, an ectomorph has to keep a foot on the brake just to keep from lurching forward. Conserving nervous energy is important. Ectomorphs need to get plenty of quality sleep on a regular schedule. Stress reduction techniques can help the ectomorph get better results as well.

## FOCUS ON WEIGHT TRAINING BUT AVOID OVERTRAINING

Ectomorphs respond best to brief, heavy, basic weight-training programmes. Daily training and high-volume workouts might even be counterproductive. The ectomorph should get in and out of the gym quickly and allow plenty of recuperation between workouts.

## KEEP CARDIO TO A MINIMUM

The big challenge for the ectomorph is gaining or even maintaining lean body weight. That's why cardio should be kept to a minimum and be done mainly for health and conditioning reasons. Twenty to thirty minutes a day, three days a week, is usually enough. Extreme ectomorphs might want to avoid cardio completely; the weight training alone will provide cardiovascular and health benefits.

## KEEP THE CALORIES HIGH AND NEVER MISS MEALS

Ectomorphs need calories – lots of them. To gain muscle, they have to hit their protein goal every day and achieve a calorie surplus. Foods with high calorie density, including moderate amounts of healthy fats, are useful. Skipping meals is a cardinal sin for the ectomorph.

## EAT CARBS

Since ectomorphs are already lean and burn up nearly everything they eat, there's rarely a reason to restrict carbs, outside of blood-sugar-related health problems. Removing carbs only makes it harder to get enough calories for a surplus. Fifty per cent of total calories from carbs is a standard baseline for *Burn the Fat, Feed the Muscle* (not carb restricted), and that works well for an ecto.

## PAY ATTENTION TO FOOD QUALITY

People with ectomorphic tendencies usually discover they can get away with eating junk food without ill effects on body composition, so they often do. However, this is not wise, because even an ectomorph should be concerned about nutrient density and food quality, not just food quantity. Choose foods for health, not just for fuel and muscle growth. Never use a naturally lean body type as an excuse to overindulge in junk food.

## MESOMORPHIC CHARACTERISTICS AND TENDENCIES

Mesomorphs (a.k.a. the "genetic freaks") are the naturally muscular and lean types. Many of them had muscle before they started working out. These are the genetically gifted ones who everyone loves to hate because they gain muscle and lose fat so easily. Heavyweight competitive bodybuilders are the prime example of the mesomorphic body type (think Arnold Schwarzenegger in his Mr. Olympia prime). Ms. Olympia figure and fitness champions such as Erin Stern and Monica Brant represent the mesomorphic body on the female side. Mesomorphs typically:

- have medium joint size
- have broad shoulders
- have a larger chest and smaller waist
- are naturally lean
- are naturally muscular
- are naturally strong
- have high energy levels
- have great carbohydrate tolerance
- tend to partition surplus calories into muscle
- have a highly efficient (fast) metabolism
- gain strength easily
- gain muscle easily
- lose body fat easily
- respond quickly to almost any type of training
- are natural-born strength and power athletes

### Mesomorphic Training, Nutrition, and Lifestyle Strategies

There's not much to say about mesomorphic training and nutrition. The ironic thing about mesomorphs is that for many of them it doesn't matter what they eat or how they train; they lose body fat and gain muscle anyway. As long as they have the basic nutrition and training fundamentals covered, they get results.

Here are two tips for the mesomorph to live by:

### DON'T COAST ON YOUR GENETICS

Although they're envied by many, mesomorphs do have their Achilles' heel. Because they get results so easily, they often coast on their genetics and don't train as hard as they could. They may cheat on their diets and skip workouts simply because they can get away with it and still look good. As a result, many never actualize their full potential.

A mesomorph with clear goals and a superior work ethic will always rise to the top and quickly become a superstar. These are the people who *can* become pro bodybuilders, fitness models, or Olympic athletes. If you recognize that you're genetically gifted for physique development, appreciate your blessing and make the most of it, even if you're not interested in sports or competition.

### PAY ATTENTION TO FOOD QUALITY

Like the ectomorphs, people with mesomorphic tendencies discover that they can also get away with eating certain foods without ill effects on body composition, so they get lax about their food choices and lower their compliance rule too far. Again, keep in mind that nutrition is not just about looking good; it's about being healthy. Gorging on junk food just because you can get away with it in the short term is not a good idea. In the best-case scenario, it will limit your development. In the worst-case scenario, it could compromise your health.

## BODY TYPE VERSUS METABOLIC TYPE

In the classic system, "somatotype" refers to the physical or external body structure, which you can appraise with a photograph or tape measure. "Metabolic type" is different; it refers to biological processes that take place internally. Another new advancement in body typing is combining these concepts of somatotype and metabolic type. For example, endomorphs are the people who have the rounder body shape as well as metabolic characteristics that predispose them to storing and holding excess body fat.

How well you process carbs and manage blood sugar is one of the most important traits to consider. People differ widely in their ability to process sugar. On the extremely unhealthy end of the spectrum, you have diabetes. In the middle, you have metabolic syndrome, which some people call "pre-diabetic." And on the normal end of the spectrum you have various degrees of carbohydrate intolerance.

These differences in metabolic type explain why some people thrive on high-carb, low-protein, low-fat diets while others get leaner, feel better, and stay healthier on high-protein, high-fat diets with lower carbs.

Although metabolic traits are numerous and complex, in the *Burn the Fat, Feed the Muscle* system, metabolic type boils down to two simple questions: Are you carb tolerant or carb intolerant? And if you're carb intolerant, to what degree? Use the body-type guidelines in this chapter, along with the information in the nutrition part of this book, and with a little trial and error experimenting with carb levels, you'll discover your tolerance quickly.

## SIZING UP YOUR TRUE NATURAL BODY TYPE

Somatotyping has fascinated bodybuilders, athletes, and fitness fanatics for decades. The classic Sheldon system did, however, have a major flaw: It was a genotypic system, which assumes that your body type is genetically fixed and can't be changed. That's only partly true. Obviously some characteristics like joint size and height are unchangeable after we're adults, but it's also obvious that our bodies do transform as a result of training, nutrition, and lifestyle change. That's the whole idea, isn't it? The ultimate goal is to start looking like a soft, round endomorph and finish looking like a lean, muscular mesomorph.

Modern body-typing science is based on a phenotypic system, which assumes that the way your body looks is a result of behaviour and environment, not just genetics. Your body changes on its own with growth and aging, and you change your body purposely with nutrition, training, and lifestyle choices.

That's why the way a person looks *now* after training may not be a reliable indicator of their true natural body type. How they looked *before* they started training is more revealing. There's an inside joke among bodybuilders who look great despite having less than ideal genes: "The harder I work, the better my genetics appear."

Another true sign of your natural body type is what happens when you stop training. Do you retain your muscle gains (mesomorphic) or do you atrophy quickly (ectomorphic)? Does the body fat stay off (ectomorphic or mesomorphic) or do you regain fat quickly the minute you stop training (endomorphic)? Recognizing these tendencies will help you maximize and customize the *Burn the Fat, Feed the Muscle* programme once you get started.

The ultimate tale of the tape is how well you respond to training and nutrition. If you grow muscle like crazy and the fat melts off with ease as soon as you start any nutrition or training programme, you have genetic gifts: You have the mesomorph's muscle-building qualities and the ectomorph's fat-burning qualities.

Body type doesn't dictate what your destiny is, but it does tell you what your tendency is and understanding your tendencies is valuable. We all have a natural body type we're born with. If we don't make a conscious effort to change the factors we control – behaviour and environment – we'll always drift back to our inherent body types.

## CUSTOMIZING YOUR PLAN FOR YOUR BODY TYPE

By now you should have a fairly good idea of your body type, and if you're still not sure, don't worry: You don't have to get it all at once. Now that you know what to look for, it will get easier to know yourself with every passing week you follow the programme and pay attention to the results. Even more important than pinpointing your exact type is to simply understand that you're unique and your programme must be fitted for your body.

If you wore the wrong suit size, it wouldn't feel right. In the same way, when you follow the wrong nutrition and training plan, it just doesn't feel right. That's why it's best to avoid programmes that aren't flexible. In the diet and fitness world, most people believe that there's only one single best way. But a one-size-fits-all approach couldn't possibly work for everyone.

Customization can be the difference between great results and no results, and this theme runs through every chapter of this book. With your new knowledge of body types, combined with the tools you'll learn in the rest of this book, customizing your plan will be easy. You'll be able to personalize your goals, calories, protein, carbs, fats, macronutrient ratios, foods, fluid intake, meal schedules, training schedules, and everything else so it fits you perfectly. And when you've got it, you'll know it, because it will feel right, just like a custom-tailored suit.

## ACCEPTING RESPONSIBILITY

Many people read about genetics or body types and get concerned about whether they've inherited "fat genes." There's no doubt that heredity dictates your ultimate potential for muscular development and plays a role in how easily you burn fat. But the primary cause of excess body fat is your own attitude, behaviour, and lifestyle. Science confirms that overweight people are more likely to be made than born and that following a healthy lifestyle can counteract gene-related risks.

Most of the factors affecting body composition are entirely under your control. No matter what your body type or genetic potential, you can always improve by consistently taking action in all these areas.

### THE FACTORS YOU CONTROL
- How much you eat
- What you eat
- When you eat
- What type of exercise you do

- How frequently you exercise
- How long you exercise
- How hard you exercise
- Your overall lifestyle
- Who you socialize with and allow to influence you
- Your mental attitude

The truth is, if you're unhealthy, you're unfit, or you have too much body fat, you're responsible. If you refuse to accept this, you'll never reach your full potential. If you want to burn fat and transform your body for good, the first step is to accept 100 per cent responsibility for where you are now.

When you're not getting the results you want, the easiest thing to do is to put the blame somewhere else and make excuses like "It's my genetics" or "I have a slow metabolism." But if you don't believe you're in control and responsible for your life, for better or worse, how do you expect to change it?

In a brief but powerful book called *As a Man Thinketh*, author James Allen wrote, "Circumstances do not make a man, they reveal him." We are not products of our environment or our heredity (our circumstances); we are products of our own thinking and belief systems.

You create positive circumstances through positive thinking and positive action, and you create negative circumstances through negative thinking, lack of action, and wrong actions. In other words, you are responsible for who you are, where you are, and what you have – and that includes the way your body looks.

## DOING YOUR BEST WITH WHAT YOU'VE GOT

Understanding your body type doesn't mean throwing in the towel if you're an extreme endomorph. It doesn't mean "I'm genetically inferior, so I won't even bother trying." Be realistic about your body type and accept the role it plays in changing your body. Don't get discouraged if you don't have Olympian genetics. You can overcome nearly any obstacle if you're willing to work hard enough. I'll show you how, no matter what your genetic endowment, you can totally transform yourself with hard work, dedication, persistence, and a positive attitude.

The late UCLA Bruins basketball coach John Wooden said, "The good Lord in his infinite wisdom, did not create us all equal when it comes to size, strength, appearance, or various aptitudes. But success is not being better than someone else, success is the peace of mind that is a direct result of self-satisfaction in knowing that you gave your best effort to become the best of which you are capable."

Don't try to become better than someone else; become better than you used to be. Instead of focusing on comparisons, focus on progress and self-improvement. Do the absolute best you can with what you've got and you'll be able to look in the mirror every day with the pride and self-esteem of a true winner.

# PART II

# THE *L.E.A.N.*
# PLAN OF ACTION

# ESTABLISH YOUR BASELINE

CHAPTER 4

# Measuring Body Composition

"Losing weight is the wrong goal. You should forget about your weight and instead concentrate on shedding fat and gaining muscle!"

    – Dr. William Evans, author of *Biomarkers: The 10 Keys to Prolonging Vitality*

## BODY COMPOSITION: MUSCLE WEIGHT VERSUS FAT WEIGHT

Beauty may be in the eye of the beholder, but let's face it: Muscle looks better than fat. Fat fills in all the lines and "cuts" that separate each distinct muscle group. It covers your muscles with a thick layer of insulation, obscuring the definition underneath, and adds a soft and doughy quality to your entire body.

Muscle is what makes your body look solid, chiselled, and athletic, but muscle has more than aesthetic value. Your goal should be to develop and maintain muscle not only for how it looks but for what it will do for your metabolism, your strength, and your health. Unfortunately, most people pay little attention to how much muscle they have, because they're obsessed with scale weight. Big mistake!

The scale doesn't tell you how much weight is fat and how much is muscle. Most dieters assume that weight loss is always a positive outcome, and weight gain, negative. But what if the loss or gain came from muscle? Another problem is that your scale weight can fluctuate on a daily basis depending on your body's water level, leading you to misinterpret your results. Losing weight is easy. Losing fat and keeping it off – without losing muscle – is a bigger challenge. If you simply wanted to weigh less, I could show you how to drop 10 to 15 pounds (4.5 to 7 kg) over the weekend with natural diuretics and other dehydration tricks. Boxers and wrestlers do it all the time to make a weight class. But what good is it to lose water weight that you'll gain back as quickly as you lost it?

If you want to get off the diet roller coaster and achieve permanent fat loss, the first thing you must lose is the preoccupation with scale weight. Instead, start judging your progress with *lean body mass* and *body fat*. Prioritizing body composition over body weight may be difficult at first, but it's essential to your long-term success.

## WHY IDEAL WEIGHT CHARTS ARE MISLEADING

One of the oldest methods for finding your ideal or healthy weight is the height and weight chart, which recommends what you should weigh based on your height alone. These charts are still popular today. They're used by insurance companies, physicians, sports teams, and the military, but they're very misleading because they don't consider body composition.

According to a height–weight chart, a 5-foot-8-inch (173-cm) male bodybuilder weighing 200 pounds (14 st 4 lb/91 kg) would be misclassified as "overweight" even though he has single-digit body fat, six-pack abs, and perfect health. On the other hand, a 115-pound (8 st 3-lb/52 kg) woman can have 33 per cent body fat and a 172-pound (12 st 4-lb/78 kg) man can have 27 per cent body fat. Both have acceptable body weights according to the charts, but if you take body composition into account, you realize they're overfat and unhealthy.

These people with low body weight but high body fat are often called "skinny fat." That term may be fitness slang, but it's a real clinical condition: Researchers call it "normal weight obesity." Today there's a new epidemic called "sarcopenic obesity." This is where men and women are clinically obese *and* overweight, but their muscle mass is so low, they're weak and nonfunctional. They're also more prone to degenerative diseases like osteoarthritis, more susceptible to metabolic disorders, and more likely to die young.

Sarcopenia by itself is a serious problem; it's the loss of muscle that happens as you age if you do nothing to prevent it. Sarcopenia has been in the news for years because health-care professionals are so concerned about how it's destroying quality of life in older men and women.

This should be a real wake-up call for people who think that strength and muscle aren't important for your health. These examples show us how losing weight and losing fat are not the same, being overweight and overfat are not the same, and there's a drastic difference between ideal weight and ideal body composition. That's why height and weight charts can't possibly tell you what your real ideal and healthy weight should be.

## FAILINGS OF THE BODY MASS INDEX

Body mass index (BMI) is another method often used to diagnose obesity. BMI is calculated with a simple formula: weight (in kilograms) divided by height (in metres) squared. You get classified as overweight if your BMI is over 25 and obese if your BMI is over 30.

Advocates of BMI say that it correlates with body composition and is a better gauge of health than your weight alone. The truth is BMI might be an acceptable screening tool for the general population, but for many people BMI is just as misleading as height–weight charts.

A "skinny fat person" could have a "healthy" BMI of 19 to 22 with a dangerously high level of body fat. A typical bodybuilder or strength athlete could have a "dangerously" high BMI of 30 and a healthy, low level of body fat. According to the BMI, almost every player in the American National Football League is overweight and some contestants in the Mr. Olympia competition are "morbidly obese," with BMIs of 40, even though there's not an ounce of visible fat on their bodies.

Here's a personal example: As a natural bodybuilder, I weighed 201 pounds (14 st 5 lb/91 kg) at my heaviest, and I'm 5 feet 8 inches (173 cm) tall. Let's plug my stats into the BMI formula and see what we come up with …

**201 pounds = 14 st 5 lb (91.17 kg)**
**1.72 metres squared = 2.96**
**91.17 ÷ 2.96 = 30.8 BMI**

Judging me according to my BMI of 30.8, my health is at risk and I need to lose some lard. Obviously, that's not the case, since I rarely hit double-digit body fat.

Shape Up America!, the anti-obesity campaign started by Dr. C. Everett Koop, published a statement years ago saying that BMI misclassifies one out of four people and should not be used by athletes who carry more muscle than most people.

Even if you're a regular fitness enthusiast who doesn't compete in strength or physique sports, you're going to be eating and training like an athlete on the *Burn the Fat, Feed the Muscle* programme. So forget about BMI and height–weight charts; the ideal way to rate your weight, check your health, and track your progress is body fat testing.

## BODY FAT TESTING:
## THE IDEAL WAY TO MEASURE YOUR PROGRESS

Weigh yourself, but don't stop there. When you measure your body fat percentage as well, you'll be able to answer two important questions about body composition:

1. How much of your weight is *body fat*?
2. How much of your weight is *lean body mass*?

Another reason you'll be measuring your body fat every week is so you can monitor your progress and get continual feedback about the effect your nutrition and training are having on your body. You'll be keeping track of what really counts – fat burned and muscle gained – not scale weight, BMI, someone else's ideal, or how much you worked out.

Many people spend hours working out each week, but they're not getting results. The real problem is they don't even know it! They mistake activity for achievement. You could be stuck in the mud (burning up calories but putting them all back) or heading in the wrong direction (losing weight but not fat). In *The 7 Habits of Highly Effective People,* Steven R. Covey points out, "Many people are climbing the ladder of success every day, only to find that it's leaning against the wrong wall."

Measuring your body fat is the only way to be sure all that activity is moving you in the right direction – toward better body composition, not just weight loss.

### What Is an Average Level of Body Fat?

Average body fat levels vary among the sexes and among different age groups. The average woman has about 23 per cent body fat and the average man approximately 17 per cent. Female hormones and child-bearing genetics cause women to carry at least 6 per cent more body fat than men. In both genders, body fat usually increases with age, while lean body mass decreases.

According to Dr. William Evans, who headed the Jean Mayer USDA Human Nutrition Research Center on Aging at Tufts University, the average person loses 6.6 pounds (3 kg) of lean body mass every decade after age 20. The rate of lean tissue loss increases after age 45. With advancing age, most people gain fat even when body weight doesn't change much; the muscle shrinks as the fat accumulates. The average male college student (age 20) has about 15 per cent body fat. The average sedentary middle-aged male has 25 per cent body fat or more.

### What Is an Ideal Level of Body Fat?

Keep in mind that the body fat levels I just mentioned are averages, not necessarily ideals. Basketball coaching legend John Wooden once said, "Being average means you're as close to the bottom as you are to the top." You can't achieve excellence if you're aiming for average. If you really think about it, when two-thirds of the population is overweight or obese, average isn't so good. Our standards have fallen.

A body fat level of 25 per cent statistically places a young woman in the average category, but 25 per cent isn't necessarily ideal; it's more like a passing grade. An optimal body fat percentage is around 16 per cent to 20 per cent for women and 10 per cent to 14 per cent for men. These ideal body fat goals will take work, but they are achievable and maintainable by almost anyone. Ideal body fat for athletes may be even lower, depending on the sport.

Everyone carries body fat differently, but at optimal levels, you'll look lean and, for the most part, fat-free. If you want the look of a *Men's Fitness* model or a figure competitor, you may need to drop your body fat even lower. Most men will start to see more muscle definition, including abs, when they hit the single digits. Women show nicely defined muscles when they reach the teens.

You're not destined to get fatter as you get older, but in the general (non-athlete) population, the average older person has more body fat. To account for this, I included ranges in my rating scale instead of single numbers. Younger people can use the low end of the range and older people can use the higher number for setting goals.

| Body Fat Rating Scale | Male | Female |
|---|---|---|
| Competition shape (ripped) | 3%–6% | 9%–12% |
| Very lean (excellent) | < 10% | <16% |
| Lean (good) | 10%–14% | 16%–20% |
| Satisfactory (fair) | 15%–19% | 21%–25% |
| Improvement needed (poor) | 20%–25% | 26%–30% |
| Major improvement needed (very poor) | 26%–30%+ | 31%–40%+ |

| Typical Average Body Fat Percentage for Athletes | Male | Female |
|---|---|---|
| Distance runners | 5%–10% | 10%–16% |
| Elite marathon runners | 3%–5% | 9%–12% |
| Sprinters | 5%–12% | 12%–18% |
| Jumpers and hurdlers | 6%–13% | 12%–20% |
| Olympic gymnasts | 5%–8% | 11%–14% |
| Bodybuilders, contest condition | 3%–5% | 9%–12% |
| Bodybuilders, off season | 6%–12% | 13%–18% |
| American football players, running backs, receivers, defensive backs | 7%–9% | NA |
| American football players, linemen | 16%–19% | NA |
| Football players | 7%–12% | 10%–18% |
| Baseball/softball players | 10%–14% | 12%–18% |

| Typical Average Body Fat Percentage for Athletes | Male | Female |
|---|---|---|
| Pro basketball players | 7%–12% | 10%–16% |
| Wrestlers | 4%–12% | NA |
| Cross-country skiers | 7%–13% | 17%–23% |
| Tennis players | 10%–16% | 14%–20% |
| Swimmers | 6%–12% | 10%–16% |

Low numbers are nice for bragging rights, but what counts is whether you're healthy and happy with how you look. You can use my charts to help you set some initial goals, but overall, I recommend using body fat percentage as a way to track your progress over time. Focus on improving yourself instead of chasing after some Holy Grail number.

## How Low Should You Go?

Competitive bodybuilders and endurance athletes such as marathon runners have been known to reach body fat levels as low as 3 per cent to 4 per cent in men and 9 per cent to 10 per cent in women. With today's obsession for leanness and the problem of body image disorders, the safety of dropping to very low body fat levels has rightfully been questioned. Being extremely lean is healthier than being obese, but trying to maintain extremely low body fat levels for too long might not be healthy or realistic, especially for women.

Many women who try to maintain their body fat levels at or below 10 per cent to 13 per cent experience health problems. Their menstrual cycles and reproductive systems become disrupted and bone density may decrease, putting them at higher risk of osteoporosis as they grow older.

For some athletes, reaching extremes of low body fat during a competitive season is simply part of the sport. Using extreme diets to get there or trying to maintain extreme low body fat is when most of the problems occur. Training and dieting in cycles so body fat levels vary between lean and competition lean is healthier and more sensible. The typical female figure or fitness competitor maintains a very lean and healthier body fat level of 14 per cent to 17 per cent for most of the year, then drops down lower for competition. Men may drop as low as 3 per cent to 5 per cent for competitions, and then maintain their body fat levels at 8 per cent to 10 per cent in the off-season.

You may have heard the term "zero body fat" thrown around. It's impossible for body fat to drop to zero because some fat is stored internally and is necessary for normal body functioning. This "essential fat" reserve is necessary for energy storage, protection of internal organs, and insulation against heat loss. Essential fat is found in the nerves, brain, bone marrow, liver, lungs, heart, and nearly all the other glands and organs of the body. In women, this fat also includes sex-related fat deposits in breast tissue and the uterus. Essential body fat is at least 10 per cent for women and 3 per cent for men.

## THE MOST POPULAR METHODS
## OF MEASURING BODY COMPOSITION

The scale, tape measure, and mirror are all helpful, but alone they're not enough. Why not go strictly by the mirror? After all, if you're happy with how you look, that's what really counts, isn't it? The problem is, when you look at yourself in the mirror every day, it's difficult to see daily and weekly changes because they're taking place so slowly; it's like watching the grass grow. It's also difficult for most people to judge their progress objectively. You rarely see changes in your own body as easily as others do. That's why you need an objective, accurate and scientific method for measuring your body composition. There are many ways to test your body fat, and in the next section I'll show you some of your options. Some are simple, inexpensive tests you can do by yourself or with a partner at home; others use high-tech equipment or require a professional to help you. Experts debate about which method is best. After weighing the pros and cons, I think you'll agree that for our purpose – tracking weekly personal progress – skinfold testing is the easiest and most practical.

### Skinfold Measurements: The "Pinch an Inch" Test

When you're choosing a method for body-fat testing, you need something that's practical, inexpensive, and easy to perform, and provides consistency over repeated measurements. The skinfold test fits the bill perfectly. Here's how it works:

Most of your body fat is stored directly beneath your skin. This type of fat deposit is called subcutaneous fat. The remainder of your body's fat is located around organs (internal or visceral fat) and inside muscle tissue (intramuscular fat). Measuring the amount of subcutaneous fat you have by pinching folds of skin and fat at several locations can give you a very accurate estimate of your overall body fat percentage.

It's ideal to have your body fat tested by a skilled technician, such as an exercise physiologist or experienced personal trainer at your gym. A friend, family member, or training partner can test you, but keep in mind there's a learning curve and the test is only as accurate as the skill of the person taking the measurements. Practice does make perfect, though.

The test is done with a vice-like instrument called a skinfold caliper. There are many brands of calipers. The Lange, Harpenden, and Skyndex are some of the most common and accurate professional models, although the cost can be high, ranging anywhere from $150 (£95) to as much as $450 (£280) for the electronic Skyndex. If someone else will be testing you at home, I recommend the Slim Guide caliper because it's one of the few inexpensive (under $20/£13) models that give fairly accurate readings.

During a skinfold test, you literally get "pinched" at several sites on your body. The jaws of the caliper clamp down on the fold of skin and fat and measure the thickness in millimetres (the larger the skinfold, the more fat you have). Then you add up the sum of the skinfolds and look up the results on the body fat estimation chart that comes with the caliper. The chart converts your skinfold thickness measurements into a body fat percentage. Computerized calipers like the Skyndex and Accu-Measure FatTrack models add up the skinfolds automatically and do the calculations for you.

There are many different body fat formulas for skinfold testing. Most have you measure at three or four different locations. Some formulas use as many as eleven skinfolds in various combinations. The standard skinfold sites are usually the abdominal, suprailiac (hip), bicep, tricep, chest, subscapular (upper back), thigh, axilla (below the armpit), and calf. Taking measurements at three or four sites is most common and is more than enough for an accurate reading.

Don't get too caught up with where your skinfolds are measured. Some people get concerned if most of their visible fat is in their lower bodies and the skinfold test measures only the upper-body sites. Body fat formulas from skinfolds will give you a very accurate estimate of your *overall* body fat using only one to four sites, even if they're all measured from your upper body.

### SKINFOLD SELF-TESTING: HOW TO MEASURE YOUR BODY FAT IN THE PRIVACY OF YOUR OWN HOME

The Accu-Measure is a skinfold caliper designed specifically for testing yourself at home. All you have to do is pinch one spot: your hip bone (the suprailiac skinfold). Since that site is easy to reach and measure, no partner is needed. A conversion chart comes with the caliper and you simply look up the skinfold thickness in millimetres to translate that into body fat percentage.

The potential margin for error with self-testing might be greater when you do it by yourself, especially when you're a newbie, but research has validated this test. A study published in the *Journal of Strength and Conditioning Research* found the Accu-Measure to be just as accurate as the sum of three skinfolds taken by an experienced tester with a professional caliper.

If you don't have access to other forms of testing, the Accu-Measure is definitely good news. Even if you're not sure about the accuracy of the body fat percentage number, the home self-test at least tells you whether your fat percentage is dropping. As long as you see the skinfold thickness dropping, it means you're losing fat!

The big advantage of the Accu-Measure is the convenience: You can use it to test your own body fat at home. Another plus is the low cost. The Accu-Measure retails for less than $20 (£13) and it's readily available online at many Internet sites.

For more details on all the different types of body fat calipers and where to find them, visit www.BurnTheFatFeedTheMuscle.com.

### ACCURACY AND CONSISTENCY OF SKINFOLD FAT TESTING

When caliper measurements are taken correctly by an experienced tester, the results are very accurate for people in the range of 15 per cent to 35 per cent body fat. For individuals with over 35 per cent body fat, the accuracy of the pinch test does go down somewhat. For lean individuals, skinfolds might be the most accurate method of all (using a multi-site test is preferable for very lean people).

Skinfold testing does require a lot of practice to master the pinching technique. The greatest errors result from not locating the right spot or from taking the skinfold improperly (for example, taking a horizontal fold when it should be a vertical fold).

Because there are so many different types of calipers and skinfold formulas, the important thing is to have the same person measure you with the same calipers and the same formula every time. Even with the most skilled tester, skinfolds are only accurate within 3 to 4 per cent.

However, if a skinfold test says you are 12 per cent body fat, it doesn't matter if your body fat is really 15 per cent. The *accuracy* is not as important as the *consistency* of repeated measurements so that you can chart your progress effectively from one measurement to the next. You'll learn more about how to track and chart progress in the next chapter, but first, let's take a quick look at some of the other body fat testing methods.

## Other Methods of Body Fat Testing

Skinfold measurement is by far the most popular way to test body fat, and it's my top recommendation for this programme. However, there are many other methods. Some of them are high-tech and extremely accurate but not as practical. Some are even more practical than skinfolds but questionable in accuracy. I want you to know about all the options available, so here are the most popular of the alternative methods.

## BIOELECTRICAL IMPEDANCE ANALYSIS

Bioelectrical impedance analysis (BIA) measures your body fat by testing the electrical conductivity of your body tissues. Lean body mass, because of its high (80 per cent) water content, is highly conductive. Fat, because of its low (15 per cent) water content, has an insulating effect and is less conductive.

The traditional impedance test is done by attaching electrodes to the skin of your right wrist and right foot. Low-amperage current is then passed through your entire body to measure resistance against muscle, bones, and fat tissue. A reading of resistance in ohms is then given to determine body fat.

BIA is a fairly reliable and valid measure of body composition, as long as the test procedures are followed properly. The results can fluctuate if you're dehydrated from alcohol, caffeine, exercise, or heavy sweating.

## BIA BODY FAT SCALES AND HAND GRIP TESTS

The most popular body-fat testing scales are manufactured by Tanita. The most popular hand grippers are produced by Omron. These scales and grippers use BIA technology, although they're not the same as the whole-body BIA test done with the electrodes on the hand and foot. New BIA scales have been developed that also have hand grippers. In theory, these hand-to-foot BIA devices should be more accurate, but there's not much evidence to verify that yet.

The advantage of using a body-fat testing scale is being able to test yourself at home; nothing beats them for convenience and ease of use. But what you gain in convenience, you might lose in accuracy. If you decide to use the body-fat testing scales, be sure to follow the test protocol to the letter. That includes a consistent time of day for the weigh-in. I've heard many reports from *Burn the Fat* readers and members saying that their morning test results fluctuated by as much as 5 per cent from their nighttime results.

If you think the scale is giving you consistent and repeatable measurements, then by all means continue to use it. However, don't be surprised if you see wild fluctuations and strange readings. Given the pros and cons for home testing, I consider these scales only a second-best choice behind skinfold testing.

## UNDERWATER WEIGHING (HYDROSTATIC TESTING)

Fat floats and muscle sinks. This simple fact is the basis for underwater weighing, also known as hydrostatic testing. Hydrostatic testing has always been the gold standard to which all other body fat testing methods are compared. However, being dunked under water is inconvenient, and you usually have to visit a hospital or university research centre to get the test done. It can also be expensive, although at some universities you can volunteer to be a guinea pig for exercise science students doing research projects. All things considered, underwater weighing is not very practical, but it's always interesting to have it done once in a while just for fun.

### THE BOD POD (AIR DISPLACEMENT)

The Bod Pod uses a technology called air displacement plethysmography. You sit in an egg-shaped fibreglass chamber and breathe into a tube, and the machine prints out your body composition results, including lean body mass and body fat. Several studies suggest that the Bod Pod has potential as another valid body fat testing tool, including in overweight and obese subjects. However, the Bod Pod has not been fully validated in all populations yet, so the jury is still out. If you're athletic, muscular, or already lean, the Bod Pod may slightly overestimate your body fat. Bod Pods can be found in many health clubs, sports medicine facilities, and some universities. The cost can vary: I've seen it range from $25 to $75 (£16 to £47) per test.

### CIRCUMFERENCE TESTING

You may have seen some of these formulas or calculators on the Internet: You simply take your measurements at one or more sites on your body, then plug them into the calculator with your height and weight, and it delivers an instant body fat estimate. The navy formula is one of the most popular methods.

A tape measure can't directly measure body fat, but there is a correlation between body circumferences, the relationship between those measurements, and your body fat percentage. These formulas are simple, convenient, and inexpensive, but there may be a larger degree of error compared to skinfold testing and hydrostatic weighing. I recommend circumference methods if you have no other testing options and you want a ballpark figure of your body fat.

It's well worth remembering, however, that there's a strong correlation between your waist circumference and your total body fat. If there's any reason you don't measure your body fat percentage, the very least you should do is to track your weight and your waist measurement. If your waist measurement is going down, your body fat percentage is almost always going down as well.

Your waist measurement is also an important health marker. Fat stored in the abdominal area is unhealthier than fat stored in the extremities. A large waist measurement is a symptom of metabolic syndrome, a precursor to diabetes, and it correlates to increased risk of heart disease and stroke. You're at risk if you're male and your waist measurement is over 40 inches (101 cm) or if you're female and your waist measurement is over 35 inches (89 cm).

**DEXA AND OTHER BODY FAT TESTING METHODS**

There are some other body fat testing methods that are high-tech, incredibly accurate, and very useful in the laboratory. Many experts consider the DEXA scan (which is also used to analyse bone density) the new gold standard. ("DEXA" stands for "dual-energy X-ray absorptiometry.") The problem is, due to inconvenience, inaccessibility, and expense, none of these methods is practical for personal home use and weekly results tracking. For example, a DEXA scan is usually available only at hospitals; it requires that you lie still for up to 20 minutes; and it can cost anywhere from $100 to $250 (£65 to £155) per test.

---

*QUICKSTART*

Not sure which body fat testing method to choose? My number one recommendation is to get an accurate skinfold test. Don't have access to caliper tests or can't get an accurate measurement? Measure your waist circumference with a tape measure and use it as a proxy for body fat percentage. Above all else, just remember, weight loss and fat loss are not the same thing.

---

## HOW TO CALCULATE YOUR FAT WEIGHT
## AND LEAN BODY MASS

By itself, your body fat percentage is nothing more than a number. The real value in knowing your body fat is to monitor your body composition progress from one week to the next. Once you know your body fat percentage, the next step is to calculate how much of your total weight is fat and how much is muscle. Then you can track your progress in total weight, fat weight, and lean body mass (LBM).

Your LBM is the total weight of all your body tissues excluding fat. This includes not only muscle but also bone and other fat-free tissues. Since muscle is the largest component of lean body mass, tracking your LBM can tell you if you've lost or gained muscle. Monitoring your LBM is one of the most useful and important purposes of body fat testing.

To calculate your LBM in pounds, you need to know two things: your body weight and your body fat percentage. First, determine how many pounds of fat you're carrying by multiplying your body fat percentage by your weight. You can then calculate your lean mass by subtracting the pounds of fat from your total body weight.

EXAMPLE:

YOUR BODY WEIGHT IS 194 POUNDS (13 ST 12 LB = 88 KG).

Your body fat percentage is 18 per cent (0.18).

Multiply your body fat by your weight to determine fat weight:

0.18 x 194 pounds = 34.9 pounds of fat

Subtract fat weight from total weight to determine lean mass:

194 pounds – 34.9 pounds fat = 159.1 pounds (12 kg) lean mass

## A SIMPLE TEST TO DETERMINE YOUR TRUE IDEAL WEIGHT

Now that you understand the importance of body fat versus body weight and you've seen the pitfalls of BMI and height–weight charts, how do you figure out your ideal weight? First of all, consider that maybe it doesn't matter what you weigh. If you were solid muscle without an ounce of visible fat on your body, and you loved the way you looked in the mirror, would you honestly care how much you weighed?

That said, it's still wise to have a weight goal in pounds as well as a body fat percentage goal. To calculate your ideal body weight, you need to know your current weight, your body fat percentage, your lean mass, and your target (desired) body fat percentage.

Enter your lean body mass (LBM) _____

Choose your target body fat % (TBF) _____

Subtract your TBF from 1 (1 – TBF) _____

Divide the difference by your LBM _____

Total = your ideal weight _____

- The ideal weight formula is: **lean body mass (LBM) ÷ (1 – target body fat %)**.
- TBF is expressed as a decimal (15% body fat = 0.15).
- You can subtract up to 2–3% more off the estimated ideal formula weight if you want to account for potential water weight losses.

## THE NEXT STEP: TRACKING YOUR PROGRESS

You now have a strong intellectual understanding of body composition and why it's so important. When it really sinks in on a practical level is after you start following the nutrition and training plan and start tracking your progress.

You'll learn more about your body by measuring and tracking your body weight, body fat, and lean body mass for just a few weeks than you will by reading about it for years. As the old saying goes, "A single accurate measurement is worth a thousand expert opinions." Recording your results, getting into a performance feedback loop, and charting your progress are steps that guarantee you'll never fail. You'll start this process in the next chapter.

# CHAPTER 5

# Tracking Progress: The Feedback Loop System That Won't Let You Fail

*"Realize that there is no such thing as failure. Keep this in mind and you will achieve all that you conceive in your mind."*

– Dr. Wayne W. Dyer, *You'll See It When You Believe It: The Way to Your Personal Transformation*

## LIFE'S DELAYS ARE NOT LIFE'S DENIALS

It was a dark and cloudy Thursday in May as I boarded a 757 for a 4:45 p.m. flight from Newark to San Francisco. I took my seat and waited for take off as I anticipated a relaxing week in northern California. Four forty-five came and went, but the plane didn't budge. At 4:55, the captain's voice echoed through the cabin over the loudspeakers: "There are level 4 and 5 thunderstorms just east of Newark and they're headed our way. These storm winds can reach tornado force, so we'll have to wait it out." We sat there on the runway for nearly two hours as fierce winds and a torrential downpour pelted the plane.

Finally, at around 6:30 p.m., the storm passed and the plane started taxiing toward the runway. Because all the planes in line were backed up, we slowly inched our way forward and had to wait our turn. At 7:00 p.m. we finally took off. With all the turbulence in the air, it was a bumpy ride on the way up. A few passengers panicked and some even looked a little sick. After about five minutes of being tossed around, the air calmed and plane levelled.

But we weren't headed toward San Francisco for long. Within minutes the plane shifted slightly off course. The onboard computer noted the plane's errant trajectory, the pilot made a small adjustment, and once again we were back on course. This process repeated itself for the entire six hours of the flight. Of course, I couldn't notice this by looking out the window, but I knew it was happening just the same because I knew how feedback systems work.

You see, an aeroplane never travels in a perfectly straight line. Even with the most sophisticated guidance systems, there's always a certain amount of drift. Using a variety of feedback such as radar, radio beacons, geographical landmarks, and aeronautical charts, the navigation equipment picks up the slight change in course. The pilot (or autopilot) then adjusts the plane's direction.

## HOW TO USE PERFORMANCE FEEDBACK TO TRACK YOUR PROGRESS AND GUARANTEE YOUR SUCCESS

The process of burning fat is a lot like the take off and flight of an aeroplane. Some people take a long time to get off the ground. Instead of patiently waiting out the storm, they quit before reaching take off speed. Others get off the ground, but as soon as they hit any turbulence, they quit and "land the plane." Some people even manage to coast comfortably toward their destination, making substantial progress. But the minute they find themselves off course, they also join the quitters instead of simply adjusting their direction.

All these people made the same fatal mistake of interpreting their results as failure. Because they believed they had failed, they gave up. Can you imagine if a pilot quit every time there was a delay, turbulence, or a slight deviation in the plane's course? No one would ever get anywhere! The key to your success starts with a mental re-frame:

**There is no such thing as failure – only feedback, only results.**

Price Pritchett, author of *The Quantum Leap Strategy*, emphasizes that what often looks like failure is actually a work in progress: "Everything looks like a failure in the middle. You can't bake a cake without getting the kitchen messy. Halfway through surgery it looks like there's been a murder in the operating room."

If you measure your body fat after a week of work and there's no change, you haven't failed; you've simply produced a result. As long as you have a goal and you're taking efficient daily action, then whatever result you produce is "performance feedback." It may not be the result you want, but it's still valuable feedback. You've learned one way that doesn't work.

If you want a different result, try a different approach. One definition of insanity is continuing to do the same thing over and over again while expecting a different result. Thomas Edison tried thousands of experiments to find a filament that would burn in the electric light bulb. When asked what it felt like to fail so many times, Edison said: "If I find 10,000 ways something won't work, I haven't failed. I am not discouraged, because every wrong attempt discarded is another step forward. Just because something doesn't do what you planned it to do doesn't mean it's useless." On the programme each week, you'll always get some kind of results. It's how you interpret your results that determine whether you'll reach your destination. Like the pilot and Thomas Edison, you need to gather feedback and change your course the instant you notice you're not heading in the right direction. You'll be like a trained pilot, course correcting your body with the tools you learn in the programme.

## THE FAT-LOSS SUCCESS SYSTEM THAT NEVER FAILS

I've developed a seven-step formula guaranteed to help you reach your goals. Because of this system's self-correcting nature, you can only fail if you stop using the system. Think of it as your own personal "navigation system." Here are the seven steps:

### 1. Know your outcome. Decide exactly where you want to go.

Knowing what you want is the first step toward success. But saying you want to lose weight is not enough. There's a science to setting and achieving goals, and it involves knowing what you want specifically, when you want to have it, and what it will look like when you do. In chapter 6 you'll learn the *Burn the Fat, Feed the Muscle* formula for goal setting. The important thing to know now is that nothing else you read in this book will be much help unless you have a clearly specified target. You might try a technique here and a tactic there, but ultimately you'll end up floundering because you won't have the direction, purpose, or motivation that come from having written goals.

### 2. Establish your starting point.

Knowing where you want to go isn't enough; you also need to know where you are now so you can chart the proper course from starting point to destination. Once you've committed your goals to writing, the next step is to take objective starting measurements, including body fat percentage, total body weight, fat weight, and lean weight, using what you learned in chapter 4. Once you have these numbers, write them down in the first row of your *Burn the Fat, Feed the Muscle* progress chart, which you can find in the appendix. (You can also download an interactive progress chart spreadsheet from www.BurnTheFatFeedTheMuscle.com.)

## 3. Formulate a plan of action.

The most efficient way to choose a plan of action is to model (copy) the physical and mental strategies used by those who have already achieved what you want to achieve. Modelling suggests that, instead of reinventing the wheel, you plug into a proven formula that already exists. You tap into the knowledge and experience of those who have gone before you and learn from their mistakes. Find successful role models, do what they did, and you'll get a similar result. Trial and error can be a long and painstaking process, and life is too short to do it the long way. Learn from the experts.

Choose your role models wisely. If you want to lose fat *permanently*, it makes no sense to model the 95 per cent of the population who lose weight only to gain it all back. Who should you follow? Model the people who have mastered the science of burning fat and maintaining muscle in a healthy way. No one fits that description better than natural bodybuilders and fitness athletes.

Modelling does have limitations. There's no guarantee that anyone can become a world-class bodybuilding or figure champion because not everyone has the same genetic potential. What modelling *will* do is help you reach the upper limits of your own genetic capabilities in the shortest time using a system that's already been proven to work. It lets you become the best *you* can be and do it as quickly as possible by bypassing unnecessary trial and error.

You're unique, so you'll always have to do some experimenting, no matter how time-tested your plan is. However, the leanest people in the world all hold certain things in common. The fundamental principles apply to everyone; there are laws of fat loss just as there are laws of gravity and electricity. People who get lean and stay lean have mastered them and you can learn them as well.

A master chef produces award-winning dishes over and over again by using the same recipe – a proven mixture of ingredients, which, when combined in the right sequence and amounts, produces a delicious dish every time. This programme is your recipe for surefire fat loss. The techniques in this book give you a guaranteed plan already tested and proven effective by the leanest athletes in the world. If you use the same recipe, it will work for you too.

## 4. Act on your plan consistently.

You can have the biggest goals and the best plan in the world, but if you don't act on them, you won't achieve a thing. A goal without action is worthless. Faith without action is dead. An affirmation without action is delusion. The bottom line is that you must put the book down, get off your butt, and get in the gym! Work at it. Deserve it.

Pay the price. Earn it. Nothing worth having ever comes without effort. It takes hard work and efficient action every single day. You must do something every day to move you closer to your goal.

### 5. Develop the sensory acuity to know if what you are doing is working or not. If it's working, keep doing it.

After putting your plan into action, you need to develop the sensory acuity to know if your plan is working. "Sensory acuity" is a neurolinguistic programming term used to describe your ability to see, feel, and notice even the smallest changes in your body. In a nutshell, it means paying attention. As long as you're taking action and tracking the results, it's okay to make mistakes. Mistakes are how we learn. The only person who makes no mistakes is the person who plays it safe and never tries anything.

The problem is some people have been making the same nutrition and training mistakes for ten years, and they still wonder why they aren't getting any results. You've got to be smarter than that. If you don't pay attention, you might be taking action but repeating the same mistakes over and over again. As Emerson once said, "A foolish consistency is the hobgoblin of little minds."

If someone asks you, "Is your programme working?" and your answer is "I don't know," then you're not paying attention and you need to develop better sensory acuity. Your programme is either working or it's not. You're either moving forward or backward. Maintenance is an illusion. You must chart your progress in writing and pay attention to the direction you're heading. If it's the wrong direction, change it quickly!

Natural bodybuilders and physique athletes are great role models to study because they've developed incredible sensitivity to the way they look and feel. They have the uncanny ability to notice the slightest difference in their bodies when they change their nutrition or training programmes. This enables them to decide whether the change was effective or not. Without this skill, your programme could be working and you might not even notice. Or worse, it might *not* be working – and you don't notice!

Sensory acuity is an art and a skill that takes time to develop, but anyone can master it. You simply need to know what to look for and then pay attention. You have already learned a major part of it – look for changes in body composition, not just body weight – and you'll learn more in this chapter. The rest comes from personal experience.

Ultimately, you need to learn how your own body responds and then make adjustments. You must become your own expert. Good coaches and trainers are always helpful, but no one knows your body like you do. Once you've locked onto a winning strategy and you're getting the results you want, don't change a thing. Stay your course, no matter what anyone tells you.

## 6. If it's not working, do something else.

The moment you realize you aren't making progress, you must immediately adjust your approach. Don't get discouraged. If you didn't get the result you wanted, remember: You didn't fail; rather, you succeeded at producing a result. You've only failed if you quit. Use the feedback as a lesson. Once you see that what you're doing isn't working and you recognize it as nothing more than feedback, then try something different. Throughout the rest of this book, you'll learn about all the options you have for changing your strategy when things aren't working the way you planned. This will become especially important if you hit a progress plateau. (Chapter 18 is devoted entirely to plateau-breaking strategies.)

## 7. Be flexible in your approach and be persistent.

Be willing to adjust your approach as many times as necessary until you reach your goal. Be willing to try as many different things as necessary for as long as it takes. Don't do what it takes for your training partner, your neighbour, your spouse, or anyone else. Do what it takes for you.

American motivational speaker and best-selling author Anthony Robbins tells the story of a man at a seminar who was extremely frustrated with his lack of business results. He said he'd tried "everything," but nothing worked.

ROBBINS: "You've tried EVERYTHING???"
ATTENDEE: "Yes, I've tried absolutely everything!"
ROBBINS: "Tell me the last HUNDRED things you tried."
ATTENDEE: "I haven't tried a hundred things."
ROBBINS: "OK, then just tell me the last FIFTY things you tried."
ATTENDEE: "I haven't tried fifty things."
ROBBINS: "All right then, tell me the last DOZEN things you tried."
ATTENDEE (getting somewhat embarrassed): "Well, I haven't tried a dozen things."
ROBBINS: "I thought you said you tried EVERYTHING! So tell me then, how many things HAVE you tried?"
ATTENDEE: (red-faced, shrinking back into his seat): "Two or three."

Ask yourself: "How persistent have I been?" Be honest. Have you quit prematurely? Did you give up at the first obstacle? How many different training and nutrition strategies have you tried? If your initial plan doesn't give you the results you want, the number of nutrition and training variations you can try is virtually unlimited. Don't be too rigid in your approach. Be flexible. It's necessary to have an action plan, but don't get married to your first plan. The more options you have at your disposal, the greater your chances for success. Leave yourself room to improvise.

## DEVELOPING YOUR OWN PERSONAL FORMULA OR PHILOSOPHY

In developing the martial art of Jeet Kune Do, Bruce Lee worked hard to create a philosophy for self-defence and personal growth. His method had four simple steps:

1. Research your own experience.
2. Absorb what is useful.
3. Reject what is useless.
4. Add what is specifically your own.

Lee explained,

> Formulas can only inhibit freedom; externally dictated prescriptions only squelch creativity and assure mediocrity ... Learning is definitely not mere imitation, nor is it the ability to accumulate and regurgitate fixed knowledge. Learning is a constant process of discovery, a process without end.

Beware of rigid programmes or dogmatic gurus who declare, "It's my way or the highway." There is no single best way. By studying, reading and modelling experts, you can quickly master all the universal principles and laws that regulate body composition. Once you've mastered the fundamentals, then through action, persistence, and sensory acuity you can do what Bruce Lee did and develop your own philosophy.

Your personal formula will unfold based on your unique body type and the way you respond to various combinations of nutrition and training. By transcending all rigid styles and systems, you'll no longer be bound by a particular way of doing things and you'll gain the freedom to reach your highest potential.

## THE TOP TEN WAYS TO GET PERFORMANCE FEEDBACK

The more feedback you get and the more ways you have to measure results, the better. Here are ten feedback tools to gauge your progress; just remember that body composition is the ideal measure:

### Ten Feedback Tools to Measure Your Progress

1. Body fat percentage
2. Skinfold thickness
3. Total body weight
4. Lean body mass (LBM)
5. Fat weight
6. How you look in the mirror
7. Before and after photographs
8. Measurements (tape measure)
9. Clothing sizes and how clothes fit
10. Other people's opinions

The mirror and photographs are useful, but they're subject to the filter of your self-perceptions. Other people's opinions will help if the feedback is honest, but they can steer you wrong if they're just being nice to avoid hurting your feelings. The fit of your clothes, especially your waistline, is a great feedback tool, but remember that growing muscles can make clothes feel tighter.

All these methods have value, so use as many as you can, but it's important to always include objective body composition measurements. Together, the skinfold caliper and scale don't lie.

## HOW TO USE A WEEKLY PROGRESS CHART

The *Burn the Fat, Feed the Muscle* progress chart in the appendix has columns for the date, body fat percentage, total weight, lean body mass, fat weight, and weekly change in each. You can also create your own custom chart on a spreadsheet. If you're using a caliper as your testing method, you may also want to track skinfold measurements (in millimetres). That will inform you about where you store most of your fat and where you are losing the most and least fat. Seeing the previous skinfold measurements also helps the tester improve the accuracy of each pinch test.

When you start the programme, weigh yourself and have your body fat measured. Then fill in the first row on your chart, including the date, your starting body weight, your body fat percentage, and your lean body mass. You can also take circumference measurements if you choose. Every week, recheck your progress and update your chart, including the change from last week.

## HOW TO WEIGH YOURSELF THE RIGHT WAY

By itself, the scale can be misleading, but together with skinfold testing to measure pounds of fat and muscle, your body weight gives you crucial information.

To get the most consistent weigh-in, always weigh yourself under the same conditions. Measure yourself on the same scale on the same day of the week at the same time of day, wearing the same amount of clothes. If you weigh yourself with shoes, then weigh yourself with shoes every time. If you weigh yourself naked, weigh yourself naked every time. Remember, your LBM and fat weight amounts will be correct only if your weigh-in is correct. Call this your official weekly weigh-in. I recommend Mondays because that tends to keep you in check on the weekends, the time that most people are liable to fall off the wagon.

Weighing yourself every day is optional for two reasons. First, you won't see significant changes in body fat on a day-to-day basis. Second, your body weight can fluctuate from day to day based on your hydration level. Daily fluctuations can range anywhere from 2 to 5 pounds (0.9 to 2.3 kg) or more from water weight alone. You'll see a statistically significant difference every seven days, so I recommend an official weigh-in once a week. If you're the analytical type, you can certainly weigh yourself daily if you want more data points. Just be sure to use that data to chart the trends or moving averages and don't get overly concerned with daily fluctuations.

## HOW TO CALCULATE MUSCLE LOSS OR GAIN

By tracking changes in your weight, body fat, and lean mass over time, you can tell if you've lost, maintained, or gained muscle. This reveals whether your exercise and diet programme is really working or if you've hit a plateau and need to make changes.

To calculate the change in your body composition over time, you simply subtract your previous weight, body fat, and lean mass from your current weight, body fat, and lean mass. Record this information on your progress chart and then decide what changes, if any, you need to make.

EXAMPLE:
WEEK ONE:
**Weight: 194 pounds (13 st 12 lb/88 kg)**
**Body fat: 21.1%**
**Fat weight: 40.9 pounds (19 kg)**
**Lean mass: 153.1 pounds (69 kg)**

**WEEK TWO:**

**Weight: 192 pounds (13 st 10 lb/87 kg)**

**Body fat: 20.5%**

**Fat weight: 39.3 pounds (18 kg)**

**Lean mass: 152.7 pounds (69 kg)**

**Change in weight: –2 pounds (0.9 kg)**

**Change in body fat: –0.6%**

**Change in fat weight: –1.6 pounds (0.7 kg)**

**Change in lean mass: –0.4 pounds (0.18 kg)**

In this example, Joe, our test subject, lost 2 pounds (0.9 kg) in one week. By taking a body fat measurement, we see that 1.6 pounds (0.7 kg) of Joe's weight loss came from fat, and 0.4 pounds (0.18 kg) came from lean body mass. This isn't ideal, because he lost a little bit of lean mass, but it's not that bad either. It's not uncommon to see an occasional drop in lean mass and it is unusual for most people (unless they're very heavy) to lose more than 2 or 3 pounds (0.9 to 1.4 kg) per week every week with 100 per cent fat loss.

## WHY YOU SHOULD WEIGH YOURSELF AND MEASURE BODY FAT ON A WEEKLY BASIS

Some experts believe that testing body fat every week is too often. They argue that weekly changes are so small, why bother? That may be a valid point, but if you don't capture performance feedback frequently, you could waste valuable time heading in the wrong direction. If a plane or ship strayed even a few degrees off course without making a quick adjustment in direction, that small deviation would grow larger over time until eventually it could end up hundreds of miles from its intended destination. Don't let that happen to you. Measure your progress weekly and make course corrections as often as necessary.

## WHAT A DECREASE IN LEAN BODY MASS TELLS YOU

As you fill out the rows in your progress chart each week, keep an eye on your LBM, especially the trend over time. Most people drop some water weight in the beginning, especially if they're restricting carbs, and this may show up in the LBM number. You can't measure water weight, muscle weight, and fat weight separately with a skinfold test, so when your start your programme, chalk up that initial LBM drop to water weight and don't be too concerned.

Water balance can affect your weight in the opposite direction too. If you eat more carbs than usual one day, and also increase your fluid or sodium intake, it's not uncommon to see an increase in body weight of 3 to 5 pounds (1.4 to 2.3 kg), especially if you were dehydrated or on low carbs. Your chart will show a several-pound gain in LBM, but obviously that overnight weight gain wasn't solid muscle. This simply reflects glycogen and water in the muscles.

This is why you must be consistent with your weigh-ins and why you shouldn't panic if you see a small or occasional drop in LBM. If your LBM continues to drop week after week in any significant amount, you may have cause for concern. A continual *downward trend over time* in your LBM number clearly shows that you're losing muscle tissue.

Also look at your ratio of fat lost to lean mass lost. If you lose more lean mass than fat, that's usually a sign that some of the weight was muscle tissue. For example, if you lose 4 pounds (1.8 kg) in one week with 1.8 pounds (0.8 kg) from fat and 2.2 pounds (1 kg) from lean mass, don't pat yourself on the back for losing more weight than average: You lost more LBM than fat.

## WEEKLY FLUCTUATIONS AND THE TREND OVER TIME

You'll rarely reach your goal in a straight line from start to finish. If you work hard, you'll see progress every week, but your rate of progress usually varies. One week you may lose 0.5 per cent body fat, the next 0.8 per cent and the next only 0.3 per cent. On some weeks you might not make any progress. Don't let this discourage you. Never panic over a one-week fluctuation. The trend over time is much more revealing.

Your progress chart is a lot like the stock market. The market fluctuates up and down in the short term, but in the long run the trend is always upward. If you're persistent – if you stay focused on the fundamentals and continue to make daily investments in your body – your progress will trend in a positive direction.

Just as you need faith in long-term market investments, you must have faith in long-term investments in your body without getting emotional about short-term results. If you look at one small segment on your progress chart, you're liable to give up or make poor and hasty decisions. Keep your eye on the big picture, keep watching the trends, and keep working hard on the fundamentals every single day.

## ANALYSING PROGRESS DATA
## AND ADJUSTING YOUR APPROACH

When you get to the chapter on how to break plateaus, it will become even clearer how important it is to track progress. The beauty of seeing the numbers on a chart is that, combined with visual assessments, you know it the instant you're stuck. By looking at the changes in body fat, weight, and lean mass, and reconciling these with your past week's training and nutrition and the trend over time, you also know exactly what to do next to get unstuck.

Your progress chart is also a great motivational tool, because nobody likes to see a blemish on their weekly "report card." Your progress chart is a tool for self-accountability as well. If you share your chart with someone else, whether that's a coach, trainer, friend, or family member, then you have double the accountability and this will help you stick with your programme even better.

After your weekly results update, look at your progress chart and, based on the past week's results, adjust your cardio, weight training, and nutrition if necessary. Each time you make a change, watch carefully for what happens every day during the following week. This will increase your sensory acuity skill. If you develop a keen eye for changes in your body based on changes to your nutrition and training, you'll eventually become a master at this, just like the fitness pros.

The more you pay attention to the weekly feedback and progress data, the better you get at applying progression and troubleshooting problems. You may reach a point when you anticipate what will happen next and you stay a step ahead of the curve, dodging plateaus before they happen and reaching your goal at the fastest possible rate.

Ultimately, you can become so skilled at this process, you won't have to track weight and body composition any more. Everything in this programme can become instinctual with enough repetition and practice.

## INTERPRETING YOUR PROGRESS CHART

There are many different results you can produce from various combinations of nutrition and training combined with your overall lifestyle. Each week, your weight, body fat, and lean mass could all rise, fall, or stay the same. This final section lists every possible outcome you may encounter on your fat-loss journey and the action steps to take when each occurs.

**LEAN MASS STAYS THE SAME AND BODY FAT DECREASES**

Fantastic! Your nutrition and training programme is working as planned and you're on your way to reaching your goal. Don't change anything. Keep up the good work!

**LEAN MASS STAYS THE SAME AND BODY FAT STAYS THE SAME**

Nothing is happening either way; you are in energy balance, so you must create a caloric deficit. First, double-check your nutrition compliance and track calories carefully. Then increase your calorie burn from cardio. You can increase intensity, duration, or frequency, depending on the volume of your current cardio programme. If you don't lose body fat within the next week, then you can reduce your daily caloric intake systematically by 100 to 200 calories at a time, provided you don't drop below your maximum allowable calorie deficit.

Keep your nutrient ratios the same unless you've been stuck for more than two weeks. If you've been on the programme for months and you've been stuck more than two weeks, you might want to experiment with reducing carbs or cycling carbs (see chapter 19 for details).

**LEAN MASS STAYS THE SAME AND BODY FAT INCREASES**

You're in a calorie surplus. You're eating more than you're burning and storing the excess as fat. Double-check your nutrition compliance and track calories carefully; you may have underestimated how much you ate. Reduce your daily caloric intake by 100 to 200 calories. Keep your nutrient ratios the same and keep your food choices as natural as possible. Recheck your body fat in one week. If it hasn't decreased, increase the intensity of your cardio. If your cardio volume is low, you can also increase the frequency or duration.

**LEAN MASS DECREASES AND BODY FAT DECREASES**

You're losing body fat, which is good, but you've also lost some lean mass. If this is the first time you've lost LBM, it may be water weight and nothing to worry about. If this is a recurring pattern and you've been losing LBM more than two weeks in a row, you're losing muscle and you need to eat more, at least temporarily. Make sure your protein intake is adequate. Increase your daily caloric intake by 100 to 200 calories, or increase your calories all the way to maintenance once every fourth day (carb cycling method) while continuing your current training programme. Be certain that your weight training is consistent and that each workout is intense, focused, and progressive.

**LEAN MASS DECREASES AND BODY FAT STAYS THE SAME OR INCREASES**

It's unlikely that your LBM will decrease and your body fat will increase in the same week. Double-check your body fat testing and scale accuracy and consider that this measurement could be an anomaly. If this outcome is confirmed, you may be in a hormonally suboptimal and catabolic state. This may occur due to overtraining, exhaustion, poor nutrition, or ignoring important lifestyle factors such as adequate sleep and stress control.

Stay on a consistent eating plan without missing meals. Make sure your protein intake is adequate. If you lost no weight, you can increase cardio slightly and or decrease calories slightly, unless your calories were already very low.

Make sure you're consistent with your weight training. Make the weight training sessions short and intense, and be sure to recover adequately from your training. Get enough sleep and consider stress management techniques.

### LEAN MASS INCREASES AND BODY FAT INCREASES

You gained muscle, which is good, but you also gained fat. This is common among off-season bodybuilders; it's called "bulking up," where the athlete gains unwanted fat while gaining muscle. If this happens, especially for more than one week, you are clearly in a calorie surplus. If your goal is to burn fat, you need to decrease calories significantly to establish a deficit. Try dropping 200 to 400 calories from your daily intake. Watch your weight during the week. Re-measure in one week. If your body fat hasn't started dropping, then repeat.

Keep your compliance level high, track calories carefully, and keep your eating relatively clean and free of calorie-dense high-fat and high-sugar junk foods. If your training volume was low, you can also increase the intensity, frequency, or duration of your cardio.

### LEAN MASS INCREASES AND BODY FAT DECREASES

This is unlikely to happen, except for beginners, genetically gifted individuals (the pure mesomorphic body type) and sometimes for ectomorphs with fast metabolisms. If you do gain muscle and lose fat in the same week, terrific! Your results are exceptional. Don't change anything. Keep up the good work; you're on your way to reaching or even exceeding your goal.

### LEAN MASS INCREASES AND BODY FAT STAYS THE SAME

Good job: You've gained muscle without gaining fat! This is the ideal outcome for a muscle-gaining programme. You are probably in a caloric surplus, at least some of the time. If you also want to reduce your body fat percentage, you'll need a calorie deficit, which you can accomplish by decreasing your calories slightly while keeping your training and activity level the same. If your cardio volume was low, you can also increase the frequency, intensity, or duration of each session.

## THE ESSENCE OF THE FEEDBACK SYSTEM:
## LET YOUR RESULTS DICTATE YOUR APPROACH

I always recommend **letting your results dictate your strategy**. If you can eat 60 per cent or more of your calories from carbs and the fat is melting off, great: Keep eating all those carbs, even if a guru told you that low-carb is more effective. If you can get lean with nutrition and weight training only and almost no cardio, fine: Don't do any cardio. Don't fix anything that's not broken! As long as everything you're doing is healthy and sustainable, the ends justify the means. The fact is the results you produce each week are the only true measure of whether you've made the right choices. Results are what count.

You are unique, and since all four elements of this programme – nutrition, cardio training, resistance training, and mental training – are customizable, customize them! Don't get locked into the freedom-restricting formulas that so many diets prescribe. When you discover an approach that works for you, develop immunity from criticism, disregard unhelpful comments from those who disagree with your approach, and judge your success only by your weekly progress.

By following this system, using body composition measurement, performance feedback, and progress charting, you will, through an evolutionary learning process, figure out your body type and develop your own personal formula quickly. Once you've discovered your personal formula, it will always be there for you for the rest of your life, whenever you want to go back to it.

---

### QUICKSTART

Want an instant increase in results? Do what all great sports coaches and business managers do: Measure everything you want to improve. Performance improves when performance is measured, so always keep score! Use the progress chart in the appendix to track your body composition, get into a feedback loop, and every week adjust your approach according to your results.

# *L*EARN:

## MENTAL TRAINING (The 1st Element)

In the previous chapters, we've been setting the stage for you to have total success on this programme. Now you're getting into the heart of the programme – starting with the first of the four elements – mental training. This piece of our four-part LEAN formula focuses on setting goals and re-programming your mind for success. Countless readers have told me that this was the missing element for them because until they mastered it, they had never been able to stay focused, stay motivated and stick with their programme, ever before. After they mastered it, they were unstoppable!

Ironically, this is the part that even the most intelligent readers are often tempted to skip, because it seems so logical that the secret lies in the food plan or workout routines, not in a motivational talk. Without fail, those who gloss over it the first time and fail to get results, eventually realize the paradox that the biggest secret to physical change is mental change. They come back to this chapter, follow the instructions to the letter and finally see the results that have eluded them for years.

I heartily suggest that you not only read chapter 6 with rapt attention and apply what you learn from day one, but that you study this material and absolutely master it. The payoff is immeasurable and goes far beyond more muscle and better abs. These techniques are transferable – they can help you become successful in every area of your life.

# Setting Goals and Training Your Mind

"The strangest secret in the world is that you become what you think about."

– Earl Nightingale

## THE SIMPLE FIRST STEP YOU MUST TAKE BEFORE YOU START ANY NUTRITION OR EXERCISE PROGRAMME

This might be the most important element in the entire programme, even though it has nothing to do with calories, proteins, carbohydrates, fats, cardio, weights, or anything else related to nutrition or training. You see, there's a simple but critical procedure you must complete before you lift a weight, jog a mile, create a meal plan, or set foot in a gym. If you successfully complete this procedure, the nutrition and training will come naturally and a lean body will soon follow. If you ignore this step, like most people, you will likely fail no matter what you do or how hard you try.

The crucial first step is setting a goal.

Much has been said about goal setting – entire books have been devoted to the subject – but the truth is most people never decide exactly what they want. Some give their goals a fleeting thought, but most never get specific and commit their dreams and desires to writing. "Most people," says Denis Waitley, author of *The Psychology of Winning*, "spend more time planning a party, studying the newspaper or making a Christmas list than they do planning their lives." According to the late Zig Ziglar, a goal-setting expert who was one of America's most respected motivational speakers, only 3 per cent of Americans have actually taken the time and effort necessary to put their goals on paper.

This is unfortunate because the number one reason for failure in losing body fat – and in life – is the lack of clearly defined, written goals. Ziglar compared not having goals to shooting at a target with a blindfold on: "How could you possibly hit a target you can't even see?" If you don't know where you're going, you'll probably end up nowhere! Action without planning is one of the biggest causes of failure.

I want to share with you the most powerful goal-achieving formula in the world. But before I do, you first need to understand the hidden reasons why goal setting is so important to your success in the *Burn the Fat, Feed the Muscle* programme.

## THE DIFFERENCE BETWEEN KNOWING WHAT TO DO AND DOING WHAT YOU KNOW

Nutrition and exercise can be confusing subjects. When you first get started, the initial challenge is that you don't know what to do. With this programme in your hands, knowing what to do is no longer a problem. However, gaining knowledge is only half the battle. The far greater challenge for most people is applying that knowledge and taking action. There's a big difference between knowing what to do and doing what you know. A goal is the bridge that spans this gap.

Goals, when properly planted in your subconscious mind, provide direction and stimulate action. Goals create energy and motivation. Goals get you out of bed early in the morning and into the gym. Goals keep you going when you feel like quitting. The secret to staying motivated all the time is to set emotionally charged goals, commit them to writing, and stay focused on those goals day and night. A goal with a purpose is the fuel that propels you forward. You might think you're in total conscious control of your behaviour, but it's really your subconscious that's running the show. If you know what to do but you can't get yourself to do it, you've probably been giving negative or conflicting messages to your subconscious mind. Repeated behaviours produced by subconscious conditioning are more commonly referred to as habits. Fortunately, you can reprogramme your subconscious mind with positive instructions and become a creature of positive habit, just as easily as you can become a victim of negative habits. It all begins with a conscious decision and written goals.

## THE POWER OF THOUGHT

After competing in dozens of bodybuilding competitions and helping thousands of people with training and nutrition programmes, I'm convinced that the most important part of getting in great shape is simply making up your mind to do it. You get in shape by setting goals and thinking about them all day long. I know that may sound a little strange, but stay with me for a minute and I'll explain.

I'm not saying you can "think yourself thin." No amount of positive thinking will help without action. Obviously you have to exercise and eat the right foods in the right amounts. What I'm suggesting is that if you don't channel your mental energies properly, even the best nutrition or training programme is useless because you will always sabotage yourself.

Did you ever wonder why you've had lapses in willpower? Or why some days you just couldn't drag yourself to the gym? Or why you fell off the diet wagon? Or why you couldn't say no to chocolate or that second helping of food? It's because negative programming in your subconscious mind was controlling your behaviour.

This is not some New Age or Pollyanna mentality: There are valid scientific reasons why goal setting works. Goals work because they harness and direct the awesome power of your subconscious mind, which guides your behaviour on autopilot.

## HOW YOUR "MENTAL COMPUTER" IS PROGRAMMED FOR SUCCESS OR FAILURE

Your mind has two components: the conscious and the subconscious. The conscious mind is the rational, logical, analytical, thinking part of the mind. It's constantly taking in information from the five senses, and then it reasons, analyses, and concludes whether the input is true or false. The subconscious is the part of the mind responsible for storing data (memory) and for automatic behaviour (habits), reflexes, and the body's autonomic functions such as digestion, breathing, and circulation.

Unlike the conscious mind, your subconscious does not think or reason. It's entirely deductive in nature, and it works like a computer. All the data programmed into your subconscious computer is accepted as a command. It doesn't matter whether the input is actually true or false; everything that reaches the subconscious is assumed to be true. Your mental programming is then carried out in the form of behaviours the same way a computer executes its programming.

Suggestions given under hypnosis or visualization during deep relaxation are quick ways to access the subconscious mind. Another way to penetrate the subconscious (although much slower) is through spaced repetition. Everything you hear, see, say, read, or think repeatedly eventually filters into your subconscious mind, especially if it's repeated with emotion. In other words, you are constantly programming your brain through conscious self-suggestion – or you are allowing your brain to be programmed through unconscious external suggestion. *That's why you must take conscious control over programming your own brain.*

The basis for positive thinking and philosophies such as the law of attraction is that the subconscious is amenable to suggestion. People who say that positive thoughts and affirmations don't work aren't using them effectively or consistently, or they're wishing for the positive while thinking about the negative.

If a captain gives an order such as "Go east," then keeps changing his mind – "No, go west … no, go north" – the ship would never get anywhere! This is also why most people get nowhere with their fitness, weight-loss, or muscle-building endeavours. Ironically, the very statement "Positive thinking doesn't work" is a negative suggestion guaranteeing that it won't work!

## THE PSYCHOLOGICAL REASON MOST PEOPLE SABOTAGE THEIR OWN EFFORTS TO LOSE BODY FAT

The conscious mind is a lot like the captain at the bridge of a ship. The captain sends a command to the engine room. The subconscious mind is like the people down in the engine room. No matter what orders come down from the bridge (conscious mind), the crew obeys, even if the orders are stupid ones that crash the ship into a rocky shore. The reason this happens is because the crew (the subconscious) can't see where the ship is going; they are simply following orders.

Like the ship's crew, your subconscious mind carries out every command it accepts from your conscious mind. Its sole purpose is to obey your orders, even if you give ones like "I'll always be fat." Frequent repetition of thoughts (mental orders) is one certain way to penetrate the subconscious mind. By constantly repeating negative commands such as "I can't lose weight," your subconscious will see to it that you never lose weight because that's its job: to follow your every command literally and without question. If you programme your mind with negative suggestions often enough, it will lead you right into cheating on your diet, skipping workouts, or some other form of self-sabotage.

Dr. Maxwell Maltz, author of the incredible book *Psycho-Cybernetics*, described the human brain and nervous system as a "perfect goal-striving servo-mechanism." This mechanism helps you achieve your goals much like a self-guided torpedo or missile seeks out its target and navigates to it. Like the torpedo, the cybernetic mechanism in your brain can only work in your favour if you've chosen a target.

Without a target, your mental "servo-mechanism" simply steers you toward your dominant thoughts. The subconscious mind is always at work 24 hours a day, whether you direct it consciously or not. Denis Waitley says, "Since we become what we think of most of the time, whatever we are thinking of now, we are unconsciously moving toward the achievement of that thought. For an alcoholic, this could be the next drink; for a drug addict, the next fix; for a surfer, the next wave. Divorce, bankruptcy, and illness are all goals spawned out of negative attitudes and thought patterns."

## THE POWER OF FOCUS

Because of how your subconscious operates, it's crucial to focus on what you want to achieve, not on what you want to avoid. This isn't just semantics; it's a vital distinction with deep implications for fat loss. If I tell you, "Don't think about pink elephants," you have to think about pink elephants because your brain can't process negation. You either think about something or you don't, and you always move toward what you think about the most, whether it's positive or negative.

Like the soil, your subconscious mind is totally impartial; it doesn't discriminate. In it will grow whatever seeds you plant there or *allow to be planted there*. Many people have perfectly good intentions, but they unwittingly allow their subconscious to work against themselves by thinking and talking about what they don't want. And as metaphysical writer Louise Hay reminds us, "The more you dwell on what you don't want, the more of it you create." Others simply pay no attention to their thoughts whatsoever, and like a garden that's neglected, soon enough, weeds start growing. Eventually the weeds take over their garden.

Here are a few examples of negative statements and self-defeating questions:

- I can't lose weight no matter what I do.
- Why can't I lose these last ten pounds?
- Why is it so hard for me to lose weight?
- I have a slow metabolism.
- I'll always be fat.
- It's not my fault I'm fat because I don't have good genetics.
- I don't want to be fat any more.
- I wish I could get rid of this gut.
- It'll never work because I love food too much.
- I don't have the willpower to get lean.
- I would work out but I don't have time.
- I just can't get myself up that early to work out.
- I hate being fat.
- I'm sick of being overweight.
- I'm tired of working out but getting nowhere.
- I'm ready to give up.
- I'll never see my abs.
- I hate cardio.
- I can't.
- I'll try.

All day long you carry on a mental conversation with yourself. Psychologists estimate that we think up to 60,000 thoughts a day and that 98 per cent of these thoughts are the same ones we had yesterday – most of them negative. In a year, that's almost 22 million thoughts! If Madison Avenue advertising giants can influence your subconscious mind to make a buying decision by repeating an ad a mere two dozen times (they can), then imagine the impact that millions of your own "thought commands" have on influencing your subconscious mind. It's staggering! That's why it's so important to take conscious control over your speech and mental dialogue and programme your brain with positive instructions.

Fortunately, the one thing in life you always have total control over is your thoughts. After all, it's *your* brain, right? If you want to be successful at getting leaner or any other endeavour in life, you must master your communication with yourself. You must take charge of your self-talk, "police" your thinking, and literally reprogramme your brain for success. If you've cluttered your mind with a lifetime of "stinkin' thinkin'," as Mr. Ziglar called it, this may be challenging at first. It will take time to overwrite the old programming, but it can be done.

The first step is to become conscious of what you are thinking and saying. Become more aware of your thoughts and your language. The instant you catch yourself in the middle of a negative thought or self-defeating question, interrupt it! Slam on the brakes like a car heading for a cliff and stop that train of thought! Mentally imagine a big rubber stamp that says "CANCEL" and stamp it out. Bob Proctor, a master success coach and creator of the Goal Achiever programme, suggests saying "NEXT" or "SWITCH" the instant you notice a negative thought, then immediately replacing it with a positive thought, affirmation, or question. Soon you'll find that your mind switches polarity and the negative thoughts pop up less.

Here are some examples of how you could change negative self-talk to positive self-talk:

- **How can I burn fat and enjoy the process?**
- **What can I do today to get me closer to my ideal weight?**
- **What can I eat right now at this meal that will help me burn body fat?**
- **How great am I going to feel after I finish my workout today?**
- **My metabolism is getting faster every day.**
- **I am getting leaner every day.**
- **I like the way I look.**
- **I am 100 per cent responsible for my results.**
- **I am doing whatever it takes.**
- **I like eating healthy foods.**
- **I love working out.**

- **Training early in the morning is exhilarating.**
- **I have time for anything I'm committed to.**
- **I am unstoppable.**
- **I like myself.**
- **I'm the best.**
- **I can.**
- **I'll do it.**

## THE MOST POWERFUL GOAL-ACHIEVING FORMULA IN THE WORLD

In the beginning of this chapter, I promised to reveal the most powerful goal-achieving formula in the world. Now that you understand the nature of your subconscious mind and why goal setting works, you're ready to learn the formula.

### 1. Set specific goals.

When I ask people what they want to achieve from their fitness programmes, I usually get vague answers like "I want to get leaner," "I want to lose weight," and "I want to build muscle." Those are good starts, but they're too general. Specific goals have a more powerful impact on your subconscious. A vague goal is like the captain of a ship saying, "Go west." The ship may be headed in the right general direction, but without a specific destination, it will probably get lost at sea.

Narrow it down. Exactly how many pounds do you want to lose? When do you want to achieve your goal? How much body fat do you want to burn off? How much do you want to weigh? What measurements would you like to have? What size clothes do you want to wear?

### 2. Set measurable goals.

You must have a way to objectively measure your progress, otherwise you'll never know if you've actually reached your goals. The mirror is a useful tool, because ultimately the only thing that matters is that you're happy with the way you look. However, because you perceive changes in your body so subjectively, it's helpful to have other ways to measure your results.

The scale is also a useful tool, but it doesn't give you 100 per cent of the feedback you need. You should be interested not so much in what you weigh as in how much body fat you carry. The ideal method to measure your progress is body composition testing. Body fat can be measured easily using a skinfold test. Chapter 4 discusses body composition testing methods in more detail, and chapter 5 teaches you how to chart your progress and interpret the results.

### 3. Set big goals.

Far too often, people shortchange themselves and make statements like "I could never look like that" and "I'm too old." Other people buy into the low expectations of well-meaning family or friends who tell them to "be realistic." Nothing great was ever achieved by being realistic! Most people get scared when setting goals and ask only for what they think they can get, not what they really want. This is a mistake, because puny goals are not motivating. Wants are motivating.

It's okay if your goal scares you a little. In fact, if your goal isn't scary and exciting at the same time, then your goal is too small. Thinking about a big goal you've never achieved before is always going to make you feel a little uncomfortable and afraid. This makes most people pull back into their comfort zones. Don't let fear of failure or the feeling of discomfort prevent you from going after what you really want. Always step forward into growth; never pull back into safety. Refuse to sell yourself short. Raise your standards. The architect Daniel Burnham said, "Make no small plans; they have no magic to stir your blood to action. Make big plans, aim high in work and hope."

Don't be afraid to think big and set your sights high, because you can only hit what you aim at! Decide what you would like to look like if you could have any body you wanted. See the picture in your mind. Make it clear, vivid, and dynamic. Dream. Fantasize. You've been endowed with an amazing creative faculty called imagination. Use it. It's the starting point of a new self-image and all lasting changes.

There are genetic limits to what each person can achieve athletically and physically. Yet, most people never reach their full potential because they don't believe it's possible, so they don't even try. It's more a question of willingness than genetics. Don't ask yourself, "Is it possible to reach this goal?" Instead ask, "How can I achieve this goal?" and "Am I willing to pay the price necessary to achieve this goal?" You can always find a way if you keep asking how, and you can accomplish virtually anything if you're willing to pay the price.

### 4. Set realistic deadlines.

"Lose 30 pounds in 30 days!" "Lose 10 pounds this weekend!" You see ads for quick weight loss like these in magazines and all over the Internet, and they sure are enticing.

But is it possible? Can you really lose weight that fast? It is possible. However, if your goal is losing that much weight in that little time, you could be making a big mistake. The real question is: What kind of weight?

Anything that dehydrates you can cause quick weight loss. You could easily drop 10 pounds (4.5 kg) over the weekend if you stopped drinking water. Of course, that would be pretty dumb and possibly dangerous, but the same thing often happens on rapid weight-loss diets: They're simply dehydrating you. Even worse, you may lose muscle as well. Your goal should be *fat* loss, not *weight* loss.

What's a realistic rate of fat loss? The American College of Sports Medicine, one of the largest and most respected health, medical, and exercise organizations in the world, has established guidelines for healthy weight loss. In their position statement "Proper and Improper Weight-Loss Programs," they recommend a weight-loss goal of 1 to 2 pounds (0.5 to 0.9 kg) per week.

It's possible to lose more than 2 pounds (0.9 kg) of pure fat per week, especially if you have a lot of weight to lose, but usually a large part of any weight loss over 2 or 3 pounds (0.9 to 1.4 kg) per week is water and lean body mass. If you lose water weight, you'll gain it back immediately as soon as you rehydrate yourself. If you lose muscle, you lose strength, your metabolism slows down, and your body starts to look soft.

Don't be afraid to set big goals. Whether that big goal is to shed 100 pounds (45 kg) of fat or to compete in a fitness competition, don't sell yourself short! But always set realistic time frames for achieving goals of this size. Usually, it's not the goal that's unrealistic but the deadline. Be patient: There are definite limitations to how quickly the human body can safely burn fat.

### 5. Set long-term and short-term goals.

As you think about what you want specifically, don't just write down one goal; make a list. Your goal list should include long-term and short-term goals. There are six types of long- and short-term goals you can include:

1. Long-term goals and your ultimate "ideal body"
2. One-year goals
3. Three-month goals
4. Weekly goals (weekly body composition test and weigh-in)
5. Daily goals (habits to develop, behaviours to do every day)
6. The goal of continually beating your personal best (personal records or "PRs").

First, set long-term goals, including your ideal body. What kind of body do you ultimately want to have? Let your imagination run wild and dare to dream. Don't listen to people who say it can't be done! You can't afford to associate with negative people who always tear you down. If you really want it badly and you're willing to work for it, then go ahead and set the goal.

Next, set a one-year goal. A one-year goal is especially important if you have a lot of body fat to lose. For example, if your primary objective is to shed 100 pounds (45 kg), that's a 12-month project for most people. If you safely and healthfully get it done faster, that's great, but if in doubt, give yourself more time for big goals like these. Then you'll be more likely to surpass your expectations, which is great for your motivation.

Probably your most important goal at any time is your three-month goal. Your three-month goal is usually the one you'll write down on a goal card and carry around with you, thinking about it and visualizing it repeatedly throughout the day. Three months is the perfect time frame for a fat-loss or muscle-building goal because it's easy to lock in your focus for that long, and a lot can happen in three months. A sensible and realistic three-month goal would be to lose about 6 per cent body fat and 18 to 24 pounds (8 to 11 kg).

The three-month goal is important because long-term goals don't have urgency. A one-year goal is so far away, you may tend to procrastinate more without the impending deadline. There's a psychological principle called Parkinson's law that says, "Work expands to fill the time available for its completion." Differently stated: "A task takes as long as there is time to do it." Deadlines are not only motivating, they're a necessity, because otherwise nothing gets done. Without time pressure, you'll rationalize missing workouts or cheating on your diet. Your brain will keep saying, "You have plenty of time, so missing this one workout won't matter." With a deadline right in front of you, you'll know that every workout and every meal count.

---

**QUICKSTART**

**The goal card is the high-achiever's secret weapon. Choose your most important, highest-priority goal for the next three months. Write it down as an affirmation on a pocket-sized card and carry it with you everywhere you go. Feel naked without it. Read it as many times a day as possible – while you eat breakfast, wait in lines, sit at traffic lights and when you're on the treadmill. It's the simplest, easiest, yet most powerful tool you can start using today to stay focused and train your mind for success. You can download a free goal card at www.BurnTheFatFeedTheMuscle.com**

---

You also need to set weekly goals to let you know if you're on track. Your weekly results provide immediate feedback to tell you whether you're moving in the right direction. Each week you should weigh yourself and have your body composition measured with a skinfold caliper. If you're getting the results you want, you simply continue doing what you've been doing. If you're not seeing the results you want, you can immediately adjust your training or nutrition to get yourself back on course. Any time you need guidance on how to adjust your approach each week, review the instructions in chapter 5. The answer always lies in the feedback loop system. If you ever feel really stuck, you can use the plateau-breaking strategies you'll learn in the final part of the programme.

To reach your weekly, three-month, twelve-month, and long-term goals, you must develop positive everyday habits. You develop positive habits by setting daily goals (action steps) and repeating them until they become behaviours as automatic as brushing your teeth or taking a shower. Write out a list of daily goals, to-dos, and action steps you need to take every day in order to reach your mid-range and long-term goals. This can include good daily habits such as eating lean protein at each meal; including fruits or vegetables with each meal; choosing mostly natural, unrefined foods; making your meals in advance for each day; and so on.

Your daily goals can also include developing a schedule or set of daily rituals such as when you're going to get up in the morning, when you're going to work out, what time you'll eat your meals, and when you'll go to sleep at night. Daily goals also include targets for each workout: how long your workout will last, how much weight you'll lift, how many reps, which exercises, how many minutes of cardio, and so forth. You should plan every workout in advance as part of your daily goals. Never "wing it."

Long-term goals are important, but if you look only at the big picture, it can be unsettling to realize how much further you have to go. There's an old saying about tackling big tasks: "The only way to eat an elephant is one bite at a time." When your larger goals are broken down into smaller parts and you focus on each little step one at a time, you won't be overwhelmed. "By the mile it's a trial, by the yard it's hard, but by the inch it's a cinch." Take baby steps. Every step you take, no matter how small, will give you a feeling of accomplishment and keep your momentum going. The important thing is that you're moving in the right direction.

The next time you feel temporarily frustrated, discouraged, or unmotivated, focus on your daily goals, not on the huge amount of work that's ahead of you. Tell yourself, "All I have is today. All I have is this moment, this workout, this meal, the next 30 minutes, the next hour. If I simply do what I know I must do today, then I know I'll reach my ultimate goal eventually." As the Zen masters remind us, concentrate on the task at hand in the present moment.

The final type of goal isn't so much a goal as it is a mind-set. If you fall into the habit of continually comparing yourself to others, this will ensure that you're perpetually unhappy and unsatisfied, no matter how much you achieve. This is called the law of contrast. There will always be people who are stronger, leaner, faster, more athletically talented, and more genetically gifted than you. Comparing yourself to them will only make you feel bad. Be inspired by others, but compare yourself only to yourself.

Set goals to *become better than you used to be*, not become better than someone else. Constantly challenge yourself. Keep aiming to beat your previous bests. Training can become fun and exciting when you always work on improving yourself. So make it fun; make a contest out of it. Go for one more rep, 5 more pounds (2.3 kg), five more minutes, or one level higher on the cardio machine. Aim for hitting your lowest body fat ever. Work on constant and never-ending improvement and make this process a fun challenge!

### 6. Make sure your goals don't conflict; prioritize and focus on your one most important goal.

There's an ancient Chinese saying: "He who chases two rabbits catches neither." One of the most common obstacles that block the way to reaching a goal is setting two or more goals that conflict with each other. Training for strength and muscle mass while preparing for long-distance endurance events is a perfect example. They're not compatible; the endurance work will interfere with the strength and muscle gains.

Many people would love to gain muscle and lose fat at the same time. That's known as "body recomposition," and it's considered the Holy Grail of fitness goals. Although it can be done, it requires a more sophisticated approach to cyclical dieting. It's also a slower and more difficult process than focusing on one thing at a time. Over a period of weeks or months, you might see a small increase in muscle with a decrease in body fat, and you'll definitely look more muscular as fat is stripped away from the muscle you already have underneath. But it's not typical to see big increases in muscle while you're also shedding fat. When it does happen, it's usually "newbie gains." That's when beginners get better results because their untrained bodies are highly responsive to exercise. As you would expect, it also happens more often in genetic superiors (the mesomorphs).

The most efficient way to get results fast is to put 100 per cent of your energy into the one goal that's most important to you. If your body fat is above average, then your number one goal should be shedding fat first, because high body fat is a health risk and it's easier to build muscle on a leaner body. Once the fat is off, you can rewrite your goals and go into maintenance mode or work on gaining lean mass. In the next chapter, where we talk about calories, I'll give you a brief introduction to how to adjust your plan for gaining muscle. (It would take another book to cover all the details about body recomposition or gaining muscle mass.)

## 7. Establish the emotional reasons why you want to achieve your goals.

Almost everyone has days when they don't feel like working out or eating the right foods. The secret to staying on track at times like these is not just having a goal; it's establishing reasons why you want that goal – the importance of it. Uncovering the reason you want to achieve something adds emotion to it. The more emotion you stir up, the more motivated you'll be to go after it. Nietzsche said that if you have a strong enough why, you can bear almost any how. Getting emotionally involved with your goal also impresses it deeper into your subconscious. Whatever idea is fixed in your subconscious will always express itself in physical form: behaviours and results.

Looking good for a wedding or vacation is an important reason why many people want to get in shape. So is being attractive to potential life partners. For others, the reason is fear of health consequences. (Their doctor tells them if they don't lose 50 pounds (23 kg) in the next six months, they'll die of a heart attack.) Some people want to get healthier so they'll live long enough to see their grandchildren grow up.

What are *your* reasons why you want to achieve your goals? To help you uncover them, answer these questions:

**I.**   What's important to you about reaching your goal?
**II.**  Why is that important to you?
**III.** What impact, specifically, will achieving this goal have on your life? (How will your life be different and better after you've achieved it?)

Answering these questions will help you discover the driving force behind your goals and add emotional impact to your goal list.

- **Who is your fitness role model?**
- **What do you want to look like?**
- **Do you want to look like a bodybuilder, an athlete, or a model?**
- **Do you want to impress anyone?**
- **Do you want to prove something?**
- **Do you want to be a role model or set an example?**
- **Do you want more energy?**
- **Do you want more mobility so you can enjoy certain sports and activities more?**
- **Do you want to win a contest or award?**
- **Do you want more self-confidence?**
- **Do you want to look great in certain types of clothes?**
- **Do you want to look good for a certain event (for example, a vacation, a wedding, a reunion, or a birthday)?**

- **Do you want to look great on the beach?**
- **Do you want to attract someone special into your life?**

## 8. Write out a goal list in the form of affirmations.

After setting your goals in terms of a specific weight, body fat, measurement, and so forth, and you know the reasons why you want them, the next step is to write all your goals on a sheet of paper or on cards in the form of positive statements called affirmations.

Here are three guidelines to follow when writing your affirmations:

### A) MAKE YOUR AFFIRMATIONS PERSONAL: USE THE WORD "I" WITH A VERB AFTER IT.

For example: I exercise, I cook, I wake up, I eat, I have, I plan, I enjoy, I lift, I get, I take, I deserve, and so on. One of the best ways to start an affirmation is to use the phrase "I AM." Your subconscious responds best to commands given to it in a personal manner. Anything you say after "I AM" has power. One of the best affirmations I've ever heard comes from Bob Proctor, and it goes like this: "I am so happy and thankful now that I am _____" (fill in your goal).

### B) WRITE YOUR AFFIRMATIONS IN THE PRESENT TENSE.

To your subconscious mind, there is no future. Your subconscious mind responds best to commands given in the present tense. It may feel strange to write a goal this way, but if you write it in the future tense (for example, "Next year I will …" or "I'm going to …"), your subconscious mind may interpret this literally and keep your goal in the future. For best results, write, think and visualize your goal as if you've already achieved it.

### C) STATE YOUR GOAL IN POSITIVE TERMS.

Your subconscious moves you toward whatever you focus on, whether it's positive or negative. Therefore, write what you want, not what you want to avoid or get rid of. For example, instead of saying, "I want to lose 20 pounds (9 kg)," say, "I weigh 130 pounds (9 st 4 lb/59 kg) with 18 per cent body fat."

## 9. Read your affirmations (your goal list) at least twice a day and always keep your goals in front of you and on your mind.

Psychologists have proven that repetition is an effective way to penetrate and programme the subconscious mind. The top 500 US companies spend billions of advertising dollars every year based on this fact. Why is it that people reach for

Coke, Pepsi, Budweiser, Marlboro, Crest, Palmolive, and other brand-name items? It's because the repetition of the advertising has penetrated their subconscious minds and moved them to action.

You can use the power of spaced repetition to influence your own subconscious and move yourself to action. After you've written out your affirmations, read your list at least twice a day, once in the morning and once at night. Read them more often if you can. If you want to amplify the effect of the affirmation technique, don't just read your affirmations; *write them out by hand every single day or record them in your own voice and listen to them regularly.*

After you've set all your goals and written your affirmations, use the power of repetition even more by keeping your goals in front of you all day long. Post your goal statements in a conspicuous place, such as on your refrigerator, on your bathroom mirror, or in your daily appointment book. Keep a goal card of your three-month goals in your pocket. Paste them onto the dashboard of your car. Set them as your mobile phone wallpaper. Stick them on top of your computer monitor or make them your desktop background and screen saver so you look at them all day long.

You may have been exposed to this affirmation technique before and shrugged it off as corny. If so, let me ask you this: Did you really give it an honest trial? Did you put it to the test for at least 28 days in a row and give 100 per cent with positive expectancy? If not, then you're denying yourself the chance of achieving everything you've ever dreamed of. Don't let the simplicity of the affirmation technique fool you. Be open-minded and don't prejudge it. Affirmations are more powerful than you can imagine, but they don't work when you just "try" them once or twice. They won't work even if you do them for a few days. They won't work if you say them and then cancel them out with negative affirmations. They work when you continue to repeat them with faith, emotion, and belief over and over again so many times that they replace your old, negative, internal dialogue.

The ultimate purpose of using affirmations is to help you permanently change the "tape" that loops in your mind every day. When you reach the point where your affirmations become your new habitual way of thinking and speaking, the results will astound you and what you've been imagining will start to materialize in your life.

### 10. Read your goals with faith.

William James, the father of American psychology, wrote, "The subconscious will bring into reality any picture held continually in your mind and backed by faith." Napoleon Hill, author of *Think and Grow Rich* and *The Law of Success*, said, "All thoughts which have been emotionalized and mixed with faith begin immediately to translate themselves into their physical equivalent." Faith, which is simply an unshakeable belief, is yet another way to plant your desires in your subconscious mind.

Faith is when you believe in what you can't see. Faith is when you know you'll eventually reach your goal, even though you look in the mirror and see that little has changed yet. The opposite of faith is doubt. Shakespeare wrote, "Our doubts are our traitors / And make us lose the good we oft might win / By fearing to attempt." The poet William Blake wrote, "If the Sun & Moon should Doubt, / They'd immediately Go Out ..." You must practise believing in yourself, or "banishing the doubt," as inspirational author Wayne Dyer calls it.

How do you cultivate this attribute of faith? Act *as if.* Read affirmation statements written in the present tense as if they were already achieved. See mental pictures of yourself as if you have already achieved your goal. When you look in the mirror every day, see what you want to become, not what is presently there. Behave as if you were already there. Speak as if you've already arrived. "Act as though I am, and I will be," says the proverb.

### 11. As you read your affirmations, mentally visualize them as already achieved.

Visualization refers to making mental pictures or movies; it's thinking without words. The brain thinks in pictures. If I ask you to think about your car, you probably don't see the letters C-A-R spelled out in your mind. Instead, you instantly get a picture of your car in your mind. Because your brain thinks in images, adding a big, bright, focused mental movie or picture of what you want will help you programme your subconscious mind faster and more deeply than if you simply read your goals.

In *Psycho-Cybernetics*, Dr. Maltz writes, "Experimental and clinical psychologists have proven beyond a shadow of a doubt that the human nervous system cannot tell the difference between an actual experience and one imagined vividly and in detail." As with affirmations, visualization is most effective when your body is in a relaxed (alpha brainwave) state, because that's when your subconscious mind is accessed most easily.

In his book *Peak Performance: Mental Training Techniques of the World's Greatest Athletes*, Dr. Charles A. Garfield writes, "Without a doubt, the most dramatic contribution to the advancement of goal-setting skills in recent years has been the Soviets' introduction of visualization. During mental rehearsal, athletes create mental images of the exact movements they want to emulate in their sport. Use of this skill substantially increases the effectiveness of goal setting, which up until then had been little more than a dull listing procedure."

Garfield goes on to talk about a startling experiment conducted by Soviet sports scientists. The study examined the effect of mental training, including visualization, on four groups of world-class athletes just prior to the 1980 Lake Placid Olympics. The groups were divided as follows:

**GROUP 1** 100% physical training
**GROUP 2** 75% physical training, 25% mental training
**GROUP 3** 50% physical training, 50% mental training
**GROUP 4** 25% physical training, 75% mental training

The researchers found that Group 4, the group with the most mental training, showed significantly greater improvement than Group 3. Group 3 showed more improvement than Group 2, and Group 2 showed more improvement than Group 1!

Dr. Maltz shared a similar account of an experiment about the effects of mental practice on improving basketball free throws. The study, published in *Research Quarterly* divided the subjects into three groups. Each group was tested for free-throw accuracy once at the beginning of the experiment and again at its conclusion.

Group 1 physically practised free throws for 20 days. Group 2 performed no practice at all. Group 3 spent 20 minutes a day getting into a deeply relaxed state and visualizing themselves shooting free throws. When they missed, they would visualize themselves correcting their aim accordingly.

The results were remarkable: The first group, which practised 20 minutes a day, improved in scoring 24 per cent. The second group, which had no practice, showed no improvement. The third group, which practised only in their minds, improved their scoring 23 per cent! Amazingly, mental practice produced results almost identical to physical practice.

What does this research on athletes have to do with losing body fat? Everything! Remember that the subconscious is the part of the mind responsible for automatic behaviour (also known as *habits*). To lose body fat, there are daily positive-action habits you must develop. By visualizing your fat loss or fitness goal as already achieved, you are giving your subconscious mind instructions that will cause you to act in a way consistent with reaching your goal. You'll go into automatic pilot mode. There will be less struggle and willpower involved.

When you're in a situation that used to tempt you, you'll suddenly notice you're no longer tempted. If you used to dread going to the gym, you'll start looking forward to it. If the idea of eating healthy, natural foods used to seem unpleasant, you'll actually begin to enjoy it. If you used to crave certain junk foods, the cravings will mysteriously disappear. Everything will seem to get easier and your workouts will become better than ever. The end result of making "mental motion pictures" is that you will get results more quickly than ever before.

All great athletes and peak performers use visualization. Jack Nicklaus said he never hit a golf shot, not even in practice, without first having *a very sharp, in-focus picture of it in his head.*

Tennis superstar Andre Agassi once told an interviewer that he'd won Wimbledon at least ten thousand times. When asked what he meant, Agassi replied, "Since I was five years old I saw it over and over and over again in my mind. When I walked on the court that day, it was my exact vision. I felt like I was stepping into the role I was made for, and I just demolished them!"

Bodybuilders and fitness athletes use visualization in many ways: They often see pictures of their bodies the way they want them to look once they've reached their ultimate goal. Arnold Schwarzenegger visualized his biceps as mountains: "When I am doing barbell curls, I am visualizing my biceps as mountains – not just big, but huge!"

As he was dieting down for competition, former pro bodybuilder Lee Labrada visualized the skin on his abs getting tighter and thinner, like cellophane wrap clinging to the abdominal muscles.

Three-time Mr. Olympia Frank Zane said that he mentally saw himself winning the Mr. Olympia *at least one million times* before it actually happened. Former Ms. Olympia Rachel McLish said, "I visualize the blood surging through my muscles with every repetition and every set I do. When I pose, I've got a mental picture of how I want to look. When you have that in your brain, the physical body just seems to respond."

Another way you can use creative visualization is to picture yourself taking the daily action steps necessary to achieve you goal. See yourself getting up early in the morning, preparing healthy meals in advance for the whole day, choosing healthy foods in restaurants, and confidently saying no to temptations.

You can also use visualization to mentally rehearse your workouts, seeing yourself training with killer intensity, breaking new records in the gym, performing exercises with perfect technique, and enthusiastically doing your cardio while the fat melts away.

Your visualization sessions could be as brief as five to ten minutes, or you can spend more time if you wish, but make it a scheduled daily discipline, preferably twice a day. You can use visualization any time, even between sets in the gym, but two of the best times are early in the morning and at night before you go to sleep. When you fall asleep thinking about your goals as already achieved, your subconscious continues to work on how to achieve them while you're sleeping, and then adjusts your actions during the next day to move you closer to your goals.

What if you're not good at visualizing? What if you can't see vivid "Technicolor pictures" in your mind? Don't worry about it: Everyone creates mental images in their own unique way. Some people see clear, vivid pictures, while others get only impressions. You'll get results either way and you'll get better with practice. It also helps to have a well-written and detailed description of your goal because words can automatically make pictures pop up into your mind.

Another great technique to improve your ability to visualize your perfect body is to flip through fitness magazines and cut out pictures of people with the body you'd like to have. Look at these pictures daily as you read your affirmations and visualize yourself with the same body.

To take it a step further, cut out a picture of your head and paste it onto the picture of someone else who has the body you want. If you know how to use photo-editing software like Adobe Photoshop, you could have a lot of fun with these "visualization photos." It might sound silly, but it's a remarkably effective technique for reprogramming your self-image.

## SOME REAL GOALS AND AFFIRMATIONS

I've given you a lot to think about, so to help jump-start your imagination, here are some ideas for how to write your goals and affirmations list. What follows is a composite list of some real goals from real people – both men and women – who successfully completed my personal coaching programmes. Use their words to generate some ideas for a list of your own.

WOMEN:

- I am so happy and thankful now that I have 13 per cent body fat!
- I am losing body fat and reaching my goal weight of 110 pounds (7 st 12 lb/50 kg) and my goal body fat of 14 per cent by June 1st.
- I am fitting into my jeans, size 10, by early November and looking so good in them when I wear them to work that I leave all the guys' jaws on the floor.
- I am becoming a fitness magazine success story. When my success story is published, one of the star fitness photographers calls me for a photo shoot and includes me in the next swimsuit edition.
- I eat natural, unprocessed foods, the way they appear in nature, as often as I possibly can.
- I fit perfectly into the slinky black suit I bought this summer, and I am wearing it to work.
- My spaghetti-strap flowered summer dress from last summer fits me perfectly and I am wearing it during my winter vacation in the Caribbean.
- I am learning enough about my body, nutrition, and exercise that I am easily staying within 2 to 3 pounds (0.9 to 1.4 kg) of my *optimal* weight for the rest of my life.

- I am celebrating the New Year with clearly visible abs.
- I wake up every morning at 6:00 to fit in my first meal and cardio before 7:00 – yes, I am a morning person!
- I eat five small, but satisfying meals a day with proper ratios of lean protein, natural carbs, and healthy fats, always on time at three- to four-hour intervals.
- I stay well hydrated and purify my body by drinking a gallon (3.8 litres) of water every day.
- I constantly improve my body and optimize my genetic potential.
- I'm grateful and proud of how good I look today.
- I deserve to be healthy and super-fit.
- I help those close to me choose healthier habits by leading through example and being a reliable source of health and nutrition information.
- I am developing clean eating and consistent exercise habits that are so ingrained into my lifestyle that they stay with me for the rest of my life.

MEN:

- I am so happy and thankful now that my body fat is in the single digits. I now have 9 per cent body fat and I look great!
- I am reaching the most aggressive weight and body fat goal possible by the programme's end (217 pounds 15 st 7 lb/98 kg and 19.3 per cent respectively) by January 1st.
- I can see all of my toes when I look down.
- By January 1st, I fit comfortably into size 32-inch (81-cm) trousers without having to inhale.
- I am surprising (and shocking) my friends and family whom I haven't seen in a while by the way I look at Christmas.
- I am keeping up these lifestyle changes when the programme is over.
- I am reaching my ideal weight and body fat composition by April so I can show off my new body in the summertime.
- I carry my goal card with me at all times and read it as often as possible (at least three times a day).
- I am reaching my goal of 15 per cent body fat and 199 pounds (14 st 3 lb/90 kg) by December 31st. I know this is a little fast but it is my dream for New Year's Eve – I can do it!
- By my 35th birthday on June 15th, I am so happy that I have lost 24 pounds (11 kg) of fat and my body fat has dropped by 6 per cent! I look awesome, I feel great, and I'm ready for some summer fun.
- I am buying all new clothes to show off my new, lean body: killer suits, nice shoes, nice casual stuff.

- I look so good by Christmastime that my wife can't stop touching and holding me.
- I am now leaner than I was 30 minutes ago (*after finishing every cardio workout*).
- Heads are turning when I take my shirt off.
- I look good with my shirt off.
- I am taking on being a bodybuilder and learning about bodybuilding (for tone and definition).
- I am continuing the programme for another three months and burning another 24 pounds (11 kg) of fat.
- I design my weekends and vacations to include healthy activities.
- I eat five moderately sized meals every day, each with a serving of lean protein and a complex, all-natural carbohydrate, and I prepare my food in advance every morning.

## WHAT YOU SHOULD DO EVERY TIME YOU REACH A GOAL

Every time you achieve a major goal you should do three things:

1. **Celebrate or reward yourself.** Great managers, great parents, and great animal trainers all have one thing in common: They know how to continually get their "people" (employees, children, or animals) to repeat the behaviours they desire. They do it by rewarding the behaviours they want repeated. You should do the same thing: reinforce your success by rewarding yourself. Did you have a great week of nutrition and training? If so, go out and splurge! Have a "free meal." Eat some pizza. Treat yourself. If food as a reward doesn't work well for you, then pamper yourself some other way. Take a vacation. Get a massage. Go shopping. Buy yourself something you've always wanted. New clothes are a great reward (you may be needing smaller sizes soon anyway!) And don't feel guilty when you really deserve it!

2. **Keep a list of your achieved goals.** It's been said that success breeds more success. That's why you should start a collection of all your successes. You will reach many small goals on your way to your ultimate goal. Write all of them down on an achieved-goal list. Any time you feel your motivation or enthusiasm flagging, go back and read your list of past successes. This is a surefire way to lift your spirits when you're feeling discouraged. Even after a few short months, you'll amaze yourself at how big your list becomes and how easily you can get motivated by reflecting on your past successes.

3. **Set new goals continually.** Goal setting never stops; it's an ongoing process, not an event. In truth, there's never an "ultimate" goal, because if there were, and you reached it, what then? When the day arrives that you no longer have goals, your life ceases to have meaning. In his book *Unleash the Power Within*, Anthony Robbins writes: "The only true security in life comes from knowing that every single day you are improving yourself in some way – that you are increasing the caliber of who you are. I don't ever worry about maintaining the quality of my life, because every day I work on improving it."

## WHY YOU SHOULD PUT THIS BOOK DOWN AND SET YOUR GOALS RIGHT NOW

To conclude this chapter, I'd like to tell you why you should put this book down this very minute and write out your goals – now!

Years ago, I read a book by peak performance coach Anthony Robbins called *Unlimited Power: The New Science of Personal Achievement*. I was so impressed that I purchased Robbin's tape series called *Personal Power* after seeing him on TV. In those tapes, Robbins discusses the importance of setting goals.

As I listened to the audio on goal setting, Robbins urged me, "Stop the tape now and do the goal-setting exercise." There was a brief pause and then Tony came back on and repeated his instructions. He said in a teasing voice, "If you just kept listening and you didn't stop the tape and write down your goals, stop the tape and do it now." Guess what I did? I just kept listening. I said to myself, "I know what my goals are; I don't need to do any corny goal-setting exercise," so I just kept listening to the rest of the tape. (Dumb, dumb, dumb!)

Eight years later I had achieved some moderate success in several areas of my life, including bodybuilding, but I was frustrated because I hadn't reached my biggest, most important goals and I couldn't figure out why. Then I thought about the Tony Robbins tape. I remembered that even though I definitely knew what I wanted, I never took the time to write it down and read it every day.

Frustrated with my mediocre results, I conceded and went back to the goal-setting exercise I blew off eight years earlier. Sure enough, within 12 months I had won two overall bodybuilding titles and within a few short years after committing my goals to writing and reading my goal list every day, I had accomplished *every single one of them*! It was amazing – almost spooky! Then I made a new list, with bigger, better goals that I am still working on to this day – and I know I will achieve them too.

Put this book down *right now*, make your goal list, and write out your three-month goal on a small card to carry with you. Don't worry if it's not perfect, just start writing. You can always go back to it later and edit. Do it now!

# $E$AT:

## NUTRITION (The 2nd Element)

Each of the four elements in *Burn the Fat, Feed the Muscle* is important, and each enhances the others, but nutrition is the foundation for everything. What you eat is the make-you-or-break-you factor. Get nutrition wrong and it can sabotage your results completely. Get it right and the rest is easy.

Nutrition is so vital it deserves extra attention. That's why I gave it more space in this book than any other topic. The detailed information in these eight chapters is what makes people call this book their nutrition bible. It's also what will make this book a reference guide for the rest of your life. Whenever you have a diet, food or nutrition question, pull this book off your shelf and you'll find the answer.

These chapters contain just enough nutrition science so you understand the rationale behind the plan, but on every page the technical is turned into the practical. There are guidelines, rules and action steps you can put to use immediately. Now dive in and start seeing your body get leaner, stronger, healthier and fitter – fast.

CHAPTER 7

# Understanding Calories

"Any discussion about optimal calorie intake is really a total waste of time – unless you are actually counting the calories! Unless you have done this in writing, and over a significant period of time (4–12 weeks), any discussion of this nature is purely academic. Don't kid yourself – get out your diary, buy a calorie/nutrient counter book, and do yourself a favour; get to really know what you are doing – and more importantly – what the result of this specific combination is."

– Ian King, Australian strength coach and author of
*Get Buffed!: Ian King's Guide to Getting Bigger, Stronger and Leaner*

## CALORIES COUNT

People talk about calories all the time, but if you ask the average guy on the street to explain exactly what a calorie is or tell you how many calories he eats and how many he burns every day, he wouldn't have a clue. What's more shocking is if you ask the average dieter, she wouldn't know either.

By the time you finish this chapter, you'll be an expert on calories. You'll know exactly what calories are, how they're stored in your body, how many you burn every day, and how many you should eat for your body size and activity level to burn fat without losing muscle. I'll also show you why not keeping track of calories might be the only thing preventing you from getting leaner. Best of all, I'll show you a simple method you can use to make calculating and tracking calories a quick and easy process.

## THE DEFINITION OF A CALORIE

A food calorie (kilocalorie) is the amount of heat required to raise 1 kilogram (1 litre) of water 1 degree Celsius. A calorie, then, is simply a measure of heat energy. Like any fuel (petrol, coal, wood, etc.), food releases energy when it's burned. The more calories that are in a food, the more energy will be released.

The word "calorie" is used to describe the amount of energy in food as well as the amount of energy stored in your body as adipose (fat) and glycogen (carbohydrate). For example, a glazed doughnut will deposit 210 calories into your body and it would take, on average, a 25-minute brisk walk on the treadmill to burn off those calories from your body's energy stores.

## CALORIES, BODY FAT, AND SURVIVAL

Body fat is like a reserve storage tank for energy. When we talk about "burning body fat," we're talking about releasing calories from your storage tank and using them to fuel your activities. If you're inactive, your body fat just sits there in storage until you need it. If you're an average 185-pound (13 st 3-lb/84-kg) man with about 18 per cent body fat, or a 135-pound (9 st 9-lb/61-kg) woman with 25 per cent body fat, you have about 33 pounds (15 kg) of adipose tissue. There are 3,500 calories in each pound of fat, which adds up to a grand total of 115,550 calories in fat storage. That's enough fuel to last you a long time!

From a survival point of view, body fat is a good thing and being too lean is a liability. But only small amounts of body fat are essential for health. In modern society, where famine is no longer the concern it was for our ancestors, excess body fat is little more than an annoying cosmetic problem. High body fat is also a health risk.

The good news is, by understanding calories and learning how to balance your energy input with your output, you can easily burn as much fat as you want and maintain a healthy and attractive body for life.

### The Calorie Bank Analogy

An easy way to understand the calorie concept is to think of your body as a living calorie bank and caloric energy as money. You can make energy (fat) deposits and withdrawals from your body the way you would make money deposits and withdrawals from the bank, depending on how high your energy costs are.

When your energy costs are equal to the calories you consume, no deposit or withdrawal of calories takes place; your balance stays the same. When your energy costs are greater than the number of calories you ingest, you make an energy withdrawal from your calorie bank and your body fat balance decreases. When your energy costs are less than the amount of calories you take in, you make an energy deposit and your body fat balance increases.

The exception to this rule is when you're on a weight training programme. In this case, a small calorie surplus can be partitioned into muscle tissue. But even when you're training hard, if the calorie surplus is too large, the excess beyond what's needed for muscle development is deposited into fat storage.

## The Law of Energy Balance

This brings us to the law of energy balance: the granddaddy of all nutritional laws, and the first nutrition fundamental you must understand and obey if you want to get super lean. The law of energy balance says that if you burn more calories than you consume, your body must withdraw stored fuel for energy to make up for the deficit and you will lose weight. The reverse is also true: If you consume more calories than you burn each day, you will deposit the surplus into fat storage and gain weight.

THE LAW OF ENERGY BALANCE:

**To lose weight, you must burn more calories than you consume each day**
**To gain weight, you must consume more calories than you burn each day**

#### THE FIRST COROLLARY TO THE LAW OF ENERGY BALANCE

There are two corollaries to the law of energy balance. The first one says that too much of anything – even healthy foods – will get stored as body fat.

Calories count! The laws of thermodynamics govern energy balance in humans just as they do in other systems. In the face of this unbreakable law, many diet programmes insist that calories don't matter. They claim that as long as you eat certain foods, you can eat as much as you want and you'll still lose weight.

For example, some foods are healthier than others because they are nutrient dense and unrefined. But eating for health and eating for weight loss are different goals. Regardless of how healthy the foods are, if you eat more calories than you burn, you'll still gain weight, usually in the form of fat.

Some diets claim that if you cut carbs, you can eat an unlimited amount of everything else (protein and fat). Not true. Even if you ate zero carbs, if you ate more calories from protein and fat than you burned in a day, you would still gain body fat. Low-carb, high-protein diets reduce hunger and make it harder to overeat. The end result is that most people *automatically* eat fewer calories.

Many people believe that eating exorbitant amounts of protein will make them gain more muscle, but even excess protein calories can be turned into fat. There's no such thing as a diet where you can eat all you want and lose weight simply by eating (or avoiding) one particular food or food group.

**THE SECOND COROLLARY TO THE LAW OF ENERGY BALANCE**

The second corollary to the law of energy balance says that if you eat fewer calories than you burn each day (i.e., you're in a calorie deficit), even if you eat unhealthy ("junk") food, you won't store it as body fat.

Corollary two is not a free licence to eat whatever you want. You might be able to get away with eating a low-calorie junk food diet without gaining weight, but if you want to stay healthy, calorie *quality* is important. When you understand this corollary, it simply takes pressure off you. It lets you relax and enjoy your favourite indulgences from time to time without feeling guilty, as long as you maintain your calorie deficit. You can have your cake and eat it, too – you just can't eat the whole thing!

## THE IMPORTANCE OF PORTION CONTROL

The law of energy balance and its two corollaries override all other weight-loss laws. Many people work out diligently, choose healthy foods, and do everything else right, but they miss the most obvious factor of all: They're simply eating too much. Sometimes the only mistake preventing you from reaching your fat loss goals is ignoring portion sizes.

Getting leaner requires the discipline and willpower to control your calories at all times, even when you eat your occasional cheat meals. Always pay attention to portion sizes. Notice how full your stomach feels and never stuff yourself. Lose the idea that you must clear your plate, especially at restaurants or when you're served by others. Instead, stop eating when you're only 80 per cent full. Even better, know your exact calorie needs and stop when you've reached your predetermined limit for each meal.

## HOW TO CALCULATE YOUR TOTAL DAILY ENERGY EXPENDITURE (TDEE)

The first step in designing your personal fat-burning plan is to calculate how many calories you need every day. This number is called your total daily energy expenditure, or TDEE. It's also known as your maintenance level, because this is the point where your calorie deposits are equal to your calorie withdrawals. TDEE is the total number of calories your body burns in 24 hours, including basal metabolic rate and all activities.

Before we do that, let's look at the six factors that TDEE depends on. All calorie formulas are estimates, but the more of these factors you account for, the more accurate and customized your estimation will be.

## Six Factors That Influence Your Daily Calorie Needs

### 1. BASAL METABOLIC RATE (BMR)

As you learned in Chapter 3, BMR is the total number of calories you burn every day for basic bodily functions. This includes digestion, circulation, respiration, temperature regulation, cell construction, and every other biological process in your body. In other words, BMR is the sum of all the energy you use, not including physical activity. BMR usually accounts for the largest part of your total daily calorie expenditure – about two-thirds.

### 2. ACTIVITY LEVEL

Next to BMR, your activity level is the second most important factor in how many calories you need every day. The more active you are, the more calories you burn. If you sit behind a desk all day and relax on your sofa all night, you don't burn much.

### 3. WEIGHT

Your total body weight and total body size are also major factors in the number of calories you need. The bigger you are, the more calories you require to sustain and move your body. This is a very important part of customizing the plan for your body. Small-framed people cannot eat as much as larger-framed people. Short and petite women make this mistake the most: If they eat like men or larger women, they won't lose and may actually gain weight.

### 4. LEAN BODY MASS (LBM)

Separating your total weight into its lean and fat components helps you calculate your calorie needs more accurately. The higher your LBM, the higher your BMR. Muscle is metabolically active tissue that requires a lot of energy to build and sustain. This means that the more muscle you have, the more calories you'll burn at rest.

### 5. AGE

Metabolic rate tends to slow with age. Therefore, the number of calories the average person requires also decreases with age. This explains why people who don't exercise but continue to eat the same amount of food as they did when they were younger find their body fat creeps up after age 35 or 40. Fortunately, you can prevent and even reverse metabolic slowdown, fat gain, and age-related muscle loss with weight training and proper nutrition.

### 6. GENDER

Men usually require more calories than women. The difference is not entirely due to gender but to body size. The average man is larger and carries more muscle mass than the average female. If not for these genetically inherited variations in BMR, a 150-pound (10 st 10-lb/68-kg) man and a 150-pound (10 st 10-lb/68-kg) woman have approximately the same calorie requirements if their activity level and lean body mass are the same.

### The Fast Way to Estimate Your Calorie Requirements

According to exercise physiologists William McArdle and Frank Katch, the average maintenance level is 2,000 to 2,200 calories per day for women and 2,700 to 2,900 calories for men. Actual calorie expenditures can vary widely and are much higher for extremely active people. Some triathletes and ultra-endurance athletes need as many as 5,000 to 6,000 calories per day just to maintain their weight. Endurance cyclists often slog down energy bars, gels, and high-calorie carbohydrate drinks on the saddle, just to keep from losing weight by the hour!

It's always best to crunch the numbers and customize your nutrition plan as much as possible, but if you're average in body size and activity level and you don't like maths, this is the fastest way to estimate your calorie requirements: Use these average ranges as your starting point.

---

*QUICKSTART*

**FOR MAINTAINING WEIGHT (TDEE):**

| | |
|---|---|
| Men (average): | 2,700–2,900 calories |
| Women (average): | 2,000–2,200 calories |

**FOR LOSING WEIGHT (DEFICIT):**

| | |
|---|---|
| Men (average): | 2,100–2,500 calories |
| Women (average): | 1,400–1,800 calories |

**FOR GAINING WEIGHT (SURPLUS):**

| | |
|---|---|
| Men (average): | 3,200–3,800+ calories |
| Women (average): | 2,300–2,600+ calories |

---

### Three formulas to calculate your customized calorie needs

Exercise physiologists have developed formulas to help you calculate your daily calorie needs. I've included three different equations you can choose from that have been real-world tested and proven to provide accurate estimates:

- The quick method (use this one for a quick estimate with the least number crunching)
- The Harris–Benedict equation (use this one if you don't know your lean body mass)
- The Katch–McArdle equation (use this one if you know your lean body mass)

## 1. THE QUICK METHOD

A fast and easy way to see how many calories you need daily is to use your total current body weight in pounds times a multiplier between 11 and 20.

> Fat loss = 11–13 calories per pound of body weight
> Maintenance = 14–16 calories per pound of body weight
> Weight gain = 18–20+ calories per pound of body weight
>
> Conversions: 1 st = 14 lb
> 1 kg = 2.2 lb

The quick method is popular, but it doesn't account for body composition or activity level, so if you're extremely active, this may underestimate your calorie needs. If you're an older adult or if your body weight is much higher than average, this may overestimate your calorie needs.

Despite these limitations, this simple formula is an excellent way for most people to get a quick ballpark estimate, as long as your activity level is average and your body fat is average or better.

## 2. THE HARRIS–BENEDICT EQUATION

The Harris–Benedict equation uses height, weight, age, and gender to determine basal metabolic rate (BMR), making it more accurate than calculating calorie needs on body weight alone. The only variable it doesn't consider is LBM. This equation is very accurate for all but the extremely muscular and extremely obese, where it may overestimate caloric needs.

> Men: BMR = 66 + (13.7 × weight in kilograms) + (5 × height in centimetres) –
> (6.8 × age in years)
> Women: BMR = 655 + (9.6 × weight in kilograms) + (1.8 × height in centimetres)
> – (4.7 × age in years)
>
> Conversions: 1 inch = 2.54 cm
> 1 kg = 2.2 lb

You are male.

You are 30 years old.

You are 5 feet 8 inches tall (172 cm).

You weigh 172 pounds (12 st 4 lb/78 kg).

Your BMR = 66 + 1068.6 + 860 – 204 = 1,791 calories/day.

Once you know your BMR, you can calculate TDEE by multiplying your BMR by an activity factor. Use the following chart to estimate your activity level. If in doubt, guess on the low side, because most people overestimate how many calories they burn each day.

| Activity Level | Multiplier | Description |
|---|---|---|
| Sedentary | BMR × 1.2 | Little or no exercise; desk job |
| Lightly active | BMR × 1.375 | Light exercise or sports, 3–5 days/week |
| Moderately active | BMR × 1.55 | Moderate exercise or sports, 3–5 days/week |
| Very active | BMR × 1.725 | Hard exercise or sports, 6–7 days/week |
| Extremely active | BMR × 1.9 | Hard daily exercise or sports and physical labour job, or twice-a-day training (football camp, etc.) |

CONTINUING WITH THE PREVIOUS EXAMPLE:

Your BMR is 1,791 calories per day.

Your activity level is moderately active (you work out three to five times a week).

Your activity factor is 1.55.

Your TDEE = 1.55 × 1,791 = 2775 calories/day.

### 3. THE KATCH–MCARDLE EQUATION

Because the Katch–McArdle equation accounts for LBM, it applies equally to both men and women and it's the most accurate method for calculating your daily calorie needs.

BMR (men and women) = 370 + (21.6 × lean mass in kilograms)

EXAMPLE:

You weigh 172 pounds (12 st 4 lb/78 kilograms).

Your body fat percentage is 14 per cent (24.1 pounds fat, 147.9 pounds lean).

Your lean mass is 147.9 pounds (67 kg).

Your BMR = 370 + (21.6 × 67) = 1,817 calories.

To determine TDEE from BMR, you simply multiply BMR by the activity factor, as shown in the following example:

CONTINUING WITH THE PREVIOUS EXAMPLE:

Your BMR is 1,817.

Your activity level is moderately active (moderate workouts three to four times a week).

Your activity factor is 1.55.

Your TDEE = 1.55 × 1817 = 2,817 calories.

The difference in TDEE as determined by both formulas is statistically insignificant (2,775 versus 2,817 calories), because the person we used as an example is average in body size and body composition. The primary benefit of including LBM in the equation is increased accuracy when your body composition leans to either end of the spectrum (very muscular or very obese).

## THE MATHEMATICS OF WEIGHT CONTROL: THREE GUIDELINES FOR ADJUSTING YOUR CALORIES

Once you know your TDEE (maintenance level), the next step is to adjust your calories according to your primary goal. The mathematics of weight control are simple:

1.   **To keep your weight the same:** Stay at your daily caloric maintenance level.

2.   **To lose weight:** Create a calorie deficit by reducing your calories below your maintenance level (or keep your calories the same and create a deficit by increasing your activity).

3.   **To gain weight:** Create a calorie surplus by increasing your calories above your maintenance level. To gain weight as lean body mass, a programme of progressive resistance weight training is mandatory.

### HOW TO ADJUST YOUR CALORIES FOR FAT LOSS

Releasing stored energy from your fat cells is a complex neuroendocrine process, but it starts with one simple condition: You create a calorie deficit by burning more than you consume. There are 3,500 calories in a pound of stored body fat. In theory, if you create a 3,500-calorie deficit per week through diet, exercise, or a combination of both, you will lose 1 pound (0.5 kg) (assuming you lose 100 per cent body fat). If you create a 7,000-calorie deficit in a week, you will lose 2 pounds (0.9 kg).

You can create the calorie deficit by reducing food, increasing exercise or preferably a combination of both.

> **EXAMPLE:**
> **Your weight is 172 pounds (12 st 4 lb/78 kg).**
> **Your TDEE is 2,817 calories.**
> **Your daily calorie deficit to lose fat is 500 calories.**
> **Your daily caloric intake for a 1-pound (0.5-kg) weekly weight loss is 2,817 – 500 = 2,317 calories.**
> **Your daily caloric intake for a 2-pound (0.9-kg) weekly fat loss is 2,822 – 1,000 = 1,822 calories.**

The "minus 500 to 1,000 method" shows you how much you would need to eat to lose 1 or 2 pounds (0.4 to 0.9 kg) per week. Depending on the individual, a 1,000-calorie deficit could be a perfectly reasonable reduction or it could be semi-starvation.

For example, if you're a large and active male with a 3,400-calorie maintenance level, a 1,000-calorie deficit means a daily caloric intake of 2,400 calories per day. That's a 30 per cent deficit, which is aggressive but well within reason. If you're a petite, inactive female with a maintenance level of 1,600 calories per day, then a 1,000-calorie deficit means a daily intake of only 900 calories. That's a 57 per cent deficit, which is semi-starvation and potentially unhealthy. As Einstein would say, that's relativity.

## *BURN THE FAT, FEED THE MUSCLE* CALORIE DEFICIT GUIDELINES

The ideal way to choose your calorie deficit is to use a sliding scale and to select a percentage deficit relative to your maintenance level. For healthy, long-term fat loss, choose a deficit between 15 per cent and 30 per cent below your maintenance level.

| | |
|---|---|
| Conservative deficit | 15%–20% below maintenance |
| Moderate deficit | 21%–25% below maintenance |
| Aggressive deficit | 26%–30% below maintenance |
| Extremely aggressive deficit | 31%–40% below maintenance |
| Semi-starvation | 50% below maintenance |

**EXAMPLE (CONSERVATIVE DEFICIT):**
Your TDEE is 2,817 calories.
Your calorie deficit is 20 per cent (0.20 × 2,822 = 563 calories).
Your optimal caloric intake for fat loss = **2,254 calories.**
Projected weight loss = 1.1 pounds (0.5 kg) per week

**EXAMPLE (AGGRESSIVE DEFICIT):**
Your TDEE is 2,817 calories.
Your calorie deficit is 30 per cent (0.30 × 2,822 = 845 calories).
Your optimal caloric intake for fat loss = **1,972 calories.**
Projected weight loss = 1.7 pounds (0.8 kg) per week

Your calorie deficit – how much you'll decrease your calories below maintenance – is one of the first places you'll customize your plan. When deciding whether to be aggressive or conservative with your deficit, you should consider not only your desired rate of fat loss (which may be influenced by whether you're under deadline to achieve a goal), but also your starting body fat level.

In an aggressive deficit, lean people tend to lose more lean tissue and retain more fat, while obese people tend to lose more body fat and retain more lean tissue. This explains why obese people can tolerate low-calorie diets better than lean people. If you have plenty of energy in storage as body fat, then you're in less danger of starvation than a very lean person.

People who are already lean but want to get even leaner (a.k.a. "ripped") have a higher risk of losing lean tissue with very aggressive calorie cuts, especially when training volume and intensity are high. That's why, if you're lean, it's wise to keep your calorie deficit moderate or conservative. If you're overweight, it's safer to make your calorie deficit more aggressive.

> ### QUICKSTART
> Want to quickly and easily figure out your ideal personal calorie intake, including your basal metabolic rate (BMR), your maintenance level (TDEE), and your optimal daily intake for fat loss? Or, do you want to skip the maths altogether and see the calorie shortcuts? Simply jump to the appendix at any time and use the *Burn the Fat, Feed the Muscle* calorie customization worksheet.

## CALORIE DEFICIT THRESHOLDS: HOW LOW IS TOO LOW?

A larger calorie deficit results in faster weight loss. But a deficit that's too large or too prolonged will eventually slow your metabolism, increase hunger, decrease energy, reduce essential nutrient intake, and cause a loss of lean body mass. That leaves you with a dilemma: How low should you go to get maximum fat loss with minimum side effects?

There's a threshold where cutting calories more triggers metabolic, health, or compliance problems at an accelerated rate. The American College of Sports Medicine's suggestions of reasonable calorie minimums are 1,200 per day for women and 1,800 per day for men. But as with all fixed recommendations, these are generalizations. It's always ideal to customize.

The best practice is to follow the *Burn the Fat, Feed the Muscle* guidelines and use a maximum calorie deficit of 30 per cent below maintenance. There are some situations where a larger deficit makes sense, but it may be riskier. Extremely aggressive deficits should not be used except by very overweight or obese patients under their doctor's orders.

## WHAT IF YOU WANT TO GAIN MUSCLE?

The initial focus of *Burn the Fat, Feed the Muscle* is burning fat off as quickly and efficiently as possible. Many people use this programme to get lean, and once they achieve the low level of body fat they want, they change their goal to gaining lean muscle. When that time comes, the principles of this programme will still apply; you'll simply need to eat more so you're in a calorie surplus most of the time. As long as you still train hard, bring up the calories slowly, and keep the surplus small, you won't have to worry about gaining back any fat.

If you have a maintenance level of 2,800 calories, then your optimal intake for fat loss would be about 2,250 calories a day – a 20 per cent deficit. If your primary goal is gaining muscle, then your optimal intake would be at least 3,220 calories per day – a 15 per cent surplus. That's a 1,000-calorie difference between a fat-loss plan and a muscle-gaining plan. You have to eat a lot more to gain lean muscle at the maximum rate.

Some people are tempted to try losing fat and gaining muscle at the same time. Advertisements in the fitness magazines have convinced many people that huge gains of muscle along with large losses of body fat are common and easy to accomplish. But you can see from the previous example how fat-loss and muscle-gain goals are on opposite ends of the calorie spectrum and why achieving both concurrently is a challenge.

High body fat is unhealthy, so if you're carrying a lot of fat, focus your goals on shedding the fat first. Once the fat is off, you can shift gears into the lifelong maintenance phase where you gradually increase your calories to your TDEE and hold it there, or you establish new goals for gaining muscle, where you set calories in a surplus.

## HOW TO RECONCILE BETWEEN THEORETICAL (ON PAPER) AND ACTUAL (REAL-WORLD) CALORIE NEEDS

The calorie equations in this chapter are surprisingly accurate, but keep in mind that they're all estimations, designed only to give you a starting point. Like all the advice in this book, the numbers on paper take a backseat to real world feedback. The only way to tell if your estimate is correct is to get started, establish a baseline, and track your weekly progress. If you don't get the results you expect, adjust your caloric intake and exercise levels and repeat the process until you do.

To help you establish a baseline and fine-tune your calories quickly, it's also a smart idea to compare your calorie calculations on paper to the amount you've been eating recently. Recall a *typical* day of eating and write down in a notebook, spreadsheet, or electronic journal everything you ate from the time you got up in the morning to the time you went to sleep at night. Don't forget the little things like sauces, condiments, mints, the milk in your coffee, the sports drink during your workout, that beer on the weekend, the late-night snacks, and the "no-calorie" sweeteners (which actually do have calories!). If your food intake varies and you never have a typical day, then write down three days' worth of recent eating, so you can add them up and divide by three to get a daily average.

Next, look up the caloric value of each food and write it down next to each food item (see p326). You may want to consider also getting a good calorie counter app, online food database, or nutrient values book such as Corinne T. Netzer's *The Complete Book of Food Counts*. Then add everything up so you can see how many calories you've actually been eating.

Once you've established your baseline, continue to adjust your calories each week based on the real-world results. You won't need to recalculate your calories often. You'll usually go back to the formulas and recalculate after a period of months when you end a fat-loss phase and transition into a maintenance or muscle-gain programme, or anytime you've had a large change in activity level or body weight.

## ADJUST YOUR CALORIE INTAKE GRADUALLY IF NECESSARY

It's sometimes inadvisable to make drastic changes to your calorie intake all at once. After you've done your calculations on paper and you've completed your typical day's food recall, compare the two numbers. If your actual caloric intake was hundreds of calories higher or lower than your new target amount according to the formulas, then you may need to adjust your calories slowly.

Cutting calories quickly and abruptly often leads to diet failure and weight regain because the change is too dramatic to sustain. On the other hand, if you crunch your numbers and see that you've been eating a lot less than you should, it's equally important to increase your calories gradually in case your metabolism is sluggish. A sudden jump in calories could cause you to gain weight at first.

The best approach is to gradually adjust your calories in small weekly increments of 100–200 calories at a time to allow your metabolism to acclimatize.

## CALORIE COUNTING MADE EASY

Some people argue that counting calories is too tedious or unrealistic for most people long term. Instead, they recommend counting portions, where you're paying attention to serving size, but you don't know the exact calorie amount. Tracking portion sizes is a start because this acknowledges the importance of energy in versus energy out. It also allows you to reduce portion size if you need to increase your deficit. The downside of counting portions is that you're only guessing at the calories.

Although a lucky few can "wing it" and guess at everything with good results, the people with the best bodies in the world are meticulous about tracking calories. They leave nothing to chance and neither should you. This is especially true at times when you're working hard to achieve a major goal with a deadline, whether it's a bodybuilding competition, a body transformation contest, or losing 6 per cent body fat for a vacation. Tracking calories is also important if you hit a plateau. If you aren't quantifying and tracking your food intake, it's almost impossible to troubleshoot stalled fat loss.

One way to make this quick and easy is to create your meal plan on a spreadsheet such as Microsoft Excel. Many apps and software programmes are also available for creating meal plans or tracking food intake. MyFitnessPal is a free app that is popular with *Burn the Fat* readers because of its extensive food database. The *Burn the Fat* Meal Planner software is available with a subscription to our members-only website at www.BurnTheFatInnerCircle.com.

Once you have your daily meal plan finished, print it, stick it on your refrigerator (or carry it in your daily planner or mobile device), and you have an eating goal for the day. If you don't want to crunch any numbers at all, you can use the *Burn the Fat, Feed the Muscle* sample meals and meal plans in chapter 14 to get you started.

All you need to get going on the road to a better body is one good meal plan, customized for your calorie needs. Eating the same thing every day makes establishing a baseline, tracking calories, sticking to the programme, and troubleshooting plateaus super-easy. If you enjoy variety, you can create a few days or even an entire week of meal plans. Using an exchange system based on food groups makes substitutions a cinch. It is a good idea, though, to include a variety of foods within each day's plan. This way you can be sure you get the complete spectrum of vitamins, minerals, fibre, and other nutrients you need for good health.

During the initial stages, weigh, and measure all your food. Get yourself a set of kitchen scales, available in the kitchen section of most department stores, and a set of measuring spoons. Make it a habit to read the nutrition facts panel on the labels of packaged foods to learn the ingredients, calories, and nutrient values. For produce and natural foods that don't come with labels (fruits, vegetables, beans and pulses, yams, potatoes, and so on), it helps to keep a calorie book, chart, or electronic database handy.

Keep up this level of tracking until you reach your goal or at least until you start to get a "sixth sense" for portion sizes and calories. You can go back to weighing and measuring food anytime in the future if you hit a plateau.

If you're not familiar with the calorie amounts in the foods you eat, and especially if you eat differently every day, I strongly recommend keeping a daily nutrition journal, either electronically or on paper, for at least 4 to 12 weeks. Keeping a food journal at least once in your life is an amazing learning experience that you'll never get from reading a book or following a pre-made meal plan.

Creating your own meal plans requires a bit of effort at first, but if you think about it, when you use the *Burn the Fat* method, you only need to count calories once in the beginning when you create your meal plans. After that, you just follow the plan. Once you've got a knack for calories from creating meal plans on paper, then you can eyeball portions and get a pretty good (and much more educated) ballpark figure.

## WHY MEAL PLANNING AND CALORIE TRACKING ARE DISCIPLINES THAT PAY

It's not necessary to write down how many calories are in every crumb you eat for the rest of your life, but it is vital to understand and obey the law of calorie balance, get familiar with the calorie counts of foods you eat often, and at least know the ballpark figure of your current daily intake. There's no better way to learn about calories than to carefully count them in the early phases when you're just getting started, otherwise you'll always be guessing.

Ultimately, how meticulously you track your food intake should depend on your results. If you're shedding fat while maintaining your lean body mass without counting anything, then keep doing what you're doing. But if you're not making the progress you want, a lack of nutritional precision might be what's holding you back.

Some people don't consider nutritional number crunching fun or easy, but tracking your food intake is a discipline and becoming disciplined about your nutrition and training habits pays huge dividends: not only great health, higher energy, more muscle, and less fat, but also great results that are steady, predictable, and completely under your control.

The best definition of "discipline" I've ever heard comes from achievement expert Brian Tracy, who said, "Discipline is doing what is hard and necessary rather than what is fun and easy and doing it when it's necessary, whether you feel like doing it or not."

If you want the best results, then do what's necessary: Get out your calorie counter, your spreadsheet, or your nutrition software and create your meal plans. Then get out your kitchen scales and start tracking what and how much you're eating.

In the upcoming chapters, you'll learn about the other numbers that are most important to track – the macronutrients – so you can cut your body fat down to super-low levels, revealing the chiselled muscle definition you've always wanted!

# CHAPTER 8

# Balancing Your Macronutrients

"Each meal should be structured to include a lean protein, a starchy carbohydrate and a fibrous carbohydrate. The protein and fibre in this combination of foods slows the digestion of the carbohydrates, consequently providing consistent energy levels, sustained endurance, and a constant supply of nutrients to your body for energy, growth and repair."

– John Parrillo, bodybuilding nutritionist

## IS A CALORIE JUST A CALORIE?

A calorie deficit is a required condition for weight loss, but if creating a healthy fat-burning nutrition plan were only a matter of calories and nothing else, then three diets at the same calorie level – the first composed of 100 per cent protein, the second 100 per cent carbohydrates, and the third 100 per cent fats – would all produce the same results. Common sense alone tells you that eating 2,000 calories of fish and vegetables (lean protein and fibrous carbohydrates) won't produce the same results as 2,000 calories of crisps and fizzy drinks (processed fat and carbohydrates).

How you divide your calories between the three macronutrients – proteins, carbohydrates, and fats – and which foods you choose from each category has a profound impact on your body and your health. Severely restricting any one of the macronutrients can lead to nutrient deficiencies and a drop in your physical performance. Your macronutrient choices can also affect your calorie intake. Some food groups have more calories per gram than others, so it's easy to overeat them. Other foods are extremely filling, so you tend to eat less.

How you split up your macronutrients can even affect your hormones. This includes hormones of hunger and metabolism, which influence how many calories you eat or burn each day, as well as hormones that influence energy partitioning. Partitioning refers to where your body sends the calories and nutrients after they're metabolized – into fat or muscle – and what kind of body mass you lose or gain as a result.

Start with calories, but don't stop there. There's more to good nutrition than calories. To achieve all your goals – not just weight loss but also fat loss, muscular growth, great health and peak performance – it's important to get the calories right *and* get your protein, carbs, and fats right. Balancing these numbers is the foundation of every *Burn the Fat, Feed the Muscle* meal plan.

## THE FIRST RULE OF MACRONUTRIENTS: EAT PROTEINS AND CARBS TOGETHER AT EACH MEAL

Before we talk about specific numbers and percentages, let's start with the most fundamental rule of macronutrients: Your nutrition programme should never consist primarily of one food type or one macronutrient; you need a proper balance between proteins, carbs, and fats.

Without breaking out spreadsheets or crunching any numbers, you can get your macronutrient ratios in the ballpark simply by having a serving of lean protein and a serving of natural carbohydrate at every meal. If you eat a lot of meals with proteins or carbs by themselves, your ratios are more likely to be out of balance for the day.

Many popular diets – such as an all-protein diet or an all-fruits-and-vegetables diet – fail to obey this rule because they overemphasize one macronutrient. Diet gurus often claim that there's magic in the special foods they emphasize. It's closer to the truth to say that restricting entire food groups is a clever way to make you eat less. Any weight lost through severe restriction is likely to return and comes at the expense of a potentially unhealthy diet that's missing major nutrients. Apart from considerations due to allergies, sensitivities, and intolerances, eliminating an entire food group is never a smart idea.

Another diet fad, which became popular through several best-selling books, is called food combining. This would be more accurately described as food separating, because it argues that certain foods, such as meat and potatoes or protein and fruit, shouldn't be eaten together. Proponents claim that improper food combinations cause poor digestion, sap your energy, put stress on your immune system, and even promote disease.

As you experiment with your food choices to customize your own meal plan, it's possible that some foods or combinations of foods might make you feel better or worse. However, there's no evidence that there are any benefits to separating carbs and protein.

In the *Burn the Fat, Feed the Muscle* programme, you combine lean proteins and natural carbs together with every meal. An example of a lean protein and starchy carb combination at breakfast is eggs (protein) and oatmeal (natural carb). A dinner example is chicken (protein) with rice and vegetables (natural carbs). There are several important reasons why we combine the macronutrients this way.

### Five Reasons to Eat Lean Proteins
### and Natural Carbs Together at Every Meal

1. **For building muscle, it's optimal to eat protein at regular intervals throughout the day.** Protein can't be stored in your body like carbohydrates. If you eat too many meals without protein, your body doesn't have the raw material it needs to build new muscle and may even break down the muscle you have.

2. **Studies have proven that protein has an appetite-suppressing effect and makes you feel fuller.** Lean proteins are also hard to overeat, while carbs are easy to overeat, so moderating your carbs and eating a lean protein at every meal is a great way to help control your calories.

3. **Out of all the macronutrients, protein has the highest thermic effect (providing a boost to your metabolism) because of the extra energy required to digest and utilize it.** A meal that has only carbs is less thermic than one that includes protein. A meal that's high in fat without protein is the least thermic of all.

4. **Muscle glycogen is the primary source of energy for weight lifting and high-intensity exercise, but your glycogen stores are limited and must be continuously replenished by eating carbs.** If you eat only protein meals, without carbs, your glycogen levels get chronically depleted, your performance declines, and your recovery suffers. Even if you have a carb-intolerant body type or you prefer carb-restricted diets, it's important to get some carbs in your meals every day to support your training.

5. **If you suffer from nagging hunger, cravings or hypoglycaemia, it's often from eating too many sugars and processed carbs by themselves.** Instead, eat natural carbs in meals that also contain fibre, lean protein, and healthy fats. This balanced combination slows the digestion of the carbs, resulting in steadier energy levels, more stable blood sugar levels, and a more controlled output of insulin.

In this programme, our definition of a complete and balanced meal is one that contains a lean protein and a natural carb. We can take this meal template a step further in nutritional quality by making sure we include vegetables in the natural carb part of most of our meals. That makes the ultimate meal combination a lean protein, a starchy carb, and a fibrous carb.

A dinner example is chicken breast (lean protein), brown rice (starchy carb), and oriental vegetables (fibrous carbs). A breakfast example is scrambled eggs (lean protein) and old-fashioned porridge (starchy carb) with spinach and mushrooms (fibrous carbs). You can add fruit into this meal template instead of (or in addition to) the vegetables (for example, eggs, porridge, and blueberries). Many dairy products are good sources of protein, so if you traded the eggs for a Greek yogurt, you'd have the same lean protein and natural carbs combination. You'll get more meal planning ideas when you get to chapter 14.

## THE POWER OF DOING NUTRITION BY THE NUMBERS

When customizing meal plans, some people get overwhelmed by the thought of crunching the numbers for all these foods. The good news is, with spreadsheets or software, it's easy. Using our lean-protein-plus-natural-carbs meal template is by itself a simple quick-start shortcut. Start each meal with that combination and your numbers will already be in the ballpark: All you have to do is tweak the protein, carb, or fat portions up or down a little if you want to hit your calorie and macronutrient targets on the bull's-eye.

Like calories, you could guesstimate your macros as long as you're getting the results you want, but if you're not satisfied with your results, it's time to get serious about tracking numbers. If you're a beginner, pre-made meal plans make it easy to get started fast. But there's nothing more powerful for understanding and customizing nutrition than doing meal plans by the numbers and fine-tuning those numbers as you go, based on your results.

Bodybuilding nutritionist to the pros Chris Aceto agrees. In his book, *Everything You Need to Know About Fat Loss*, he writes, "I feel that number crunching is a very important part of learning about nutrition. You will never be able to build an exact diet, one that really works, and one that is built especially for you, without knowing how to count calories, carbohydrates, protein and fat."

Creating meal plans by the numbers gives you the kind of nutritional precision that puts you in complete control of your results. It enables you to easily troubleshoot plateaus, accelerate your fat loss, or dial yourself into peak condition on the date of your choosing. This is how the leanest people in the world do it.

Your ratios must be customized, but as you'll learn shortly, there is a sensible place – a baseline – where *everyone* can start.

## MACRONUTRIENT PERCENTAGES DEFINED

A macronutrient ratio is simply the percentage of your total calories that come from protein, carbohydrate, and fat, respectively. To create a meal plan by the numbers, you start with your daily calorie goal, which you calculated in the previous chapter. Then you choose your macronutrient goals and divvy up the calories. Think of it as slicing a pie. For example, if you sliced your daily nutritional "pie" into three equal portions, the ratios would be 33⅓ per cent carbohydrate, 33⅓ per cent protein, and 33⅓ per cent fat.

How do you define a low-carb or high-carb diet? When is a nutrition programme considered high-protein? What does a high-fat diet really mean? Drawing a line is difficult, but for the purpose of our discussion, let's clarify what we're talking about when we refer to high, medium and, low macronutrient percentages.

## CARBOHYDRATE DEFINITIONS

| Carbohydrate Level | Percentage of Total Calories |
| --- | --- |
| Very high carb | 65%–70%+ |
| High carb | 55%–60% |
| Moderate carb | 40%–50% |
| Low carb | 25%–35% |
| Very low carb | Less than 20% |

## PROTEIN DEFINITIONS

| Protein Level | Percentage of Total Calories |
| --- | --- |
| Very high protein | 45%–50%+ |
| High protein | 35%–40% |
| Moderate protein | 25%–30% |
| Low protein | 15%–20% |
| Very low protein | Less than 15% |

## FAT DEFINITIONS

| Fat Level | Percentage of Total Calories |
| --- | --- |
| Very high fat | 40%+ |
| High fat | 30%–40% |
| Moderate fat | 20%–30% |
| Low fat | 10%–20% |
| Very low fat | Less than 10% |

How do you know what percentage is ideal? There's no best way for everyone. One tip is to avoid extremes. For improving body composition, the best approach for most people is moderate carbs, moderate fat, and moderate to high protein. That's what you call balance! From this starting point, you can modify and customize based on how you respond.

Ironically, in the diet world, it's the extremes that often attract the most attention, especially low carb and low fat. Before we talk about finding the ideal baseline in the sensible middle, let's look at these two extremes.

## VERY LOW FAT

In the 1980s and early '90s, the most popular trend was the low-fat diet. This came with very high carbs. Some of the best-selling programmes at that time recommended macronutrient ratios of around 70 per cent carbs, 20 per cent protein, and 10 per cent fat. They're not as popular today, but plenty of diets still promote the very low-fat approach. Proponents believe that fat makes you fat and that dietary fat causes heart disease and other health problems, so fats are said to be the "bad macronutrient." These ideas have all been challenged.

If you keep your calories in a deficit, you will lose weight on very low-fat, high-carb diets. If the carbs are carefully chosen and include nutrient, phytochemical and fibre-rich fruits, vegetables, whole grains, and natural starches, this could also be a healthy way for some people to eat. But problems always exist with extreme diets of any kind. Potential problems with the very low-fat approach include falling short on essential fatty acids, being too low in protein for serious strength training (which doesn't support your efforts to build muscle), and having too many carbs for carb intolerant people (which doesn't support your efforts to burn fat or maintain good health).

## VERY LOW CARB

At the other extreme, you have the very low-carb diets. Some are high in fat and protein. Others, like the ketogenic diets, are very high in fat and lower in protein. The amount of carbs in a low-carb diet can vary from as high as 35 per cent to as low as 10 per cent and occasionally you hear about the ultra-extreme zero-carb diets. Supporters claim that carbs are driving obesity because carbs stimulate insulin and insulin causes fat storage. Therefore, carbs are said to be "the bad macronutrient." Like the low-fat diet, these ideas have also been challenged.

There are legitimate concerns about excessive carb intake. Many people are getting an overdose of sugar and not enough lean protein or healthy fat. Unfortunately, the concerns about carbs have been blown out of proportion, creating unwarranted fear. Carbs are not fattening outside of the easy calorie overload they cause if you're not careful with portions. Also, not every body type has trouble metabolizing carbs. Most athletes thrive on them and exercise can improve anyone's carb tolerance and insulin sensitivity. Carb restriction can be a good way to accelerate fat loss, but that's not saying carbs make you fat.

## THE ORIGINAL BODYBUILDER'S DIET

The 60–30–10 nutrient ratio is the programme I originally used when I first started bodybuilding. When I began competing, it was the early 1990s, right in the middle of the fat phobia era. My nutrition plan was high in natural carbs and low in fats simply because that diet was in vogue and widely accepted.

So I conformed and did what everyone else was doing. It worked. The 60–30–10 ratio was effective for fat loss and I felt strong and energetic. That shouldn't be surprising, because I was tracking my calorie deficit, the protein was adequate, and I found that my body type handles carbs fairly well. I later discovered that one small adjustment improved my results even further.

It wasn't until the late 90s that I really began to reach my best physical condition, winning multiple overall bodybuilding titles and looking my absolute best ever. For years I turned myself into a human guinea pig, experimenting with every diet imaginable from very high-carb, zero-fat diets to high-fat, zero-carb ketogenic diets, and I finally stumbled onto a formula that worked beautifully.

With this change, I gained more muscle in the off-season, burned more fat in the contest season (dropping below 4 per cent body fat at my all-time lowest) and stayed leaner year round, maintaining a 9 per cent body fat percentage without much difficulty. I also moved up a full weight class. I was stronger. My energy was better. My mental focus was sharper.

What was this adjustment? Believe it or not, I ate more fat. I dropped the carbs by 10 per cent and replaced it with healthy fat sources such as nuts (like almonds and walnuts), natural peanut butter, fatty fish like salmon, flaxseed (linseed) oil, and extra virgin olive oil. I also allowed myself some red meat and one or two egg yolks a day (instead of only egg whites, the bodybuilder's staple protein).

In the next chapter, you'll learn everything you'll ever need to know about dietary fats. For now it's enough to say that adding some "good fats" is vitally important for optimizing your health and improving your body composition.

## *BURN THE FAT* BASELINE NUTRITION: YOUR STARTING POINT

My small adjustment to 50 per cent carbs, 30 per cent protein, and 20 per cent fat not only worked well for me, it also worked for the majority of my training clients and coaching protégés over a period of many years. My personal experience and the results from my clients, combined with what the research said, convinced me that this was a good place to start and it became the baseline of the *Burn the Fat, Feed the Muscle* programme.

Do your goals include burning fat and transforming your body? Do you want to achieve these goals in a healthy, balanced way without losing muscle or energy? Are you already training or planning to start training? If so, it's hard to go wrong with 50 per cent carbohydrates, 30 per cent protein, and 20 per cent fat as your starting point as well.

The 50–30–20 macronutrient split is not a rigid prescription. Five per cent either way won't make that much difference, but you might want to adjust your starting numbers slightly depending on your goals, preferences, past experience, and body type. Highly active athletes might start at 55 per cent carbs. For endomorphic or carb-intolerant types, they might find 45 per cent carbs is a better starting point. Many strength and physique athletes start at 35 per cent protein because they believe it supports the intensity of their weight training better.

Some people make adjustments purely for personal preference reasons. For example, they might find their meals more enjoyable, their hunger reduced, or their energy levels higher when eating more fat, so they might start with 5 per cent more fat than the baseline.

Once you're off and running, you'll probably make even more adjustments over the weeks and months you're pursuing your goal. The most common is to reduce the carbs and increase the lean protein (and sometimes the healthy fat) when you want to accelerate fat loss or break a plateau. But before you can make any of these types of changes, you need to establish a baseline plan and get some feedback on how it's working.

## ESTABLISH A FOUNDATION FIRST, THEN EXPERIMENT, ADJUST, AND CUSTOMIZE

Whenever you want to master a new subject or acquire a new skill, you must learn the basics first. If you have a shaky foundation, then nothing else you do will matter; your castle will crumble. As Emerson wrote, "The height of the pinnacle is determined by the breadth of the base."

Remember the 80–20 rule. That's the efficiency principle, which says that 20 per cent of your actions – the vital few – will produce the majority of your results. The other 80 per cent – the trivial many – is minutiae. Most people are wasting their time on the small stuff. They're constantly chasing after magic food combinations, exotic fat-burning berries, or weird diet hacks, all the while missing the simplest and most obvious factors that would make the biggest impact on their physiques.

On *Burn the Fat, Feed the Muscle* you'll do the opposite of the quick-fix diets: You'll nail down the fundamentals first. It starts with calories and macronutrients. You'll establish a baseline for those numbers and measure the results. If the baseline nutrition produces good results, you don't have to change anything. If not, then you start to experiment, tweak, and adjust.

If you want to experiment with the little details, from macronutrient ratios to food substitutions or eliminations to meal timing tweaks, you should. It's the fine-tuning you do over time that helps you customize your plan and squeeze out that extra few per cent in results that most people leave on the table.

But skip the weird stuff and don't jump into anything too advanced, aggressive, or restrictive until after you establish a baseline of fundamentals, get into a feedback loop, and start charting your results. With real-world progress data, you can see how your body is responding to all the variables and make the right adjustments at the right time.

## Adjustments for Nutrient Ratios by Body Type

The right macronutrient amounts can vary depending on your body type, your goals, and your training volume and style. Bodybuilders, for example, thrive on more protein than people who are sedentary. Endurance athletes sometimes require calorie and carb intakes that start where the average person's end. Although competitive bodybuilders and endurance athletes represent the far ends of the fitness spectrum, they help illustrate how important it is to customize.

### MESOMORPH

The mesomorph could probably follow almost any nutrient ratio and still get results. I know some mesomorphs on the 50–50 diet: 50 per cent McDonald's and 50 per cent pizza. They still grow muscle like weeds and have ripped abs. I'm not endorsing this approach, just making a point. If our genetically gifted mesomorph friends would be more meticulous with their macros and choose more nutritious foods, they would get even better results. The baseline plan – 50 per cent carbs, 30 per cent protein, and 20 per cent fat – would work as well as any.

**ECTOMORPH**

The ectomorph usually isn't concerned with losing body fat. Usually his goal is to gain muscle, and for gaining muscle the baseline plan with 50 per cent carbs, 30 per cent protein, and 20 per cent fat is also a good starting point. An ectomorph rarely needs to restrict carbs. Sometimes eating more fat (snacking on nuts, for example) helps ectomorphs hit their surplus, because dietary fat is calorie dense.

**ENDOMORPH**

It's the endomorph who needs to pay the most attention to macronutrient ratios, especially the carbs. Overweight endomorphs are usually more carb intolerant than the general population and have a natural tendency for less activity, so reducing carbs is their most common food adjustment. Some endomorphs might want to start closer to 40 per cent to 45 per cent carbs, then consider whether to cut more based on their weekly results.

### Adjustments to the Baseline Ratios for Accelerating Fat Loss

For short periods when maximum fat loss is the goal, the macronutrient ratios can be shifted to more protein and less carbs. In physique sports, where you see some of the leanest bodies in the world, 40 per cent carbs, 40 per cent protein, and 20 per cent fat is one of the most popular macronutrient splits during the fat-loss phase.

Reducing carbs and increasing protein can give you some measurable advantages when it comes to fat loss. It increases metabolism through the thermic effect of food, helps reduce hunger, makes calorie control easier, and protects lean body mass when the calorie deficit gets aggressive.

The best way to do it is to cut sugar as much as possible and reduce your intake of calorie-dense starches and grains (pasta, bread, rice, potatoes, cereal, and so on). That leaves the less calorie-dense fibrous carbs (such as green vegetables and salads), lean proteins, and healthy fats.

When carb restriction is too extreme, there's an increased risk of side effects such as hunger, low energy, loss of lean tissue, and the dreaded "brain fog." Fortunately, even a small reduction in carbs can help accelerate fat loss without the side effects of extreme low carbs. Carb cycling strategies help as well. We'll take a closer look at how to accelerate fat loss with these advanced techniques in chapter 19.

*QUICKSTART*

**If you're metabolically healthy and active, aim for 50% carbs, 30% protein, and 20% fat as your baseline. If you're an endomorph or you want to accelerate fat loss, decrease the carbs and increase the protein (40% carbs, 40% protein, and 20% fat is super-popular among fitness models and physique athletes). Using nutrition tracking spreadsheets or software makes calculating your macronutrient ratios a cinch! But if you make sure to eat a lean protein, a fibrous vegetable and a natural starchy carb with every meal, your numbers will be in the ballpark, automatically!**

## THE SPREADSHEET METHOD FOR MEAL PLANNING

A simple way to estimate your nutrient ratios for an individual meal is to follow the 3–2–1 rule. Imagine your plate divided into six sections like slices of a pie. Fill up three slices (3/6, or 50 per cent) with natural carbs like potatoes, yams, oats, whole grains, fruits, and vegetables. Fill up two sections (2/6, or 33 per cent) with lean proteins like egg whites, chicken, and fish. Finish with one section of fat (1/6, or 17 per cent). This easy method puts you very close to the optimal ratios and you don't need to be a maths whizz to figure it out.

The best and most accurate technique for meal calculations is free, and you probably already have it on your laptop or desktop computer: It's a plain old spreadsheet like Microsoft Excel.

These days, there's also no shortage of nutrition apps and software for creating meal plans, including our own custom-made *Burn the Fat* Meal Planner, which is available with a subscription to our members-only Inner Circle community at www.BurnTheFatInnerCircle.com. These tools make meal planning easy because the spreadsheets are built in and they do all the maths for you; all you have to do is set your goal numbers and choose the foods you like. They're also convenient because they have large food databases and they're compatible with mobile devices or smartphones.

To calculate your ratios, take your total calorie goal for the day (which you calculated in the previous chapter) and multiply it by your target percentage of each macronutrient. Then, divide the calories from each macronutrient by the calorie content per gram. You'll need to know the following three conversions, also known as the Atwater factors, to calculate your ratios:

**1 gram of carbohydrate = 4 calories**
**1 gram of protein = 4 calories**
**1 gram of fat = 9 calories**

I've crunched the numbers for you in the two examples below. These represent the typical man or woman. These numbers are a good starting point, but you'll need to customize based on your own personal calorie needs.

For men, here is an example of a 2,300-calorie-per-day fat-loss plan:

| Macronutrient Type | Percentage of Total Calories | Conversion to Grams |
|---|---|---|
| Carbohydrates 50% | 0.50 × 2,300 calories = 1,150 calories from carbohydrates | 1,150 carb calories ÷ 4 calories per gram = 288 grams of carbs |
| Protein 30% | 0.30 × 2,300 calories = 690 calories from protein | 690 protein calories ÷ 4 calories per gram = 173 grams of protein |
| Fat 20% | 0.20 × 2,300 calories = 460 calories from fat | 460 fat calories ÷ 9 calories per gram = 51 grams of fat |

For women, here is an example for a 1,600-calorie-per-day fat-loss plan:

| Macronutrient Type | Percentage of Total Calories | Conversion to Grams |
|---|---|---|
| Carbohydrates 50% | 0.50 × 1,600 calories = 800 calories from carbohydrates | 800 carb calories ÷ 4 calories per gram = 200 grams of carbs |
| Protein 30% | 0.30 × 1,600 calories = 480 calories from protein | 480 protein calories ÷ 4 calories per gram = 120 grams of protein |
| Fat 20% | 0.20 × 1,600 calories = 320 calories from fat | 320 fat calories ÷ 9 calories per gram = 36 grams of fat |

If you hit your targets at every meal, then your entire day will take care of itself, but you don't have to worry about making every meal have the same amount of carbs and total calories. It's okay if your meals vary in size. For example, your post-workout meals may be larger and contain more carbs. Or if you're a big breakfast eater like I am, your first meal may have more carbs and calories as well.

Your primary goal is to come as close to your macronutrient target as possible *when you add it all up for the day*. Don't worry about being perfect. If you try to micro-manage your macronutrients, you'll probably just drive yourself crazy. If your protein, carb, and fat numbers are within 5 per cent or so of your target in either direction, that's close enough. Your daily totals may not add up to exactly 100 per cent either. Nutrient information in databases and on food labels is usually estimated and often rounded off, so if you ever see your daily totals add up to only 98.7 per cent, for example, it doesn't mean you made a mistake.

## COUCH POTATO NUTRITION VERSUS
## MUSCLE-BUILDING NUTRITION

The recommendations in this chapter are designed to support people involved in resistance and cardio training programmes. Some conservative or traditional nutritionists might tell you that the protein is too high. They might say that the government-mandated guidelines are sufficient. They might insist that the protein should be set at only 15 per cent. That's couch potato advice. It has nothing to do with you if you're training hard and pursuing a body transformation goal.

Your success with *Burn the Fat, Feed the Muscle* will be based on how well you consistently combine all four elements of the programme: nutrition, cardio training, weight training, and mental training. If you're not training hard, you're not following the programme. If you're training hard, your nutrition needs are different from those of couch potatoes.

When you see nutrient recommendations for the general population, keep in mind that the average person is not training and that minimum and optimum nutrition needs are two different concepts. If you want to get lean and muscular, then do what lean and muscular people do, and at the same time listen to your body so you can make the right adjustments for you.

## THERE'S NO ONE-SIZE-FITS-ALL PRESCRIPTION

Although it's wise to pursue a healthy balance between macronutrients, a single perfect ratio for everyone doesn't exist.

✓ No ratio has any magical fat-burning or muscle-building properties.
✓ No ratio will override the law of calorie balance. Any impact nutrient ratios have on weight loss is minimal compared to the effect of calorie levels.
✓ No nutrient ratio will prevent metabolic slowdown if your calories are too low, too long.
✓ No nutrient ratio will prevent you from gaining fat if your calories are too high.
✓ No nutrient ratio will enable you to gain muscle if your calories are too low.
✓ No nutrient ratio will work for everyone. Optimal nutrient ratios depend on goals, differences in body type and carb tolerance.

Macronutrient ratios aren't the singular key to fat loss, but they do give you a great way to set up your daily meal plans and ensure that you get optimal amounts of the major essential nutrients. Always remember, regardless of whether you eat high carb, low carb, or anywhere in between, if you eat too many calories, you won't burn fat.

Start with the baseline and then experiment to find what works best for you. If you think high carbs are problematic for you, then drop the carbs and increase the protein and fat. If you think you're extremely carb intolerant, or you want to get ripped for a fitness competition, then bring down the carbs even lower, which bumps up the protein ratio, and see what happens.

## TRUSTING YOUR NUTRITION INTUITION

Did you ever notice how some people gravitate toward a certain style of eating without anyone telling them to do it? Why do some people instinctively become vegetarians while others are heavy meat eaters? Why do some people avoid wheat and dairy? Why do some people crave certain foods? The reason is their bodies tell them so, and wisely, they listen.

I'm not vegetarian, but if your body tells you to not eat much meat, I believe you should listen and explore other protein sources. If your body tells you you're carb intolerant, listen. If you think your carbs are too low, listen. If a certain food disagrees with your stomach, listen. Listen to your body and pay attention to your results each week.

If you navigated *only* by intuition, that would not be intelligent. You need a plan that's carefully structured. On the other hand, blindly following a programme without the flexibility to make adjustments along the way is also a recipe for failure. Making the right weekly adjustments requires a scientific approach, real-world feedback, as well as a keen intuition. The people with the leanest and best bodies in the world are the ones who train hard, eat properly, track their results, and do what their bodies tell them to do. This is true with macronutrients as it is with individual foods.

In the next three chapters, we'll take a closer look at each one of the macronutrients. You'll learn everything you need to know about proteins, carbohydrates, and fats to get leaner, healthier, and more muscular.

# CHAPTER 9

# Good Fats, Bad Fats

"Unfortunately for the much maligned lipid, fats and oils have been lumped together in the minds of most people as having the same properties, with the result of people trying to avoid ALL fats and oils for fear of adding body fat and looking like the Pillsbury dough boy. Well, I am here to tell you that fats have gotten a bad rap. There are good fats and there are bad fats. The difference between the two is substantial and of great importance."

– William D. Brink, author of *Priming the Anabolic Environment:*
*A Practical, Scientific Guide to the Art and Science of Building Muscle*

## THE MISSING LINK DISCOVERED: A DOSE OF "HEALTHY FATS"

In the last chapter I revealed how, after a long period of practically zero fat dieting, I took my results to a higher level with one small change: I ate more fat. But not too much fat, and not just any fat. As dietary fat expert Dr. Udo Erasmus says, "There are fats that heal and fats that kill."

Adding the *wrong* kind of fats can clog your arteries, promote weight gain, and wreak havoc in your body. Adding the *right* kind of fats can turbocharge your energy, burn more fat, boost muscle-building hormones, improve blood sugar control, strengthen your joints, and enhance your skin tone.

With benefits like these, good fats may sound like some kind of wonder drug, and in many respects the effects *are* almost drug-like. Surprisingly, you can get these miraculous results simply by eating small amounts of foods or oils rich in the healthy good fats while reducing or avoiding the unhealthy bad fats.

## THE ERA OF FAT PHOBIA

The first time I picked up a barbell was in 1983, the heart of the "fat phobia" era. During the 1980s and early '90s, the magazines, television, and nearly all the media pounded the message into our brains that fat was bad. No distinction was made between types of fats; the message was black-and-white: "Fat is unhealthy and fat makes you fat."

This spawned an entire industry of fat-free foods such as frozen dinners, processed meats, sweets, ice cream, yogurt, and nearly every other treat you can think of. This was the age of fat-free biscuits and cakes, and almost all of us partook of these deliciously sweet and seemingly guilt-free goodies. We ate them without fear and believed it was healthy, since the labels said "zero grams of fat"!

Even though dietary fat consumption decreased dramatically over the two decades that followed, a very strange thing happened: Waistlines and health problems continued to increase. According to US government statistics, the adult obesity rate rose from 15 per cent in 1980 to 32 per cent in 2004. Today, two out of three adults are overweight or obese; heart disease and diabetes are still two of the biggest killers; and it seems there's no end in sight to these epidemics.

If we cut down our fat intake so much in the '80s and '90s, then why did we continue getting fatter and sicker? Part of the answer is so obvious it's almost embarrassing:

## Fat-free doesn't mean sugar-free or calorie-free!

What happened is that many people cut the fat calories and simply replaced it with sugar calories. Even foods that always were fat-free suddenly started sporting new labels that proudly proclaimed, "No fat!" A food may say "fat-free" on the label but it could be 100 per cent sugar! If you eat too much sugar, it doesn't matter how little dietary fat you eat: You'll still gain body fat. You'll probably get sick too.

Most people have been conditioned to believe that eating fatty foods is the primary cause of health problems such as high cholesterol and heart attacks. There's no question, certain types of fats *are* unhealthy. What most people don't realize is that processed carbs and sugar can be even more harmful to your health and are every bit as responsible for climbing disease and obesity. The real culprit is an overload of processed foods, not one macronutrient.

## WHY A NONFAT DIET IS NOT THE BEST WAY
## TO A NONFAT BODY

Previously, we defined a very low-fat diet as anything under 10 per cent of total calories. On 2,300 calories per day, that's 26 grams or less. On 1,600 calories, that's only 18 grams of fat per day. I've consulted with clients who were proud of eating only 10 or 15 grams of fat per day. A few even boasted with excitement that they were eating almost zero grams! Ironically, they came to me because they were stuck and they couldn't get any leaner.

I taught them not to fear all fats, to distinguish between the good fats and the bad, and to include small amounts of healthy fats in addition to their lean proteins and natural carbs. When they started eating the good fats, almost like magic, they had more energy, more strength, and better workouts, and the fat loss started coming again.

Fat phobia is still so ingrained into dieting consciousness that most people are reluctant to add fat back in. To break free from fear of fat, it helps to understand the reasons why cutting it all out may do more harm than good.

The biggest problem is that by trying to eat a nonfat diet, many people inadvertently cut out the healthy fats along with the unhealthy ones. A deficiency in essential fatty acids can cause a long list of health issues, including skin and hair problems, joint pain, fatigue, depression, cardiovascular diseases, and reduced metabolism. Nonfat diets are also correlated with low testosterone levels. You need a little bit of fat – even the saturated kind – to maintain normal anabolic hormone levels.

When you eat pure carbs and no fat, this can also aggravate blood sugar problems in those who are susceptible, develop into metabolic syndrome, and eventually lead to type 2 diabetes and cardiovascular disease. Eating healthy fat (and fibre) slows digestion, which helps control blood sugar and insulin more effectively. This makes fats especially important for people who are carb intolerant.

Most surprising to many, eating nothing but nonfat, high-carb meals can sabotage your fat-loss goals by increasing hunger. After eating carbs without fibre or fat, your blood sugar peaks and quickly crashes, leaving you with that shaky, empty I-have-to-eat-now-or-I'm-going-to-pass-out feeling. It's more than an emotional craving for a specific food; it's physical hunger and it's hard to resist.

Cutting out all fat is not the answer. You need to eat fat. On the other hand, you don't want too much.

## THE TRUTH ABOUT HIGH-FAT DIETS

Most people believe that a low-carb diet is a high-protein diet, but that's not always the case. Ketogenic low-carb diets are actually high in fat, with modest amounts of protein and of course very few carbs. Despite being extremely unbalanced in macronutrients, these controversial diets attract a lot of interest. Advocates say that the metabolic state of ketosis produces greater fat loss than other diets. That claim has never been proven. They also claim a high fat intake is not inherently unhealthy. On this point, they're not entirely wrong.

The Greenland Inuit diet is mostly meat and fat (60 per cent), but the Inuits stay perfectly healthy. The cardio-protective omega-3 fatty acids in the marine foods they eat (fish and whale blubber) may explain their low incidence of disease. That's a far cry from the high-fat diets of modern Americans, which include factory-farmed meats, hydrogenated oils, baked goods, fried foods, refined cooking oils, and other processed fats, often eaten in combination with refined grains and sugar.

Conventional wisdom says that everyone should follow a low-fat diet. But some people are going against the grain of convention and it seems to be working for them. People do lose weight on ketogenic and other types of higher-fat diets. The real question is which type of programme is ideal for transforming your body? All it takes to lose weight is a calorie deficit. It takes a lot more to develop a great body and maintain it.

There's little or no evidence that high-fat, low-carb diets are better for fat loss than balanced diets or less extreme low-carb diets. They clearly fall short in the muscle-building department. Ketogenic diets that are low in carbs and high in fat still have an enthusiastic cult following in the mainstream weight-loss world. But they've never been the nutrition plan of choice in the physique world, where training is such an important part of the lifestyle.

For high-intensity training, muscle glycogen is your body's preferred and most efficient fuel. Glycogen is restored by eating carbs. If you eat too much fat, it displaces your carbs and depletes your glycogen, which may make your training suffer. If your training suffers, your muscle gains suffer. Even worse, studies have shown that training in a glycogen-depleted state has catabolic effects on muscle and decreases protein synthesis.

There are good fats that we benefit from eating in small amounts, but we don't need that much! It's also the quality of fat, not just the quantity that matters. In the next section you'll learn which fats you should eat more of, which you should eat less of, and which you should avoid completely. To choose your fats properly, you need to understand the differences between them.

## THE TWO MAJOR CATEGORIES OF FATS

Fatty acids are made from chains of carbon and hydrogen atoms linked together. The differences in their molecular structure give each fat its unique properties, such as its melting point, its "stickiness" in the blood, and how it affects your health. The structure of every fat or oil is either saturated or unsaturated.

### 1. Saturated fat

Butter, cheese, dairy fat, chocolate, egg yolk, meat fat, shortening, palm oil, palm kernel oil, milk fat and coconut oil are all saturated fats. With the exception of the tropical oils (palm, palm kernel, and coconut), saturated fats are primarily animal fats.

Saturated fats, with the exception of the tropical oils, are solid or semisolid at room temperature (think butter or animal fat). Saturated fats have historically been considered the least desirable because they can raise blood cholesterol.

The long-standing traditional advice has been to reduce saturated fat intake. However, without looking at each different type of saturated fatty acid individually and within the context of your genetics, health status, lifestyle, quantity eaten, and overall diet, it's overly simplistic to say that all saturated fats are bad for you or should be completely avoided. Saturated fats do, however, lack the essential fatty acids you need, so you must balance them with the unsaturated fats.

## 2. Unsaturated fat

Unsaturated fats are subdivided into polyunsaturated and monounsaturated fats and they come primarily from vegetable and plant sources. They are mostly liquid at room temperature (think olive oil). Generally, they tend to lower levels of blood cholesterol and have other health benefits or cardio-protective effects. The polyunsaturated fats contain the healthy essential fatty acids (EFAs)

| Saturated | Unsaturated (Poly) | Unsaturated (Mono) |
|---|---|---|
| Beef fat | Fish oil | Olive oil, olives |
| Poultry fat | Flaxseed oil | High-oleic sunflower oil |
| Other meat fats | Sunflower oil | High-oleic safflower oil |
| Butterfat | Safflower oil | Avocado |
| Coconut oil, coconut | Rapeseed oil | Rapeseed oil (contains both) |
| Cocoa butter | Sesame oil | Peanuts, peanut butter |
| Palm oil | Primrose oil | Cashews |
| Palm kernel oil | Borage oil | Pecans |
| Shortening, lard, tallow | Walnut oil, walnuts | Almonds, almond butter |
| Single cream | Hemp oil, hemp seeds | Brazil nuts |
| Milk fat | Soybean oil | Pistachios |
| Cheese fat | Corn oil | Macadamia nuts |
| Cream cheese | Pine nuts | Hazelnuts |

## ESSENTIAL FATTY ACIDS

Like other essential nutrients such as amino acids, essential fatty acids are those that your body can't make on its own, so they must be supplied through your diet in the right amounts and in the right ratios. The two primary EFAs include:

**Omega-3 (alpha linolenic, or LNA)**
**Omega-6 (linoleic acid, or LA)**

According to Artemis P. Simopoulos, author of *The Omega Diet: The Lifesaving Nutritional Program Based on the Diet of the Island of Crete*, human beings evolved on a diet that was not only free of manmade trans-fatty acids and lower in saturated fat than the modern diet, it also contained roughly equal amounts of omega-3 and omega-6. The modern Western diet today is very high in omega-6 fatty acids as compared to omega-3 with a ratio of 20:1 or even higher (optimal is more like 2:1).

One of the reasons for this imbalance is our increased consumption of refined grains and decreased consumption of omega-3-rich fish, as well as the industrial production of animal feeds containing grains high in omega-6 fatty acids. Since animals are what they eat, their meat becomes high in omega-6, unlike the leaner and higher omega-3 wild game that our ancestors once ate.

As we consume high-omega-6 meats and refined grains, we lose the natural balance we once thrived on and begin to suffer from inflammatory and cardiovascular diseases that were once unheard-of. By increasing your intake of omega-3 fats, you obtain a long list of health benefits, restoring you to the balance that nature intended.

### The Amazing Benefits of Essential Fatty Acids

Most people don't get enough omega-3 fatty acids, and their omega-3-to-omega-6 ratio is skewed badly in favour of the pro-inflammatory omega-6. Here are some of omega-3's most important functions in your body:

✓ EFAs improve insulin sensitivity.
✓ EFAs are required for absorption of fat-soluble vitamins.
✓ EFAs are essential for joint health.
✓ EFAs are required for energy production.
✓ EFAs are required for oxygen transfer.
✓ EFAs maintain cell membrane integrity.

✓  EFAs suppress cortisol production.
✓  EFAs improve skin texture.
✓  EFAs promote muscle growth.
✓  EFAs increase your metabolic rate.
✓  EFAs help burn fat.

It takes only a small amount of EFAs to prevent a deficiency, but if you want to maximize fat loss, muscular development, and physical performance, your goal is to get optimal amounts of every nutrient, not just to avoid deficiency. You can achieve this by adding at least one rich source of omega-3 into your meal plan every day.

Fatty fish is the best source of the omega-3 fatty acids eicosapentaenoic acid (EPA) and docosahexaenoic acid (DHA). You get protein at the same time, making it a true "superfood." Eating fatty fish at least two or three times per week is recommended by almost every major health authority. Omega-3 fats are also found in rich amounts in plant sources including flaxseeds and walnuts. Small amounts are found in dark leafy greens like kale, cabbage and broccoli, and spinach and some other types of seeds.

Ground flaxseed is another way to get omega-3 fats and it's also a great source of fibre (about 3 grams per tablespoon). Flaxseeds (or ground milled flaxseeds) can be used as an ingredient in baking, cooking, and special healthy recipes. You can mix flaxseeds in protein shakes, stir them into porridge, or sprinkle them on salads. It's best if you grind the seeds so you can fully digest them. It takes about 3 tablespoons of ground flaxseeds to equal the amount of EFAs in one tablespoon of oil.

**RICH SOURCES OF OMEGA-3 ESSENTIAL FATTY ACIDS:**

**Salmon**

**Sardines**

**Herring**

**Mackerel**

**Rainbow (lake) trout**

**Albacore tuna**

**Flaxseeds**

**Walnuts**

**Fish oil**

**Krill oil**

**Flaxseed oil**

### Essential Fatty Acid Supplements: Fish Oil and Flax Oil

It's possible to get all the healthy fats you need from food, but omega-3 fats are so important, many people take a supplement to be certain they're getting optimal amounts on a daily basis. Two of the most popular are fish oil and flax oil. Supplements can never take the place of whole foods. However, if you take an essential fatty acid supplement, meal planning is easier because you don't need to stress over whether you included an omega-3 whole food every day.

Research on fish oil suggests that 1.5 to 2.0 grams per day of combined DHA/ EPA is the ideal dose for supporting fat-loss programmes. A big guy might go with as much as 3.0 grams. There are studies that tested higher doses for specific health ailments, but the American Heart Association warns against taking more than 3.0 grams of combined EPA/DHA per day without a physician's supervision because of potential side effects, including increased bleeding time. I recommend consulting your doctor before taking any supplements.

Flaxseed oil is the richest plant-based source of omega-3, with twice the omega-3 content of fish oil. The type of omega-3 fat in flaxseed oil is alpha-linolenic acid, which requires conversion in your body to the usable forms, EPA and DHA. There's been debate about how well your body makes this conversion and whether flax oil is better than fish oil. Over the last decade, mounting research has made fish oil the darling of the health and fitness world and the most popular choice for a healthy fat supplement. In any case, flax is an extremely rich source of omega-3 fat and it's the top choice for vegetarians or anyone else who doesn't eat fish.

One tablespoon of flax oil per day is a typical dose; unusually large or active people might take more. Flaxseed oil is sensitive to heat, so it's not meant for cooking. However, you can add it to foods after cooking as well as to salads or protein shakes. Flaxseed oil goes rancid quickly, so buy it refrigerated, keep it refrigerated, and use it quickly once you open the container.

Like all whole food sources of fats and oils, essential fatty acid supplements have calories. If you use any supplements, be sure to add the calories and grams of fat into your daily totals.

## INCLUDE SATURATED FATS IN MODERATION

Cutting out all saturated fats isn't necessary, but they should make up only a small portion of your total calories and total fat intake. This leaves room for the other macronutrients and other types of fat, respectively. Most health and nutrition organizations recommend limiting saturated fat to 10 per cent of your daily calories and splitting the remainder between 10 per cent mono- and 10 per cent polyunsaturated fats. By following the food suggestions in this chapter, you won't need to worry about crunching those numbers: They will automatically be in the ballpark.

Small amounts of saturated fat tag along with your protein when you eat meat and poultry. You can keep the fat and calories to a minimum by picking the leanest cuts possible. If you eat red meat for your protein meals, it will also include some fat. Grass-fed beef is popular because it's leaner, it's lower in calories, it's lower in saturated fat, and it has a better omega-3-to-omega-6 ratio than grain-fed beef.

Eggs are another protein food that also contains fat (in the yolk). Many bodybuilders are known for eating egg whites when they want more protein with fewer calories. However, the idea that you shouldn't eat any whole eggs because they raise cholesterol and cause heart disease has been strongly challenged in recent years. There's a growing body of evidence that eating one or two whole eggs per day has no negative effects on cholesterol. Eating larger amounts of whole eggs may increase blood cholesterol, but research shows that the good HDL cholesterol goes up with the bad LDL, it doesn't alter the ratio, and the type of larger LDL particle that does go up is the less harmful kind. Other studies have failed to find a cause-and-effect link between egg consumption and heart disease.

Egg yolks also contain valuable nutrients including zeaxanthin and lutein, which help protect you from macular degeneration. Some eggs are higher in omega-3 fat because of what they feed the hens (flaxseed meal or marine algae). Omega-3-enriched whole eggs aren't a replacement for fatty fish, but they can give your omega-3 intake a little bump. Whole eggs are also filling. Research from the University of Connecticut found that eating whole eggs at breakfast stabilized blood glucose, reduced levels of the hunger hormone ghrelin, and reduced calorie intake for the day.

Saturated fats are also found in dairy products. Many people avoid dairy completely because they have a hard time digesting it. However, if you tolerate dairy products well, you can use them on a fat-loss programme. In fact, recent research links eating dairy products with better body composition. Dairy products are also an excellent source of calcium and two very high-quality proteins: whey and casein. If you want to minimize saturated fat, limit the calories, and get more protein, choose fat-free or reduced-fat dairy products.

Butter is best kept to small amounts because it provides lots of calories but no essential fatty acids. There are now many lower-calorie substitutes for conventional fats, such as butter-flavour sprinkles, low-calorie butter-flavour sprays, reduced-fat butter spreads, fat-free dressings, cooking spray, and so on. These can all save you calories while keeping some flavour. (Read the labels carefully, though, because not all low-calorie products or fat substitutes are good for you.)

Unrefined extra virgin coconut oil has become increasingly popular, shedding its past reputation as a fat to avoid. Many enjoy it because you can cook with it and use it to add flavour to recipes. Coconut oil sometimes gets promoted as a health food and even a weight-loss aid. While you can certainly include it as part of your daily fat intake, there's no evidence it will help you lose weight. If you're not careful, the calorie density of oils can actually sabotage your weight loss.

## CONTROL FAT TO CONTROL CALORIES

Many fats and oils have healthy properties, but they're all calorie dense, with more than twice the calories per gram than protein or carbs. Extra virgin olive oil, for example, contains phenolic compounds that are powerful antioxidants, making it a healthy choice (great for salad dressings and low- to medium-heat cooking). However, olive oil is a high-calorie food. One tablespoon will set you back about 130 calories and 14 grams of fat.

If you need to save calories, using cooking spray is more calorifically economical than pouring oil in your pan because it takes a 15-second spray to equal the calories in 1 tablespoon of oil.

Nuts are little nutrition powerhouses. They give you fibre, vitamins, healthy phytonutrients, and good fats (walnuts are high in omega-3). But if you eat large amounts of walnuts, almonds, macadamia nuts, cashews, or peanuts as snacks without keeping track of calories, you could be hundreds or even a thousand calories over your optimal fat-burning level!

Ironically, a common reason for fat-loss plateaus is eating too much healthy food, and healthy fats are a prime culprit. Keeping your meal plan lower in fat overall helps you to control your calories and that makes it easier to get leaner. You simply need to dole out enough healthy fat so you get the nutrition you do need without calories you don't need.

## FATS TO AVOID: HYDROGENATED, PARTIALLY HYDROGENATED AND TRANS-FATTY ACIDS

Oils are, by nature, unstable substances that go rancid quickly with exposure to light and air. Hydrogenation and partial hydrogenation are industrial processes that food companies use to prolong the shelf life of their products and make cheap spreadable products such as margarine. They also make baked goods moist and flaky. Udo Erasmus calls hydrogenated oils "a manufacturer's dream: an unspoilable substance that lasts forever."

Unfortunately, hydrogenation turns a natural, healthy fat into an unnatural, unhealthy fat. You could say that hydrogenated oil is a processed fat, the same way that white flour is a processed carbohydrate. Partially hydrogenated oils contain large amounts of chemically altered fats known as trans-fatty acids, one of the unhealthiest foods you can eat.

Some trans-fatty acids are found in meats and dairy products, but those are the naturally occurring variety. Industrial trans fats are found in hydrogenated oils, margarines and spreads, baked goods, and fried foods. Food companies can be sneaky when it comes to trans fats. Labels may say "no cholesterol" or "low saturated fat", but the products may be loaded with harmful trans fats. A prime example of this is margarine. Many people switch from butter to margarine, thinking they are doing themselevs good by avoiding saturated fat. What they don't realise is it's full of trans fats!

Piles of convincing research has proved how dangerous these fats are, but as yet the UK government has not changed food labelling laws and trans fats continue to sneak into products without us noticing. Do read labels carefully and regard anything labelled as "low saturated fat" with suspicion.

### Where Are the Trans-fatty Acids?

- Fried foods (fried chicken, chips, fried onion rings, etc.)
- Biscuits
- Crackers
- Pies
- Pastries
- Icings
- Doughnuts
- Tortilla chips
- Taco shells
- Shortening
- Partially hydrogenated vegetable oils
- Refined vegetable oils
- Packaged baked goods (croutons, crackers, biscuits, cakes, some breads)
- Margarine

### What Trans-fatty Acids Can Do to Your Body

Trans-fatty acids cause numerous health problems, including heart disease. A 2 per cent increase in calorie intake from trans fats is associated with a 23 per cent increase in cardiovascular disease risk. Trans-fatty acids in hydrogenated oil also raise bad cholesterol (LDL) and triglyceride levels, while reducing good cholesterol (HDL). Trans fats may also slow down the fat-burning process in more ways than one.

The American Heart Association recommends a maximum of 2 grams per day, but some experts say there's no safe amount of trans-fatty acids. Referring to hydrogenated oils, Dr. Erasmus says, "If you see the 'H' word on the label, get the 'H' out of there!"

### 12 Destructive Effects of Trans Fats

- Trans fat raises LDL (bad) cholesterol.
- Trans fat lowers HDL (good) cholesterol.
- Trans fat increases blood triglycerides.
- Trans fat decreases insulin sensitivity.
- Trans fat increases insulin response to glucose.
- Trans fat hampers immune system function.
- Trans fat interferes with your liver's detoxification processes.
- Trans fat may cause cancer.
- Trans fat can increase risk of type 2 diabetes.
- Trans fat causes inflammation in the body.
- Trans fat interferes with EFA functions.
- Trans fat makes your platelets stickier.

## WHAT THE LEANEST PEOPLE IN THE WORLD DO

Most mainstream medical, health, and nutrition organizations have published position statements with similar opinions on dietary fat intake. For good health and weight control, the most common recommendation is to keep your dietary fat intake between 20 per cent and 35 per cent of total calories.

When it comes to dietary fat, physique athletes follow the conventional wisdom fairly closely, though they tend to stay on the lower end of the range. That leaves them more room for lean protein and natural carbs. They're also meticulous about choosing the highest-quality fats with the most nutritional value. Based on my research and real-world experience with physique athletes, I've found that most people get the best results with about 20 per cent of their daily calories from fat.

You may need to adjust for your goals and experiment to see what suits your body type the best. Naturally, people who are carb intolerant fare better on fewer carbs and more fat. If you use a reduced-carb approach for accelerated fat loss, a slightly higher fat intake often makes sense. Some people report more energy or less hunger with a slight bump in fat. Others have a personal preference in one direction or the other and they find it helps them stick to their meal plan better. If you choose your fats carefully, there's no reason you couldn't take your fat intake to 25 per cent to 30 per cent of your total calories and you'd still be in the range.

On a practical level, hitting these numbers means you'll need to check your meal plans and make sure you've included some fats every day. If you're accustomed to nonfat diets or you prefer low-fat foods in general, sometimes you have go out of your way to add fat back in alongside your lean proteins and natural complex carbs. That could be as easy as taking an EFA supplement. It could also include adding fatty fish to your meal plans, making recipes with extra virgin olive oil, having a whole egg or two, stirring flaxseed into your porridge, putting avocado in your salads, snacking on a handful of nuts, or eating a tablespoon of natural peanut butter.

Nonfat and very low-fat diets are not the answer for maximizing fat loss or muscle growth. High-fat diets are not the answer either. If you eat a moderate amount of fat, and you eat the right kinds of fats, then you'll be on your way to a body that's healthy, muscular, and lean.

In the next chapter, you'll learn about the macronutrient that fitness enthusiasts, bodybuilders, athletes, and almost anyone who has ever hit the gym is more fascinated by and concerned with than any other: protein!

## *BURN THE FAT, FEED THE MUSCLE* ACTION SUMMARY: FAT

- Aim for 20 per cent to 30 per cent of your total calories from fat.
- Eat fatty fish such as salmon, trout, mackerel, sardines, and herring at least two or three times a week.
- Eat nuts and seeds, provided you stay within your calorie limits (nuts are healthy but calorie dense).
- Eat avocados and olives, provided you stay within your calorie limits.
- Reduce fats in general to help you control your calories during deficit eating.
- Use an essential fatty acid supplement such as flaxseed oil or fish oil if you don't get enough healthy fats from whole foods.
- Avoid trans fats, including foods with "hydrogenated" on the label.
- Avoid any foods that are deep-fried in oil.

**QUICKSTART**

Getting enough good fats and avoiding the bad fats is easy! All you have to do is follow the eight simple guidelines in the *Burn the Fat, Feed the Muscle* Action Summary punch list every week. Even without crunching any numbers, you'll automatically be eating the right fats in the right amounts.

# CHAPTER 10

# Protein, the Muscle Builder and Metabolic Stimulator

"Individuals habitually performing resistance or endurance exercise require more protein than their sedentary counterparts ... [H]igher protein diets have consistently been shown to result in greater weight loss, greater fat loss, and preservation of lean mass as compared with 'lower' protein diets."

– Dr. Stuart Phillips, Exercise Metabolism Research Group,
Department of Kinesiology, McMaster University, Hamilton, Ontario

## WHY YOU ARE WHAT YOU EAT – LITERALLY

Heraclitus, the Greek philosopher, said, "You cannot step in the same river twice." A river may look the same every day, but it isn't the same because of the never-ending flow of new water running through it. The same is true of the human body. Although your body appears solid, it's in a constant state of flux as old cells die and new ones replace them.

You are continually replacing old blood cells with new ones. Every month you produce a new skin as dead cells are shed and new cells grow underneath. Parts of your skeleton are completely remodelled every four months. Every six weeks, all the cells are replaced in your liver. You have a new stomach lining every five days. The proteins in your muscles are continually turned over as old tissue is broken down and new tissue is synthesized. Every cell in your body is constantly being recycled.

From a molecular point of view, you're not the same person you were a year ago. It makes you realize that the maxim "You are what you eat" can and should be taken literally. Once you've grasped this concept, it makes you think twice about what you feed your body every day.

## PROTEIN: THE RAW BUILDING MATERIAL FOR THE BODY

If your body is constantly creating new cells, the question is: Where do all these new cells come from? The answer, of course, is: from your food – specifically, protein foods. Proteins play many roles in your body. They serve as enzymes, hormones, antibodies, and nutrient transporters. But proteins are best known for their structural functions: They are literally the raw construction material for body cells as bricks are for a building.

Body structures made from protein include skin, hair, nails, bones, connective tissue, and, of course, muscle. Next to water, protein is the most abundant substance in your body, making up approximately 15 per cent of your weight. Of most interest to those who want a better physique is that 65 per cent of all the protein in your body is located in your skeletal muscles.

## AMINO ACIDS: THE BUILDING BLOCKS OF PROTEIN

The smallest units of a protein are called amino acids. Just as glycogen is formed from the linkage of glucose molecules, proteins are formed from the joining of numerous amino acids. Bricks are building material that can be cemented together into a nearly unlimited number of structures, such as a brick house, a brick wall, a brick road, and a brick chimney. In the same way, your body takes individual amino acids and "cements" them together with peptide bonds into various configurations to create muscle tissue and other body proteins.

There are 20 amino acids the human body requires for growth. From these 20 amino acids, tens of thousands of different protein molecules can be formed. Each protein is assembled from the bonding of different amino acids into various configurations. Growth hormone, for example, is a protein chain of 156 amino acids. The muscle protein myosin is formed from the linkage of 4,500 amino acid units.

## ESSENTIAL VERSUS NONESSENTIAL AMINO ACIDS

Of the 20 amino acids, your body can make 11. These are called the nonessential amino acids (also known as dispensable amino acids). The other nine amino acids are called essential amino acids (or indispensable amino acids). Essential amino acids are those that can't be manufactured by your body and must be supplied from your food.

| Essential (Indispensable) Amino Acids | Nonessential (Dispensable) Amino Acids |
| --- | --- |
| Histidine | Alanine |
| Isoleucine* | Arginine |
| Leucine* | Asparagine |
| Lysine | Aspartic acid |
| Methionine | Cysteine |
| Phenylalanine | Glutamic acid |
| Threonine | Glutamine* |
| Tryptophan | Glycine |
| Valine* | Proline |
| | Serine |
| | Tyrosine |

* Leucine, isoleucine, and valine are known as branched chain amino acids, or BCAAs, which are metabolized mostly in muscle and play an important role in protein synthesis. Glutamine is known as a conditionally essential amino acid because under conditions of stress or trauma, you may require more of it than your body can produce.

## WHY YOU MUST EAT COMPLETE PROTEINS EVERY DAY

Foods that contain all the essential and nonessential amino acids in the exact ratio and amounts required by your body for growth are called complete proteins. For your body to synthesize muscle, all the essential amino acids must be available simultaneously. Any nonessential amino acids that are in short supply can be produced by your liver, but if an essential amino acid is missing, your body must break down its own proteins to obtain it.

Proteins can't be stored to any significant degree. There's only a very small and transient amino acid pool in the blood and tissues, making up only about 1 per cent of all the protein in your body. To maintain the ideal environment for muscle growth and prevent muscle breakdown, complete proteins must be eaten every day, and ideally with every meal.

Protein has the highest thermic effect of all the macronutrients. Up to 30 per cent of the calories are burned off to digest and absorb the protein. The thermic effect of carbohydrate is 10 per cent or less, so replacing a portion of your carb calories with protein gives you a metabolic advantage. High-quality complete proteins such as chicken, beef, fish, eggs, and dairy products increase that advantage even more than low-biological-value proteins like beans or wheat. One study published in the

*American Journal of Clinical Nutrition* found that the number of calories burned was 2 per cent higher when the subjects got their protein mostly from meat rather than soy.

## PROTEIN QUALITY: COMPLETE VERSUS INCOMPLETE PROTEINS

Protein quality refers to how well your body can digest and utilize a particular protein.

Scientists have many ways to rate protein quality, such as testing for biological value, protein efficiency ratio, or protein digestibility. The important thing for you to know is that the highest-quality proteins come from animal sources such as milk, eggs, fish, and meat. These are complete proteins that contain all the essential amino acids in the exact amounts and proportions your body needs.

### ARE PROTEIN SUPPLEMENTS BETTER THAN PROTEIN FOODS?

The protein industry is large and lucrative, so the advertisements make protein drinks seem like muscle-building miracles. But protein supplements – powders, ready-to-drink shakes, and pills (amino acids) – are not better than whole foods and they're not mandatory. If you get enough protein from whole food sources, there's no need for a supplement. If you often fall short of your daily protein goal from food, then supplements can be helpful.

One real advantage is convenience. When you're busy, instead of a sit-down meal that takes time for food prep and cooking, you could whip up a high-protein meal-replacement shake and it only takes minutes. If you learn some tasty smoothie recipes, that might even make your meal plans more enjoyable and easier to follow. You can use straight protein powder in whole-food recipes too. For example, you could stir vanilla whey protein in your porridge and add a pinch of cinnamon, and you have a delicious three-minute breakfast. Try chocolate whey protein mixed in plain Greek yogurt with 1 tablespoon of natural peanut butter and you have a two-minute snack that tastes like dessert.

Remember that the human body was not designed to process liquids all day long; it was designed to digest food. Whole foods contain biologically active nutrients that interact with one another in the whole-food matrix and in our bodies in ways that isolated nutrients do not. Use protein supplements occasionally as you see fit, but focus on whole foods first.

## COMPLETE LEAN PROTEIN FOODS

✓ Eggs (whites and whole eggs)
✓ Dairy products (semi-skimmed or skimmed milk, cheese, cottage cheese, and yogurt)
✓ Milk, egg, casein, and whey protein powders
✓ Lean beef
✓ Venison, and other game meats
✓ Chicken breast
✓ Turkey breast
✓ Lean pork (tenderloin)
✓ Fish
✓ Shellfish

One issue with animal proteins is that many of them also contain large amounts of calories and saturated fat. If you want to control calories, reduce the amount of animal fats you consume by going with the leaner proteins. This is easy to do by choosing lean meats such as turkey and chicken breast, only the leanest cuts of red meat (topside, lean sirloin, bison, or game meats), egg whites (instead of only whole eggs), and low-fat or fat-free dairy products instead of whole-milk dairy products.

Many vegetables, beans, nuts, pulses, grains, and other plant-based foods contain substantial amounts of protein, and it all counts toward your total daily protein goal. However, the protein in these foods is usually not considered complete because it's low in one or more of the essential amino acids (known as a limiting amino acid). Beans, for example, are high in protein with about 15 grams per 175 g (6 oz). However, they are low in the essential amino acid methionine. Grains lack the essential amino acid lysine.

In general, proteins from plant sources are lower in quality and digestibility. However, combining two incomplete sources of plant-based protein gives you all the amino acids you need to build muscle. Complementary protein combinations such as rice and beans are how vegetarians can improve their overall daily protein quality. It's not mandatory to eat a lot of animal proteins to get lean and muscular, but it is mandatory to eat complete proteins and meet your total protein requirement every day.

## CAN A VEGETARIAN FOLLOW *BURN THE FAT, FEED THE MUSCLE*?

Yes. This programme can easily be adapted for lacto-, ovo-, or pesco-vegetarians. There's no doubt that vegetarians who eat dairy products, eggs, or fish can build great physiques. Meat is a favourite bodybuilder's food, but it's not mandatory. Bill Pearl was well-known for giving up red meat, but he did get complete proteins from eggs and dairy products. With his semi-vegetarian approach, Pearl won the Mr. America and Mr. Universe titles and became a legend in the bodybuilding and fitness world.

What about vegans? Yes, even people who eat no animal products at all can achieve low body fat levels and sculpt highly fit physiques. However, this more restricted approach does require greater attention to make sure calorie, amino acid, and nutrient needs are met. Without including at least some complete proteins in the form of eggs, dairy, fish, or milk-based protein powders, vegans may find their muscular development falling short of their maximum potential.

A vegan having a hard time hitting the minimum protein targets could supplement with vegetarian protein powders such as soy, pea, rice, and hemp (hemp contains not only plant protein, but also fibre and valuable omega-3 fats). Exercise physiologists William McArdle, Frank Katch, and Victor Katch, the authors of *Sports and Exercise Nutrition*, suggest that vegetarians could also benefit by increasing their total protein intake by 10 per cent above standard recommendations to adjust for the less efficient digestion and lower quality of plant proteins.

## SHOULD YOU EAT SOY PROTEIN?

Among the plant-based proteins, soybeans have a respectable amino acid profile (some soy isolate supplements are even fortified with methionine), although soy is only 78 per cent digestible, whereas milk and egg proteins are 97 per cent digestible. Soy is promoted for lowering cholesterol and reducing symptoms of menopause, but at the same time criticized for negative effects. Soy contains plant chemicals called phytoestrogens, a concern for men who worry about feminizing effects.

The health pros and cons are still being debated, but a small amount of soy protein shouldn't have any major downsides, even for men. However, unless you're allergic or intolerant to milk products or you're a vegetarian, there's little reason to depend on soy as a major protein source when your goal is more muscle and less fat. Recent research shows that the milk proteins, whey and casein, are superior to soy for stimulating protein synthesis, and research on soy foods and weight loss says there's no difference either way.

## HOW MUCH PROTEIN: WHAT THE LEANEST PEOPLE IN THE WORLD DO

The US government has provided official recommended daily intake (RDI) nutrition guidelines from the National Research Council. The RDI for protein is based on total body weight and is set at 0.8 grams per kilogram of body weight (0.36 grams per pound of body weight). For a 172-pound (12 st 4-lb/78-kg) person, that's only 62 grams per day. Many traditional nutritionists say this paltry amount is enough for everyone.

Bodybuilders and fitness athletes say it's not even close to being enough, because the RDI was developed for the average sedentary person to avoid deficiency, not for people training hard to burn fat and build muscle. Minimum and optimum protein levels are two different numbers. Among the leanest, most muscular people in the world, 1 gram per pound of body weight per day has been a rule of thumb for years. The science suggests they're right.

Dr. Peter Lemon, director of the exercise nutrition research laboratory at the University of Western Ontario, has been studying protein requirements since the 1980s. His research indicates that strength athletes not using anabolic drugs need approximately 0.8 grams of protein per pound of body weight just to maintain an anabolic state. To support new muscle growth, Dr. Lemon said, "Certainly in the range of 0.9 grams per pound of body weight is where to start, though optimal intakes might be higher." If we add a little margin for safety, that's right in line with the bodybuilder's 1-gram-per-pound rule.

---

*QUICKSTART*

**Eat a high-quality protein food with every meal (lean meat, fish, eggs, or dairy products) and aim for approximately 1 gram of protein per pound of body weight per day, and your protein nutrition is covered!**

---

## DOUBLE-CHECK TO BE SURE YOU MEET YOUR DAILY PROTEIN QUOTA

The macronutrient percentage method is an easy way to set up your meal plans by the numbers and figure out how many grams of carbs, protein, and fat to eat. If you do your calorie calculations properly and choose the right percentages – which you learned how to do in previous chapters – you should automatically land within the ideal range for grams of protein.

EXAMPLE 1:

YOU ARE A FEMALE, 130 POUNDS (9 ST 4 LB/59 KG), VERY ACTIVE

Your optimal calorie intake to lose fat is 1,700 calories per day

To determine your protein intake, multiply your calorie intake by 30 per cent.

1,700 calories per day × 0.30 = 510 calories from protein

510 protein calories ÷ 4 calories per gram of protein = 127.5 grams of protein

EXAMPLE 2:

YOU ARE MALE, 190 POUNDS (13 ST 8 LB/86 KG), MODERATELY ACTIVE.

Your optimal calorie intake to lose fat is 2,600 calories per day.

To determine your protein intake, multiply your calorie intake by 30 per cent.

2,600 calories per day × 0.30 = 780 calories from protein

780 protein calories ÷ 4 calories per gram of protein = 195 grams of protein

If you set your protein at 30 per cent of your total calories, that usually comes very close to the 1-gram-per-pound-of-body-weight rule. However, getting enough protein is so important for achieving your body composition goals, you should double-check your protein intake in grams to be sure you don't underestimate. Sometimes, you may need to bump your protein to a higher percentage of calories to hit your gram quota.

On the other hand, if someone is overweight, with high body fat, the 1-gram-per-pound-of-body-weight rule may overestimate protein needs. A 250-pound (17 st 12-lb/113-kg) woman with 35 per cent body fat doesn't need 250 grams of protein: Extra protein isn't required to support extra body fat tissue. In this case, she could use 1 gram per pound of *lean* body weight, which would be only 162 grams of protein. For men over 20 per cent body fat and women over 30 per cent body fat, I'd recommend checking your daily protein quota in grams per pound of lean body weight.

In some special cases, there may be advantages to eating even more protein than one gram per pound. These include:

1. When your goal is gaining muscle and your training is demanding.
2. When your goal is getting lean and your calories or carbs are low.

## PROTEIN INTAKE AND GAINING MUSCLE

To gain lean body weight, you must increase your calories into a surplus. A 190-pound (13 st 8-lb/86-kg) male with a 3,000-calorie maintenance level needs a surplus of approximately 15 per cent. That's an extra 450 calories, for a total of 3,450 calories a day. Thirty per cent of that is 1,035 protein calories or 259 grams of protein a day. That's a lot of protein – more than 1.3 grams per pound of body weight. Is it too much?

In the *Journal of Sports Sciences*, protein researcher Dr. Kevin D. Tipton speculated that protein intakes as high as 1.1 to 1.4 grams per pound of body weight might be the best recommendation when the goal is muscle growth and training is demanding. If that's more than the muscles can use for growth, the excess will simply be oxidized.

As long as other important nutrients aren't displaced, at the very least, eating more protein won't hurt.

There's not enough evidence to say for sure whether more than 1 gram per pound of body weight will increase muscle growth. Most of the research we have is the in-the-trenches kind from the experience of bodybuilders and fitness athletes. Also, extra protein alone doesn't guarantee more muscle. It takes adequate protein, surplus calories, and progressive weight training – combined with proper recovery – to stimulate muscle growth.

So why eat more protein? If your goal changes from burning fat to gaining muscle, you're going to need a lot more calories. Those surplus calories have to come from somewhere. The alternative is to eat more fat and carbs. If you go overboard with any food, the excess can be stored as fat. But in a surplus, dietary fat is the macronutrient most likely to be converted into body fat first. Carbs and fat are also a lot easier to overeat. All things considered, when you increase your calories to gain muscle, it's reasonable to raise your protein along with your calories.

## PROTEIN INTAKE AND LOW-CALORIE/LOW-CARB DIETING

If your goal is to get super-lean, show off six-pack abs, achieve fat loss at the fastest rate possible, or break a fat-loss plateau, you'll sometimes get more aggressive with your calorie cuts or carb restrictions. If you want to burn more fat, one way or the other, your calorie deficit must increase. However, your protein requirement does not decrease. If anything, as your calorie intake goes down, your protein needs go up. That's why it makes so much sense to increase a deficit by cutting carb calories specifically and leaving that precious protein intake high.

You could simply cut all calories across the board, and as the law of energy balance dictates, you'll still lose weight. But if you hold the protein steady, or even increase the protein, it's more likely that all the weight you lose will be fat. Maintaining muscle isn't the only advantage: Protein also suppresses hunger and increases metabolism more than any other macronutrient. That makes three major advantages to keeping protein high when calories are low.

Most people pursuing advanced fat-loss goals will optimize their results by getting about 40 per cent of their calories from protein. This usually falls in the 1.1- to 1.3-grams-per-pound-of-body-weight range. By definition, this is a high-protein intake, which is more than enough to give all the fat-loss advantages. Bodybuilders in serious training and in a calorie deficit are known to take in as much as 1.4 to 1.5 grams per pound of body weight. When they're training for fat loss and their deficit is aggressive, that can sometimes be as much as 45 per cent to 50 per cent of total calories – a very high protein ratio.

Not surprisingly, many mainstream nutritionists question whether it's necessary to eat so much protein if the excess simply gets converted into glucose and burned off. Bodybuilders argue that even if it does, it isn't a bad thing. Metabolizing protein burns calories, so physique athletes consider this a slight edge in achieving the ripped look.

In that sense, you could say that a high-protein diet is not only a muscle builder, it's also a metabolic stimulator. The metabolism advantage may be small, but when combined with the hunger-reducing and muscle-preserving effects, a higher protein intake beats lower protein for fat loss every time.

## HOW OFTEN SHOULD YOU EAT PROTEIN?

There are two high-priority protein goals in *Burn the Fat, Feed the Muscle*. The first and most important is to hit your total daily protein target, including high-quality proteins that supply all the essential amino acids. The second is to eat protein with every meal.

When you eat protein is not as important as hitting your total daily quota, but scientists say there's evidence that spreading your daily protein intake over several meals helps optimize muscle growth. Protein also helps control hunger, so there are benefits on both the fat-burning and the muscle-building sides.

Donald K. Layman, PhD., a protein researcher from the University of Illinois, says that the average American eats over 65 per cent of his daily protein in a single large dinner meal, leaving less than 35 per cent distributed among the other meals (as little as 10 grams or less at breakfast). In his research papers on protein metabolism, he points out that this meal pattern is not optimal for a variety of reasons. "Vitamins and minerals can fulfil nutrient needs on a once-per-day-basis, but for protein, the body has no ability to store a daily supply … To stimulate protein synthesis, adults need at least 25–30 grams of protein and at least 2.5 grams of (the BCAA) leucine per meal … Dietary patterns that provide adequate protein at only one meal produce an anabolic response only after that meal."

Among bodybuilders and fitness athletes, eating four to six times per day has always been the best practice and that's the model we follow. In *Burn the Fat, Feed the Muscle*, our baseline plan has you eating five times per day. If it's feasible, eat a protein at every one of those meals or snacks. At the minimum, eat protein three or four times per day if you want to optimize the muscle-building response. This also makes it easier to hit your daily protein goal without overloading your stomach all at once.

There's no reason you can't eat more in one sitting: Your body will still digest a big steak with 60 grams of protein. But there's no point to eating more protein at one meal, hoping it will turn into more muscle. The research shows that protein synthesis caps out around 30 or 40 grams and that spreading out your protein is better. If you spread the protein evenly, it usually averages out to about 25 to 30 grams per meal for women and 35 to 40 grams per meal for men during fat-loss programmes (maybe a little more for big, tall, or highly active people).

## SOME FINAL THOUGHTS ON PROTEIN RULES

It's impossible to set carved-in-stone rules about protein intake. Protein needs vary from person to person based on goals, body size, training intensity, calorie intake, and whether the goal is burning, building, or maintaining. The range of recommended intakes is very broad, which is good, because it gives you plenty of room to customize and you don't have to worry about hitting one number as long as you're in the acceptable ranges.

That said, the 1-gram-per-pound-of-body-weight rule is a no-brainer guideline for any healthy person doing resistance training and pursuing fat loss. The low end of the range is around 0.8 to 0.9 grams per pound. Some strength or physique athletes doing intense training or serious dieting might get optimal results with as much as 1.1 to 1.4 grams or more.

This doesn't mean you should try to duplicate Mr. Olympia's meal plan or go crazy and eat as much protein as you can. Too much of any food will get converted into fat, including protein. Too much of any nutrient can also be unhealthy, especially if it pushes out other important nutrients. But when you weigh all the evidence, from the viewpoint of getting leaner and more muscular, it's better to err on the side of too much protein than too little.

There's a final macronutrient to talk about – one that's even more controversial than protein. Carbohydrates! Are carbs your friends or your foes? You'll find out in the next chapter.

## *BURN THE FAT, FEED THE MUSCLE* ACTION SUMMARY: PROTEIN

- Aim for a daily protein target of 1 gram per pound of body weight, give or take 0.1 to 0.2 grams.
- As a baseline, set up your meal plans with approximately 30 per cent of total calories from protein.

- When your calorie deficit is aggressive, you may increase your protein to approximately 40 per cent of total calories or 1.1 to 1.3 grams per pound of body weight.
- If you're in serious training for muscle growth, you may (optionally) increase your protein to or above 1.1 to 1.4 grams per pound of body weight.
- Eat a high-quality complete protein with every meal.
- Aim for about 25 to 40 grams of protein per meal: women and smaller individuals toward the lower end of the range, men and larger individuals toward the higher end.
- Eat protein before and after your weight training workouts.

# CHAPTER 11

# Clearing Up Carbohydrate Confusion

"Carbohydrates get a bad rap. Eat carbs. Enjoy them. In fact, 'earn' more of them through exercise. The more you exercise, the more carbs your body will use. And eat most of your carbs from colourful fruits and veggies. When you do eat grain based foods, focus on fibre!"

– Chris Mohr, PhD, RD, founder of MohrResults.com

## PINPOINTING THE PERFECT CARBOHYDRATE INTAKE

In previous chapters, you learned that extreme diets, including extremely low- or high-carb diets, are not the best way to get lean and stay lean. That leaves a lot of room in the middle. In this chapter, I'll help you narrow this gap and pinpoint the perfect carbohydrate intake for you based on your goals, your training, and your body type.

You'll also learn about the different classes of carbs, including which ones are best for energy, health, and fat loss. You'll discover that some carbs are healthful and some are harmful. You'll find how to distinguish processed from natural carbs, fibrous from starchy carbs, and simple from complex carbs. You'll read about the dangers of refined carbs and the virtues of natural carbs as well as the difference between calorie-dense and nutrient-dense carbs.

To shed fat, build muscle, optimize your health, and increase your energy, the key is to learn the differences between the categories of carbs, choose the right types, and eat them in the right amounts at the right times. This plan shows you how.

## CARBS: PREMIUM FUEL FOR BODY AND BRAIN

Unlike proteins, which are used as building materials, carbs are used for energy. Sports nutritionist Dr. Michael Colgan calls carbs "premium fuel." I've never heard a better definition. Protein can be broken down into glucose and used for fuel, but that's an inefficient process, and you never want to sacrifice your muscle protein. Fats are also used for fuel, but even fats don't burn as efficiently as carbs.

It's a common misconception that fat is a *more efficient* fuel. It's not; it's simply a *more concentrated* fuel (nine calories per gram for fat versus four calories per gram for carbs). Carbs are your body's preferred and most efficient energy source for intense training. Scientists tell us that, under normal conditions, your brain needs 100 to 130 grams of glucose per day. If you cut carbs too much, your physical performance and even your mental sharpness usually take a nosedive.

Fat is stored in your body as a backup energy source. A 135-pound (9 st 9-lb/ 61-kg) woman with 25 per cent body fat has 118,125 calories stored in her "reserve fuel tank." Your body can also store carbs (as glycogen), but in much more limited quantities. About 1,600 calories of glycogen can be stored in your muscles and approximately 400 calories in your liver.

Your body is always burning a mixture of carbs and fat for fuel, but the fuel mix changes based on demand. During low-intensity, long-duration exercise, most of your energy comes from fat. Most of your energy also comes from fat while you're at rest. During shorter bouts of high-intensity exercise, such as sprinting or weight lifting, carbs are the main fuel.

Your primary energy source can also change depending on which fuel is more readily available. If carbs are restricted, your body can easily use fat for fuel. However, carbs are the limiting factor in exercise performance. Intense exercise burns up muscle glycogen quickly, and if you fail to replace it by eating enough carbs, you "hit the wall," or "bonk," as athletes like to say. Within about three days of a severe carb cutback, your muscle glycogen will be significantly depleted. Reducing carbs may make fat loss easier, but since cardio and weight training are such important elements of *Burn the Fat, Feed the Muscle*, cutting carbs completely is not recommended.

Ultimately, all the carbs you eat end up in your bloodstream as glucose (blood sugar), but you can't lump all carbs together into one category, because they're not all the same. Some carbs are good and some are bad. The good carbs are your friends: they supply you with energy and nutrients and help you get leaner and more muscular. The bad carbs are your foes; they have a greater propensity for fat storage, contribute to health problems, and are nutritionally empty.

## SIMPLE CARBS

Structurally speaking, there are two broad categories of carbs: simple and complex. Simple carbs consist of a single sugar molecule (monosaccharide) or two sugar molecules linked together (disaccharide).

Monosaccharides include fructose, glucose, and galactose. The two you hear about the most are fructose and glucose. Glucose is found naturally in food, or your body can produce it by breaking down complex carbs. Fructose is the type of simple carb found in fruit.

Disaccharides are formed by the combination of two monosaccharide molecules. Examples include sucrose (table sugar), which is formed by the combination of fructose and glucose, and lactose (dairy sugar), which is composed of galactose and glucose.

In general, simple carbs are digested quickly and cause a rapid rise in blood sugar, especially when you eat a lot of them alone or in meals with no fat, fibre, or protein. When there's a blood sugar spike, there's a large release of insulin from the pancreas. The insulin quickly clears the sugar from the bloodstream, leading to a blood sugar dip known as hypoglycaemia. You probably recognize low blood sugar by its common symptoms: low energy, shakiness, weakness, mood swings, and hunger. The hunger leads you back to more sugar and perpetuates a vicious cycle of ups and downs throughout the day.

When you hear about simple carbs, you usually think about white sugar and white flour products. These processed carbs are well-known as the "bad" kind. They're the ones that cause your blood sugar to spike and crash; they come with lots of calories but no nutrition, and they contribute to obesity, diabetes, and other diseases. But not all simple carbs are bad for you. Foods that contain natural sugars are fine if you eat them in balance with the other macronutrients and stay inside your calorie limits. Some of them are very nutritious and actually help you lose fat.

## IS FRUCTOSE REALLY FATTENING?

Fructose, the natural sugar in fruit, has been wrongly accused as a bad guy to the point of alarmism. Many people claim that fructose is fattening and unhealthy but they don't distinguish between the natural fructose in fruit and high-fructose corn syrup (HFCS), also sometimes called glucose/fructose syrup. HFCS is a refined sugar used to sweeten soft drinks and other processed foods. It delivers large amounts of calories with no nutritional value. Fruit is a natural, nutritious, low-calorie whole food.

Another reason for the "fruit-is-fattening" myth is because fructose is processed differently in the body than other carbs and most people misunderstand how that works. Fructose restores liver glycogen preferentially over muscle glycogen and your liver has a limited storage capacity. Beyond about 50 grams daily, fructose can be converted to fatty acids. But a typical piece of fruit has only about 5 to 10 grams of fructose. At that dose, it would take a huge amount of whole fruit for any conversion of fructose into fat.

On the other hand, you could easily hit 50 grams of fructose in a day if you drink fizzy drinks or other drinks sweetened with HFCS or sucrose (which is 50 per cent fructose). Just two 12-fluid ounce (350-ml) soft drinks can provide up to 50 grams and 200 calories of fructose.

Health and fitness professionals have always urged people to eat more fruits and vegetables, but between 1970 and 1997, intake increased by only 19 per cent, providing a mere 2.5 grams per day increase in naturally occurring fructose. During the same time frame, HFCS consumption increased by 26 per cent per capita, from 64 grams per day to 81 grams per day, an average daily intake of 324 calories from added fructose. Clearly, refined sugars and too many calories are the real problems, not natural sugars.

## EVIDENCE THAT WHOLE FRUIT HELPS WITH FAT LOSS

Ironically, amidst all the fructose fears, there's evidence that fruit actually helps with fat loss. Studies from the University of Navarra in Spain examined the effect of fruit on both health and weight loss. One group of women ate a low-calorie diet with 5 per cent fructose from fruit, while a second group ate a diet with 15 per cent fructose from fruit. There were no differences in weight loss. However, the higher fruit group retained more lean body mass. In the group with the higher fruit intake, LDL (bad) cholesterol decreased and there was less oxidative stress.

Whole fruit is a healthy food because it contains vitamins and minerals as well as carotenoids, flavonoids, and polyphenols, which are natural compounds with health-promoting properties. Most fruits also have a low-calorie density. This comes from the high-fibre and high-water content, a combination also known to increase the feeling of fullness after a meal. Fruits also contain fibre, and some, such as raspberries, are extremely high in fibre.

Like many ambitious bodybuilders, I cut fruit from my pre-contest diets in the early days of my career because the diet gurus told me to. I got super-lean. I later put the fruit back in moderate amounts (one or two pieces every day). There was no difference: I still got super lean. The research confirms my experience, but to this day, certain corners of the fitness community still can't shake the stigma that fruit is fattening.

For physique athletes heading toward single digit body fat, every little bit counts, so many bodybuilding and figure competitors still choose to minimize fruit even if it's just to make room for more fibrous vegetables and lean proteins. The idea of limiting fruit for fat loss also appears often in the low-carb community. But don't misconstrue any of this as meaning that "fruit is fattening."

The bottom line: Whole, fresh fruit is not the bad guy; it's an innocent casualty of bodybuilding tradition, low-carb dogma, and misunderstanding of human physiology. If you're eating fruit while consistently staying in a calorie deficit, you're going to lose body fat and gain health benefits. High-fructose corn syrup and added sugars, on the other hand, deserve the bad rap and should be avoided.

## LACTOSE AND DAIRY PRODUCTS: DO THEY BELONG IN A HEALTHY FAT-BURNING PROGRAMME?

Dairy products contain protein and carbs. Lactose is the natural sugar found in dairy products. In recent years, dairy products have become almost as controversial as fructose. Some people wonder whether dairy products are fattening. Others are concerned that milk products might be unhealthy.

Physique athletes and others who want extremely low body fat have traditionally removed the dairy from their diets, at least before competitions or photo shoots. Some bodybuilders believe that dairy products are more easily converted to body fat because of the simple sugars they contain. Many swear that dropping dairy from their diets gets rid of bloating and puffiness, revealing more muscle definition. It might make a difference at the competition level, but calorie for calorie, there's no reason to believe that lactose or dairy products are more fattening than other types of carbs.

What's most likely to undermine fat loss is the high-calorie density of full-fat dairy products. Full-fat cheeses, for example, can add an enormous number of calories to your meals. There's an easy solution: Use low-fat or fat-free versions of cheese, milk, cottage cheese, and yogurt. Some people consider shop-bought milk to be a processed food or they worry about hormones and antibiotics. If these are concerns for you, there's a solution for that as well: Choose organic.

As long as your digestive system can handle them, dairy products can be a part of any fat-loss programme. They add variety and flavour to your meal plans while giving you another superb source of high-biological-value protein in addition to your lean meat, fish, and eggs. Vitamin D and calcium are bonuses.

Not everyone can stomach dairy products. People with lactose intolerance don't have the enzyme necessary to digest lactose, so they experience gas, bloating, abdominal cramps, or diarrhoea when they eat certain dairy products. In those with minor intolerance, the symptoms can be subtle. Those with severe intolerance pay the price if they as much as touch the stuff. Products like Lactofree may help, but if you're one of the many who can't drink milk or eat dairy products, don't worry: This programme works with or without dairy. It's your choice.

## COMPLEX CARBS: FIBROUS VERSUS STARCHY

The second major carb category is complex carbs, also known as polysaccharides. Most complex carbs contain fibre and they provide sustained energy without the highs and lows you get after eating simple carbs. They're usually more filling as well, making you feel more satisfied on less food. Complex carbs from natural sources are also more nutrient dense, whereas simple carbs from refined sources are nutritionally void. Complex carbs include grains, starchy vegetables, and fibrous vegetables.

Starch is the storage form of energy in plants. Starchy carbs include potatoes, yams, cereals, grains, bread, pasta, rice, oats, wheat, pulses, and beans. Your body is able to completely absorb and digest all the calorie energy in starches, so starchy carbs are more calorie dense than fibrous carbs.

Fibre is the indigestible portion of the plant, so it passes through your digestive tract without all the calorie energy being absorbed. Fibre gives bulk to the intestinal contents, promotes healthy digestion and elimination, speeds the transit time of food through your digestive tract, and protects you from gastrointestinal diseases and colon cancer. You could say that fibre is "nature's internal cleanser."

A study from Tufts University said that the average fibre intake in the United States is only 15 grams per day. Most dieticians and health organizations recommend about 25 to 35 grams per day. A customized fibre formula was published by researchers at the University of Kentucky in the journal *Nutrition Reviews*. They recommended 14 grams of fibre per 1,000 calories per day of energy expenditure. For a female at 2,100 calories of TDEE per day, this is 29 grams of fibre. For a male at 2,800 calories of TDEE, it's 39 grams of fibre per day.

Some people think that a programme high in protein must be low in fibre, but that's not true with *Burn the Fat, Feed the Muscle*. You eat optimal amounts and sometimes high amounts of lean protein on this plan, but you also eat lots of greens and fibrous vegetables. The combination of fibrous carbs with lean protein is what makes this programme so healthy in addition to being so effective for reducing hunger and burning fat.

You won't even have to count grams of fibre, unless you want to, because simply following the meal plan template (in chapter 14) and including the fruits and vegetables with each meal will automatically assure you of getting optimal amounts of fibre.

### HOW FIBROUS CARBS HELP YOU BURN MORE FAT

Fibre can also help with fat loss. Fibrous foods take more time to chew and swallow, add bulk to your meals (filling up your stomach), slow down gastric emptying, and may even decrease appetite-stimulating hormones. The big advantage of fibrous carbs such as leafy greens and other nonstarchy vegetables is the low calorie density. It's nearly impossible to overeat green vegetables and fibrous carbs. You would get tired of chewing before you ate too much.

For example, 350 grams (12 ounces) of rice (a starchy carb) contains more than 400 calories, while 312 grams (11 ounces) of broccoli (a fibrous carb) contains only 60 calories. The volume (the space it takes up on your plate – and in your stomach) is the same, but there is almost a sevenfold difference in calorie density!

## COMMON TYPES OF COMPLEX CARBS
## (STARCHES AND FIBRES)

Starches such as oats, beans, rice, potatoes, and whole grains do contain fibre. However, in this programme and throughout the world of bodybuilding nutrition, we use the phrase "fibrous carbs" to describe a separate category of leafy greens and other nonstarchy vegetables such as broccoli, asparagus, cauliflower, and salad leaves.

Combined with lean protein, fibrous carbs are your secret weapon in the war against fat.

That's why a fat-burning nutrition programme should always be high in fibrous carbs and why it's important to know the difference between these two categories:

| Starchy Carbs (Grains and Starchy Vegetables) | Fibrous Carbs (Nonstarchy Vegetables) |
| --- | --- |
| Potatoes | Broccoli |
| Sweet potatoes | Spinach |
| Yams | Asparagus |
| Oats | Cucumber |
| Beans | Tomatoes |
| Brown rice | Cauliflower |
| Lentils | Brussels sprouts |
| Chickpeas | Celery |
| Black-eyed beans | Onions, spring onions, leeks |
| Green peas, other peas | Peppers (red or green), hot peppers |
| Corn | Bok choy, cabbage |
| Pumpkin | Kale |
| Barley | Mushrooms |

| Starchy Carbs (Grains and Starchy Vegetables) | Fibrous Carbs (Nonstarchy Vegetables) |
| --- | --- |
| Winter squash (acorn, butternut) | Aubergine |
| Quinoa | Courgette (summer squash) |
| Millet | Carrots* |
| Whole wheat | Runner beans, green beans* |
| 100% whole grain bread, cereal, or pasta | Lettuce and all leafy salad leaves |
| Other whole grains and starchy vegetables | All other nonstarchy vegetables, greens, and herbs |

* Carrots are technically a starchy vegetable, but they're low in calorie density and high in fibre, so they're are often included in lists of fibrous carbs. Green beans are also technically starchy carbs (legumes) but also have low calorie density, so they appear on fibrous carb lists as well.

---

**QUICKSTART**

**If you cut out refined carbs including sugar-sweetened beverages, white sugar, and white flour products, you're 90 per cent of the way there. To accelerate your fat burning to the next level, learn the difference between the fibrous carbs and the starchy carbs. Fill up your plate with more fibrous carbs (right next to your lean protein) and less starchy carbs, and watch in amazement as the fat drops off your body.**

---

## HIGH-GLYCAEMIC VERSUS LOW-GLYCAEMIC CARBS

It is easy to classify carbs under two major categories, "complex" and "simple," but it's an admittedly imperfect concept. The basic principle is that complex carbs are digested and released into the blood slowly, while simple carbs are digested and released into the blood quickly. Therefore, to maintain blood sugar levels, stay healthy, and burn fat, you should go for more of the slow-release complex carbs. That's not bad general health advice. But the way carbs are processed in the body isn't (pardon the pun) that simple.

Each carbohydrate food may be released at different rates, regardless of its complexity. The glycaemic index (GI) is a scale from 1 to 100 that was developed to measure how a carbohydrate food affects blood sugar. Surprisingly, some complex carbs, such as potatoes, break down into blood glucose very quickly. These are high-GI foods. Some simple carbs, such as apples, are converted into blood glucose more slowly. These are medium- or low-GI foods.

The GI was initially created to help diabetics manage their blood sugar and it also has some applications in sports nutrition. Many weight-loss diets base their carb recommendations entirely on the GI, claiming that high-GI foods are fattening and low-GI foods are not. However, at least a half a dozen studies found that, when all else is equal, eating low-GI foods does not increase fat loss.

Like the concept of complex and simple, the GI has drawbacks that limit its usefulness. The GI scale was developed based on the effects of eating a fixed amount of carbs (50 grams) alone in a fasted state. When you eat carbs throughout the day in mixed meals that contain protein, fat, and fibre, that slows the release of sugar into the bloodstream. For example, if you combine potatoes with salmon and broccoli, the GI of the entire meal is much lower than potatoes alone. Many dieters ditch the potatoes, carrots, and other high-GI foods, thinking that "slower-burning" carbs will lead to better fat loss. This is unnecessary, because fat loss is not about glycaemic index, it's about energy balance.

White potatoes, a high-GI food, may even satisfy your hunger better. In a study published in the *European Journal of Clinical Nutrition*, researchers found that potatoes had the highest satiety index score of all the foods tested by far, revealing that potatoes make you feel fuller than other foods. To say that foods like potatoes are fattening and avoid them simply because they're high on the GI is a mistake. Both research and real-world results confirm it. I've eaten white potatoes every day during competition prep and had no trouble reaching single-digit body fat.

If managing blood sugar is a concern, then GI is a factor you might consider. You may want to take it a step further and look into glycaemic load (GL). GL overcomes one limitation of the GI by factoring in the amount of carbohydrate as well as the GI. Consult a doctor or a registered dietician for any clinical nutrition questions you have. For healthy people wanting to get leaner, there are far more important factors, including whether your carbs are natural or refined, high or low in calorie density, and high or low in nutrient density.

## NATURAL VERSUS REFINED CARBS

For good health, the most important distinction you can make about carbs is the difference between natural and refined. The ultimate test for whether a carbohydrate is natural is to ask, "Did this food come out of the ground or off the tree or plant this way?" If the answer is yes, then it's a natural, unrefined food. Vegetables and fruits are on the top of that list.

Whole grains and unprocessed starches have an important place in muscle-building nutrition. Within your calorie and macronutrient limits, these natural carbs give you energy and help you get the most out of your training. But the more human hands meddle with them and process them to make them sweeter, more palatable and longer lasting on the shelf, the more they lose their positive qualities and gain negatives. Refined grains and starches are not recommended, at least not as daily staples (that includes white pastas, white breads, pretzels, crisps, crackers, and bagels).

Of all the nutritional bad guys, refined-sugar products (white sugar, sweets, pastries, soft drinks, and so on) are arguably the worst. An overdose of refined sugar and processed carbs is probably more responsible for poor health and excess body fat than any single factor. If you did only one thing starting today – reduce your refined sugar intake – the improvement in your health, energy, and body fat levels would astonish you!

You might wonder, "Can refined sugar really be that bad?" If your calories are under maintenance, what harm could a little biscuit or chocolate bar do? If you kept your intake to "a little" consumed occasionally, you'd be right: It probably wouldn't impact your health or your physique at all. In fact, I encourage you not to eliminate your favourite foods completely unless you have a good reason. But "a little" consumed every day habitually adds up over time. According to the US Department of Agriculture, the average American consumes 156 pounds (71 kg) of refined sugar every year. It's best to avoid processed carbs as much as possible.

**TEN REASONS TO AVOID PROCESSED CARBS**
1.  Processed carbs can increase body fat.
2.  Processed carbs can increase triglycerides.
3.  Processed carbs can decrease good HDL cholesterol.
4.  Processed carbs can suppress your immune system.
5.  Processed carbs can deplete your body of important minerals.
6.  Processed carbs can increase insulin.
7.  Processed carbs can cause reactive hypoglycaemia.
8.  Processed carbs can cause tooth decay.
9.  Processed carbs can promote diabetes.
10. Processed carbs are linked to depression.

## HOW TO GET THE PROCESSED CARBS OUT!

Processed sugars are easily missed, because small amounts are hidden in foods you might never think of, such as fat-free salad dressings, steak sauce, tomato sauce, cranberry sauce, sliced processed meats, ketchup, mayonnaise, soup, canned fruits, wholemeal bread, whole grain cereals, and too many others to mention. If you eat a lot of these items every day, it can add up.

It would be difficult for most people to eliminate 100 per cent of the sugar. Fortunately, you don't have to. If you get your calorie, protein, and micronutrient priorities in order, you don't need to give up your favourite sweet stuff completely. Simply cut back as much as you can, save for the occasional cheat meal, and do it gradually if necessary. Cold turkey doesn't work well for everyone. Start with the obvious calorie-dense culprits such as sweets, biscuits, pastries, doughnuts, desserts, sugary cereals, granulated sugar, and soft drinks.

How strict to be with your sugar cutbacks is up to you. The American Heart Association suggests that men set a "prudent" daily upper limit of 150 calories of added sugars and women an upper limit of 100 calories. The most successful people on this programme usually keep their sweet treats and other "cheat meals" down to about twice a week. They don't let eating refined carbs and sugar become a daily habit.

## HOW TO SPOT REFINED SUGARS BY READING FOOD LABELS

Don't judge a food entirely by the grams of carbs or even the grams of sugar on the nutrition facts panel because that doesn't tell you what kind of sugar it is. Dig a little deeper and inspect the ingredients list to see if refined sugars have been added, then make your decisions based on the calories, total carbs, and type of carbs.

For example, on the nutrition facts panel of one popular brand of sugar-free, fat-free yogurt, it says that out of 15 grams of carbohydrates, 9 grams are sugar. But if you look at the ingredients, you'll see that there are no added sugars. The 9 grams of sugar come from lactose, the *naturally occurring* simple sugar in dairy products.

Added refined sugars can be found in the list of ingredients under different names, including high-fructose corn syrup, glucose-fructose syrup, corn syrup, rice syrup, glucose syrup, sucrose, dextrose, brown sugar, demerara sugar, and invert sugar. By law, the ingredients have to be listed in the order of their precedence, so if refined sugar is listed as one of the top two or three ingredients, that's not a food you want to eat in large amounts or on a daily basis.

## THE CALORIE DENSITY PRINCIPLE

For fat loss, one of the most important distinctions you can make about carbs is calorie density – the number of calories per unit of volume. Dietary fats have the highest-calorie density of all the macronutrients, at 9 calories per gram, but a lot of refined carbs and sugars are surprisingly calorie dense. They're also highly palatable and easy to overeat. With 270 calories per 140 g (5 oz), pasta is a prime example. Most people are more likely to have 420 g (15 oz) of pasta than 140 g (5 oz). That's 810 calories, not including what you put on it or what you drink with it.

Pasta, bread, bagels, and cereal are complex carbs, but all of them are processed. (You've never seen a bagel tree, have you?) Milling, refining, and bleaching the grains decreases the nutritional value while increasing the calorie density. Whole grain varieties are better, because they retain some of the nutrients and fibre, but even these are somewhat processed and may be high in calories.

You should also be cautious of "natural" sugars. Many people swear off white sugar and look for natural alternatives. While sweeteners like honey, agave nectar, maple syrup, and treacle are less refined and may have nutritional value, they're still calorie dense and they're still sugar.

In "natural" cereals or baked goods, you often see sweeteners like evaporated cane juice, which is called "a healthy alternative to refined sugar." It's easy to feel righteous shopping in a health food store and choosing the "natural" product instead of the one with white sugar. Just remember, "natural," "healthier," or "more nutritious" do not always mean "low-calorie." It's possible to get fat on high-calorie natural carbs. If you want to keep high-calorie sugars to a minimum and you want to avoid artificial sweeteners, consider the herb stevia as a natural low-calorie sweetener.

## THE NUTRIENT DENSITY PRINCIPLE

If you want to get leaner and healthier, focus on calorie quantity and quality, not one or the other. You can still lose weight while eating sugar if you're in a calorie deficit, but this doesn't mean a low-calorie Twinkie (Mini Roll) diet is good for you, especially over the long haul. It's important to hit your calorie target, but the ideal plan is to choose foods that give you the maximum nutritional value from every calorie you eat. The fewer calories you eat, the more important this is.

A food that has a large amount of vitamins, minerals, phytochemicals, and other nutrients per unit of volume is known as having high "nutrient density." Fibrous vegetables and whole fruits top the carb list. When you're on a calorie budget, these nutrient-dense carbs are the best place to spend your calories first. The natural starches and grains are also high in micro-nutrition; these carbs simply come with more calories, so watch the quantities.

Always be aware of the nutritional value of everything you eat, given how many calories it's costing you. Think of every food – and especially sugar – the way you think of money when you're on a tight budget. Ask yourself, "Is it worth spending my calories on this?" White sugar, for example, has no vitamins, no minerals, no amino acids, just pure empty calories.

## HOW MANY CARBS? WHAT THE LEANEST
## PEOPLE IN THE WORLD DO

Most of the traditional health and nutrition organizations recommend getting about 55 per cent of your calories from carbs. That's not a bad carb guideline for active, metabolically healthy people, provided the quantity is right and quality is high. The baseline for carbs on *Burn the Fat, Feed the Muscle* is 50 per cent of total daily calories. That's just slightly lower than the conventional recommendations, which allows for a slightly higher protein intake. This is a sensible starting point because it's balanced, maintainable, and nonrestrictive, and it supports hard training.

In the example below, you'll see what a typical baseline would look like on a fat-loss programme (for maintenance or muscle-gain programmes, all these numbers would be higher).

**BASELINE CARB RECOMMENDATIONS FOR WOMEN:**

1,600 CALORIES PER DAY:

1,600 calories × 50 per cent = 800 calories from carbs

There are 4 calories in each gram of carbs.

800 carb calories ÷ 4 = 200 grams of carbs per day

**BASELINE CARB RECOMMENDATIONS FOR MEN:**

2,300 CALORIES PER DAY:

2,300 calories × 50 per cent = 1,150 calories from carbs

There are 4 calories in each gram of carbs.

1,150 carb calories ÷ 4 = 288 grams of carbs per day

For carbohydrates, more than any other macronutrient, it's absolutely vital to customize, because one rigid prescription doesn't account for individual goals, sugar tolerance, activity levels, or type of training. After you establish your baseline and see how you respond, you can make carb adjustments based on your results.

This is where the physique athlete method is superior to rigid low-carb diets or high-carb diets. *Burn the Fat, Feed the Muscle* is not high-carb or low-carb, it's carb customized. You have lots of room to adjust your carb intake on this programme. In fact, the lean protein and healthy fats often remain fairly steady and it's the carbs that get tweaked up or down the most.

When you want to accelerate fat loss or break a fat-loss plateau, you might drop the total amount or ratio of carbs. Occasionally, you may even use the counterintuitive strategy of spiking your carb calories. These techniques are so effective for stubborn fat and end-stage fat loss (those last 10 pounds/4.5 kg) that bodybuilders have developed an entire system of reduced-carb dieting with carb cycling. You'll learn about that in the last section of the book, which focuses on accelerating your results.

For now, focus on getting your baseline nutrition in order; clear out all those processed carbs and replace them with natural, nutrient dense carbs. When the time comes, those advanced carb manipulation techniques will be there, and they can unlock a whole other level of lean for you.

### BURN THE FAT, FEED THE MUSCLE
### ACTION SUMMARY: CARBOHYDRATES

- Eat natural, unprocessed carbs; reduce processed, refined carbs as much as possible, especially the "whites": white sugar, white flour.
- Learn the difference between starchy carbs and fibrous carbs. (Memorize the lists!)
- Eat a starchy carb and a fibrous carb with each meal (along with your protein).
- Eat fruit every day with meals or as snacks. If you don't have a fibrous vegetable with a meal, have a fruit.
- Aim for 25 to 35 grams of fibre per day or 14 grams per 1,000 calories of energy expenditure. If you follow the *Burn the Fat* meal templates (chapter 14), you'll easily hit your fibre goal automatically.
- As a baseline, aim for approximately 50 per cent of your total calories from natural carbs. (Follow the meal templates and you'll come close to this amount automatically.)
- Customize your carb intake based on your activity, body type, and results.

# CHAPTER 12

# Hydrate Like an Athlete and Burn More Fat

"If you dehydrate your body, it's like dehydrating your plants. Who wants to have a wilted body?"

– Dr. Lawrence E. Lamb, author of *The Weighting Game: The Truth About Weight Control*

## THE MOST ESSENTIAL NUTRIENT OF ALL: DO YOU TAKE IT FOR GRANTED?

Fitness enthusiasts looking for an edge tend to focus on what's new and sexy in nutrition science, so it's no surprise that something as simple and ubiquitous as water is easily overlooked. But ignoring proper hydration is a costly mistake. If you want a leaner and more muscular body, you need to eat like an athlete and train like an athlete. If you train like an athlete, you need to hydrate like an athlete.

Dr. Bob Murray, founder of Sports Science Insights, says, "From an athlete's standpoint, or anybody who is physically active, hydration is the number one nutritional intervention for protecting performance, making us feel good during exercise and recovering afterwards. There is no cheaper, easier and more effective way at getting the most out of our bodies and improving performance."

Water is the most abundant compound in your body, making up 60 per cent to 70 per cent of your weight. Your blood is about 90 per cent water. Your muscles are 70 per cent water. Even your bones are 20 per cent water. Water is necessary to regulate your body temperature, transport nutrients, build tissues, and remove wastes from cells. Water is required for joint lubrication, brain function, digestion, circulation, respiration, absorption, and excretion. Without water, nothing in your body works properly.

## HOW DEHYDRATION AFFECTS YOUR ENERGY, STRENGTH, AND PHYSICAL PERFORMANCE

Did you ever wake up in the morning feeling so groggy it almost felt like a hangover? Guess what? You may have been dehydrated. In fact, a hangover – headache, dry mouth, tiredness, and fatigue – is partially caused by the diuretic effects of alcohol. Do you usually enjoy excellent workouts, but some days your butt is dragging by the end – or, worse, you can't get started? Guess what? You were probably dehydrated.

The effects of dehydration creep up on you. By the time you feel the full impact, it's too late: You're already dehydrated. If it's not particularly hot, you might not link the symptoms to lack of water. You might think you're just overworked, you didn't get enough sleep, or you're coming down with something.

As you become dehydrated, your body's core temperature increases. This adversely affects your cardiovascular function and reduces your physical work capacity. As it gets more severe, your risk of heat cramps, heat exhaustion, and heat stroke increases.

Even mild dehydration equal to 1 per cent of your body weight can impair exercise thermoregulation. For a 200-pound (14 st 4-lb/91-kg) person, that's only 2 pounds (0.9 kg), but can occur in as little as 30 to 60 minutes of sweaty training. A study from the *Journal of Strength and Conditioning Research* found that a 1.5 per cent loss of water weight reduced bench press strength by 5.6 per cent. With a 3 per cent loss, muscle strength can decrease by 10 per cent. When you lose 4 per cent to 5 per cent or more of your body weight in water, muscular and aerobic endurance can decrease by 20 per cent to 30 per cent. If you lose more than 10 per cent of your body's weight as water, you could die.

## HOW MUCH SHOULD YOU DRINK?

Making general recommendations for water intake is challenging because individual needs vary dramatically, especially with exercise and heat stress. You can lose water in sweat at rates over 3 litres per hour, and total daily fluid requirements are known to range from as low as 2 litres to 10 litres per day or more.

Among the general public, the most common guideline is "drink eight 8-fluid ounce (225-ml) glasses of water per day" (8 × 8 or 64-fluid ounces; approximately 2 litres per day). In the bodybuilding world, 'drink a gallon a day' (3.8 litres or 128-fluid ounces) is not uncommon advice.

In recent years, there has been a re-evaluation and major debate over water guidelines. Several nephrologists reviewed all the research, said they couldn't figure out where the 8 × 8 rule came from and claimed there was no evidence to back it up. Before you knew it, fitness writers and bloggers were telling people the opposite: "8 × 8 is a myth! Stop drinking so much water!" (I know, so confusing, right?)

No doubt, the profitable bottled water industry has a vested interest in the "Drink more water" message, but that doesn't mean it's a myth or a conspiracy. If I were you, I wouldn't be so quick to drop your water intake without evaluating your individual needs and considering adequate versus optimal.

The origin of 8 × 8 seems clear: It corresponds with the original recommendations made by the US National Research Council to consume at least 1 millilitre for every calorie burned. That puts 8 × 8 at the *minimum* recommended level.

These doctors and journalists who appeared intent on debunking the "Drink more water" message were mainly reminding us that water guidelines include *total water* (which includes water from other beverages and moisture in food), not just *drinking water.* They were also only questioning 8 × 8 as a rigid rule. The truth is 64 fluid ounces (about 2 litres) of total water each day might be inadequate for many people, especially those who work out.

## HOW TO FIND YOUR PERSONAL CUSTOMIZED WATER INTAKE

A basic principle of *Burn the Fat, Feed the Muscle* is to customize everything and avoid one-size-fits-all mind-sets, programmes, and recommendations. This goes for water intake just as it does for calories, protein, carbs, and other nutrients.

Large people need more water than smaller people, and active individuals need more than inactive folks. Climate is a huge factor. If you work or train in the heat, your water needs are much higher. If you follow a high-protein diet, it's also smart to slide to the higher side of the recommended water range.

In 2004 the Institute of Medicine in Washington, D.C., convened to set new dietary reference intakes (DRIs) for water. The recommendations were based on experimental and observational human research. Although they made it clear that water needs can vary dramatically and this number was only a median, they concluded that *a daily total water intake of 3.7 litres for adult men and 2.7 litres for adult women covers the majority of individuals.*

| INSTITUTE OF MEDICINE GUIDELINES FOR WATER (DRI) | |
|---|---|
| Men | Women |
| 3.7 litres (125 fl oz) per day | 2.7 litres (91 fl oz) per day |

If you want a customized guideline, you can use the US National Research Council's recommendation: 1.0 to 1.5 millilitres per kilocalorie expended per day. (You calculated your total daily calorie expenditure in chapter 7: Women burn an average of about 2,100 calories per day and men burn approximately 2,700 calories per day.) Use the high end of the required water range if you're active or you train in the heat.

| NATIONAL RESEARCH COUNCIL GUIDELINES FOR WATER INTAKE | | |
|---|---|---|
| **Calories Expended** | **Water Required** | **Water Required** |
| 2,000 | 67–101 fl oz | 2.0–3.0 litres |
| 2,500 | 84–126 fl oz | 2.5–3.75 litres |
| 3,000 | 101–152 fl oz | 3.0–4.5 litres |
| 3,500 | 118–177 fl oz | 3.5–5.25 litres |
| 4,000 | 135–202 fl oz | 4.0–6.0 litres |

Note: One gallon = 128 fluid ounces or 3.8 litres.

---

*QUICKSTART*

**Men; drink approximately 3.5 litres of water a day. Women: drink approximately 2.5 litres of water per day. Follow this tip and your hydration needs will be covered under all normal conditions, with room to spare. Drink more water if you get extremely active, and even more if you're training in the heat.**

---

## SHOULD YOU COUNT THE LIQUIDS FROM FOODS AND BEVERAGES TOWARD YOUR WATER INTAKE?

These recommendations are based on total water, so all fluids do count. Almost all foods contain water. Fruits and vegetables are 75 per cent to 90 per cent water. Even meat is at least 50 per cent water. Milk, coffee, tea, and sports drinks are mostly water. Caffeine has a mild diuretic effect, but not enough to cancel the hydration provided from caffeinated liquids. (Don't use caffeinated drinks for rehydration, however.)

It's difficult to determine the exact amount of water you're getting from food, so don't bother. In general, the average person gets about 20 per cent of their water intake from food, provided they eat fruits and vegetables every day.

It's not uncommon for bodybuilders to use the *total water* guidelines as their daily target for *drinking water*. I do. My calorie expenditure is about 3,200 per day, so that's at least 3.2 litres or usually closer to a gallon (3.8 litres) – well over 8 × 8. I drink that amount in pure water every day.

My method puts you on the high side when you add water from all sources, but it doesn't hurt. It offers an extra margin of assurance that your water intake is more than adequate and perhaps is closer to optimum. Personally, I feel better, train harder, and have more energy when my water intake is on the high side rather than the low side. I've heard this sentiment echoed throughout the fitness industry for decades.

## CAN DRINKING MORE WATER INCREASE FAT LOSS?

Many health experts outside the athletic community focus on deficiency prevention. They're mostly concerned with finding the minimum amounts needed for maintaining health or avoiding illness in average or sedentary people. Instead of finding out how little you can drink before your results suffer, why not search for what's optimal and see if your results improve?

It's clear that dehydration decreases your performance and becomes dangerous as it progresses. It's also clear that with all nutrients, there's a difference between deficiency and adequacy. Could there be an optimal level for water, beyond adequate, that improves your fat loss? We don't know for sure because there's a lack of strong evidence to confirm it. However, drinking water can help your fat-loss efforts in many ways, and some of them make a huge difference.

The most controversial theory is water-induced thermogenesis. Experiments at the German Institute of Human Nutrition found that drinking cold water increased metabolic rate in adults by 24 per cent to 30 per cent for 30 to 60 minutes. An Israeli study published in the *International Journal of Obesity* reported similar results in children: a 25 per cent increase in resting energy expenditure lasting for over 40 minutes. Some people speculate that when the water is cold (3 to 4 degrees Celsius), your body must heat it up, and that burns calories. Other scientists say the mechanism has to do with sympathetic nervous system stimulation or improved cellular metabolism.

The big question is whether this small, short-term metabolism boost continues and adds up to body fat loss over time. If it does help, it's a small effect. The Israeli scientists said that simply following the standard water drinking guidelines theoretically adds an additional weight loss of about 2.6 pounds (1.2 kilograms) per year. The most optimistic projection is about 5 pounds (2.3 kg) in a year. Not much either way, but considering how easy it is to do, my guess is that you'll take every extra bit of fat loss you can get.

Drinking water before or during a meal also helps. Water may not be a true appetite suppressant (in the hormonal sense), but water can increase stomach fullness and reduce calorie intake at a meal. In a 2008 study from Virginia Tech, subjects drank 500 millilitres of water about 30 minutes before breakfast. Calorie intake decreased by 13 per cent. In a 2010 follow-up study, 500 millilitres of water was consumed before every main meal, and weight loss was 4.4 pounds (2 kilograms) greater over a 12-week period.

There's not much research on long-term effects, but a twelve-month study was conducted at the Oakland Hospital Research Institute. Increases in drinking water were associated with significant fat loss and loss of body weight in overweight subjects. An obvious reason was because they swapped calorific drinks for water. Even after accounting for this, the water drinkers still showed increases in weight loss – about 5 pounds (2.3 kg) in a year.

A lot less controversial (this one's a sure thing) is the replacement strategy. Cutting something out cold turkey creates a void that begs to be filled, so it helps if you think in terms of replacement rather than removal. Every time you get the urge to reach for a fizzy drink or another calorific drink, tell yourself, "I'll have water instead." Within a few weeks, you'll have a positive new habit installed. The average person saves at least 200 calories per day with this one simple swap. On paper, that's 20.8 pounds (9 kg) of fat gone in one year. If you've been drinking sugar-sweetened beverages every day, this could be the best bang-for-your-buck fat-loss tactic in the entire book.

As you can see, there's plenty of evidence showing a variety of ways that water is your friend for fat loss as well as for health, energy, and performance. Drinking water may also be tied strongly to other healthy behaviours. Healthy habits come in clusters: drink more water, and you automatically start doing other healthy stuff.

Many people snub their noses at increasing their water intake, complaining that it's too much trouble or drinking when you're thirsty is good enough. But if you're serious about sports or fitness, is it really?

## THIRST: IS IT A GOOD SIGNAL FOR HYDRATION?

Your body has an exquisite homeostatic thirst mechanism that guides you to rehydrate and restore water balance on a day-to-day basis. The problem is that thirst isn't a good indicator for maintaining hydration, especially for athletes. By the time your body registers the sensation of thirst, you may already be underhydrated. This becomes truer as you get older, when the thirst mechanism doesn't work as well as it used to.

Most people don't drink purely based on thirst; they drink in response to other stimuli, such as mealtimes, walking past a fountain, or when drinks are offered during social events. Instead of waiting until you're parched or otherwise prompted, the proactive strategy for optimal hydration is to drink water throughout the day, before training and during training, even when you're not thirsty.

In addition to thirst, urine colour and body weight are two other practical ways to monitor your hydration level. Your urine should be clear to straw-coloured and odourless. If it's a deep or dark colour with a strong odour, you're dehydrated. (Note: Some vitamin supplements and medications can darken urine colour.) If you sweat heavily during exercise, check your weight before and after each workout. Replace any weight lost during an exercise bout with water.

## CAN YOU DRINK TOO MUCH WATER?

Science and health organizations have not set a tolerable upper intake level (UL), probably because water intoxication is so rare. You see it mostly in athletes (especially females), who replace heavy sweat losses after long endurance events with copious amounts of plain water without the needed electrolytes. This leads to hyponatraemia, a low concentration of sodium in the blood, which can lead to swelling of the brain; this can be fatal. Hyponatraemia is rare outside the endurance sports world, but one case was publicized after a water drinking contest sponsored by a radio station in California ("Hold your wee to win a Wii").

Bodybuilders and competitive athletes have been known to take their training and nutrition not only seriously, but to extremes. They're often perfectionists, not satisfied until they reach 100 per cent on their nutritional scorecard. This is admirable, but sometimes can lead to a more-is-better mentality, and more of a good thing is not always better. "Drink as much as you can tolerate" is not good advice, even though sports nutrition organizations have given it in the past.

Don't forget practical considerations as well. If you buy bottled water, there's extra expense, plus an impact on the environment (from production, transportation, and disposal). And if you drink so much that you must be a few steps from a bathroom 24-7, you're probably overdoing it.

## A SIMPLE HYDRATION SCHEDULE FOR
## PEOPLE WHO WANT THE OPTIMAL "BURN"

You can drink water whenever you want, but there are a several times when drinking can be especially helpful. Following a schedule also helps turn the behaviour into a habit, making it something you don't have to think about.

First, drink immediately when you wake up in the morning because you haven't had fluids all night. Suggestion: Keep a glass of water by your bedside so it's waiting for you when you wake up. Pre-breakfast water intake may help with your daily calorie control efforts and it also sets a good, healthy tone for the day.

Second, drink before your workouts. Shoot for about 500 millilitres (17 fluid ounces) anywhere from 2 hours to 20 minutes prior to training (with or apart from a meal).

Third, drink during your workouts. Most sports nutritionists recommend about 200 to 250 millilitres every 15 minutes. Water is the best drink for strength and general fitness workouts of an hour or less. Sophisticated strength and physique athletes sometimes experiment with amino acids during the workout, but this isn't mandatory and benefits are not conclusive, given adequate protein intake from food. If you're an athlete with endurance training bouts longer than one hour, be certain to consult your coach or a sports nutritionist for advice on water, carbohydrate, and electrolyte replacement.

Fourth, drink after your workout. The goal is to begin rehydrating immediately after the workout to replace any water weight loss before the next session. A half a litre (500 millilitres) of water represents about 1 pound (0.5 kg) of body weight lost.

Fifth, drink when it's hot and you're sweating, even if it's not during a formal workout.

On your nontraining days, you don't need as much water, but remember to drink up in the morning and keep drinking throughout the day, as you won't be prompted by your training session. Mealtime is a great cue: Two of the easiest fat-loss strategies are drinking water before meals and drinking water during meals (in place of calorific drinks).

## THE DARK SIDE OF LIQUID CALORIES

Barry Popkin, professor of global nutrition at the University of North Carolina, said, "Perhaps nothing has contributed more to our weight gain than the clash between our drinking habits and our biology." There's no doubt about it: Calorific drinks are keeping a lot of people fat.

In the United States, the primary source is sugar-sweetened beverages, with cola and other soft drinks leading the way. Now a close second are speciality and dessert coffees. A Starbucks Frappuccino can cost you 500 calories or more. A Dunkin Donuts Frozen Mocha Coffee Coolatta has 360 calories – and that's the small size with skimmed milk! The large one with cream will set you back 1,050 calories! That's two-thirds of a typical female's daily calorie intake on a fat-loss programme.

Energy drinks high in sugar and caffeine round out the top three, and I'm sure you know someone who practically lives on those things. Whereas a 12-fluid-ounce

(350-ml) can of fizzy drink usually runs you 140 to 160 calories, many of the popular energy drinks come in 16-, 20-, or 23-fluid-ounce (400- 570- or 655-ml) sizes and clock in at 220 to 345 calories.

Many people think that fruit juice is an improvement over fizzy drinks, but whole fruit is better. Whole fruit gives you fibre, contains fewer calories, and satisfies your appetite more. Unless you're an athlete with very long workouts or events, skip the sports drinks, too: They're sugar water with electrolytes, not fat-loss food. Whether or not it's "natural," liquid sugar makes calorie control much more difficult.

Sugar-sweetened beverages have a high calorie density, and they require no chewing, so they can be consumed more quickly than solid food. They also have a low satiety value. Scientists recently confirmed that, compared to whole foods, liquid calories produce a smaller increase in satiety hormone GLP-1 and a smaller decrease in the hunger hormone ghrelin.

At no time in our history have we had access to such large amounts of liquid calories. Alcohol may have been around as far back as 5000 BC, but even that is a blip on the evolutionary calendar of humanity. What did our ancestors drink? As infants, breast milk. As adults, water. As a result, our genetic code never developed the physiological mechanisms to properly register the calories in liquids the way it does when we eat whole foods.

If you counted calories carefully and made sure you hit your calorie target for the day, there would be little or no difference in weight loss regardless of whether you ate your calories or drank them. The trouble is most people are terrible at tracking their calorie intake. Hunger gets the best of them and they drink calories in addition to their usual food intake, not instead of it.

Bottom line: The best strategy to beat body fat is to cut out all sugar-sweetened beverages.

## WHAT ABOUT DIET FIZZY DRINKS AND OTHER NO-CALORIE DRINKS?

Diet fizzy drinks, diet tea, flavoured waters, and other diet drinks are artificially sweetened, so they contain few or no calories. Artificial sweeteners, however, have been burned at the stake in the court of public opinion, especially aspartame. Sucralose (brand name Splenda) doesn't generate as many complaints, but artificial sweeteners have become controversial and unpopular in general.

Let me first point out the obvious: Diet soft drinks contain absolutely nothing healthy. But does that mean they're toxic? A basic premise of toxicology is that the dose makes the poison. There's little reason to believe that light or infrequent use of diet drinks is harmful. If you drink them by the six-pack every day, who knows? I don't recommend that.

Second question: Can diet drinks cause weight gain? As paradoxical as it sounds, some people believe they do. However, the idea that "diet fizzy drinks make you fat" confuses correlation with causation. If you survey overweight people about their beverages, you might discover that as a group they drink a lot of diet fizzy drinks. Is it more likely that the calorie-free fizzy drink *caused* them to gain weight or that they started drinking the diet fizzy drink because they were trying to lose weight they'd already gained? Rest assured that diet drinks by themselves do not cause weight gain. If a drink doesn't have calories and it doesn't stimulate appetite or trigger excess food intake, it can't make you fat.

It is possible, however, that diet drinks sharpen your sweet tooth. They also might create a false sense of security and entitlement to eat something else because of the calories you saved from the drink. Remember that using drinks with no calories is not a free pass to eat extra calories elsewhere or pay no attention to your deficit.

All things considered, I recommend drinking mostly water and keeping artificial anything to a minimum. If you want an occasional diet drink, go ahead and have it, just like you might have an occasional glass of wine or a cheat meal. You'll never find diet fizzy drink stockpiled in my refrigerator, but a diet cherry cola once in a while sure takes the edge off a strict diet, and I've never seen a shred of hard evidence that diet drinks slow down fat loss if all else remains equal.

## COFFEE AND TEA

If you read the health headlines, it seems like one year experts say coffee is bad for you, the next it's good, and the year after that it's bad again. Drives you crazy, doesn't it? Many nutritionists and trainers suggest avoiding caffeinated beverages, and there's a negative vibe about caffeine in the health and fitness world in general. Ironically, caffeine increases thermogenesis and lipolysis, plus many people find it helps as a pre-workout stimulant. Coffee also provides antioxidants and some research shows it may lower risk of type 2 diabetes.

However, caffeine is not entirely benign. It can elevate heart rate and blood pressure. Large doses may acutely affect your blood sugar and insulin, and it may disrupt your sleep if you have it late in the day. Some people are more sensitive than others, but condemning coffee without discussing dose and context is silly. The problem is not coffee, it's the abuse of caffeine or other stimulants. Truth be told, I love my Starbucks. The difference between me and folks who don't have abs is I drink coffee black, with only a splash of skimmed milk and maybe a no-calorie sweetener. They drink mochas and Frappuccinos.

The calories you put in your coffee will add to a surplus or chip away at your deficit. Even a little cream and sugar in your coffee adds up if you drink a lot, and these are the kind of calories most people forget to count. If you don't drink your coffee by the pot or with a lot of added calories, there's no reason to believe it will harm your health or halt your fat loss. It might even help.

Unsweetened tea is another great beverage for fat-loss programmes. But take heed: Sugar-sweetened tea drinks are not. One popular brand of bottled green tea made the *Men's Health* list of the 20 worst drinks in America, with 240 calories and 61 grams of sugar in one 20-fluid-ounce (570-millilitre) serving.

Arguments over which tea is healthiest abound, as many contain bioactive compounds such as polyphenols, carotenoids, and flavonoids. If there are no calories, I suggest you simply drink whatever type of tea you enjoy. My favourites are antioxidant-rich green tea and Captain Picard's choice: Earl Grey. Hot.

## WILL ALCOHOL MAKE YOU FAT?

An occasional glass of wine or a couple of beers will probably do no harm to your health or waistline, provided you budget for the calories. Red wine has been associated with some health benefits, such as increasing good HDL cholesterol. Excessive alcohol, on the other hand, can easily derail your performance and slow your fat loss.

Your body has no storage capacity for alcohol as it does for carbs and fats. Alcohol must be detoxified as quickly as possible (which is why some people consider it a poison). As a result, the oxidation of alcohol takes priority over other macronutrients. In other words, while your liver is busy metabolizing those beers you drank, the use of fat for fuel is almost entirely suppressed.

## THE HIGH-CALORIE DENSITY/LOW-NUTRIENT DENSITY PROBLEM

Alcohol is not converted directly into body fat; it's metabolized by your liver. However, this doesn't mean it doesn't contribute to fat gain. With 7 calories per gram, alcohol is calorie dense and the calories add up with the food you eat. It's a poor way to spend your calories, because those calories have almost no nutritional value.

Red wine contains healthy compounds like polyphenols and some alcoholic beverages provide traces of vitamins or minerals. But considering that you get a wide variety of antioxidants and micronutrients from fruits and vegetables, it's foolish to recommend beer or wine as a source of nutrition. In fact, alcohol interferes with digestion and absorption of many vital nutrients, including the B vitamins niacin, thiamin, and zinc.

## ALCOHOL AND YOUR HEALTH

Excessive alcohol use is linked to numerous health problems, including heart disease, high blood pressure, stroke, cardiomyopathy, abnormal heart rhythms, liver disease, stomach problems, cancer, decreased resistance to infections, gout, and hypoglycaemia. And don't forget alcoholism and all the troubles that come along with addiction.

Although alcohol is liquid, it's a potent diuretic. It pulls water from the cells and increases water loss through the kidneys, leading to all the negative effects of dehydration.

Heavy drinking suppresses testosterone, one of the main muscle-building hormones. And alcohol is like other liquid calories: You don't compensate properly for the extra calories. Good-bye, abs; hello, beer belly. Basically, booze can ruin your health, make you fat, and rob you of muscle if the drinking gets out of control.

### Five Tips for Drinking Sensibly Without Compromising Your Results

There are plenty of food cops who will tell you to never let a drop of alcohol cross your lips, but if you're a wine or beer lover, I think it's better to enjoy your drink if you can do it moderately and sensibly. I also believe that for long-term success, it's important that you're happy and that your nutrition programme is socially acceptable. Here's the best way to approach it:

#### 1. REDEFINE MODERATION.

"Moderation" is a fuzzy word in nutrition circles, but in the case of alcohol it's usually defined as one drink for women and two for men. Doing this daily could add up to 14 drinks per week. That's not moderation in my book. I strongly urge you to avoid daily drinking (or daily junk food eating, for that matter), because behaviours repeated daily become habits. Habits are hard to break and habitual drinking can escalate. Save the drinking for weekends, or even less often – only for holidays and special occasions (you might enjoy it more that way).

Binge drinking has no place in a fitness lifestyle, and hangovers aren't conducive to good workouts. If you drink frequently or in large amounts, don't complain about your fat-loss plateau. Look in the mirror and admit the truth: "I'm not that serious about getting in shape. It's not a high priority right now. I don't want it that bad." At least you're being honest with yourself.

## 2. ALWAYS COUNT THE CALORIES AND STAY WITHIN YOUR DEFICIT.

In the final analysis, weight loss is calories in versus calories out. If you count your alcohol calories and stay within your limits, you'll still lose weight. The problem is most people forget to add up the calories in all their drinks, and alcohol can increase your appetite. Men in particular are not good at compensating: They tend to eat in addition to drinking, while women usually drink instead of eat. Alcohol can also lower your inhibitions. The more you drink, the easier it is to say, "To heck with this diet!" The next thing you know, two drinks turn into six and you top it off with midnight pizza.

I'm often asked, "What's the best alcoholic drink when you're dieting? Best answer: none. Second-best answer: the drink with the least calories. Mixed drinks with high-calorie additives such as milk, juice, sugar, or tropical drink mixes can completely undermine your fat-loss goals. A light beer contains about 95 calories. An 8-fluid-ounce (230-ml) margarita packs about 500 calories. And if you like piña coladas, you'd better like hours of cardio, because a big one can cost you up to 640 calories. Two of those isn't moderation, it's diet sabotage.

## 3. GET TO BED EARLY AND DON'T COMPROMISE YOUR SLEEP.

Drinking and late nights often go together. Partying until the wee hours of the morning can mean abnormal sleeping patterns, less sleep, and lower sleep quality. Your body needs rest and thrives on structure and schedule. Disrupted sleep patterns often mean missed meals, poor workouts, and poor recovery.

Scientists have discovered that inadequate sleep can wreak havoc on the hormones that regulate appetite, metabolism, and the anabolic/catabolic balance in your body. Sleep deprivation can increase ghrelin, decrease leptin, increase cortisol, and decrease insulin sensitivity.

If this isn't enough, how about losing your hard-earned muscle while dieting? A Dutch study found that sleep curtailment (5.5 hours versus 8.5 hours) decreased the amount of weight lost as fat by 55 per cent. This came with increased hunger, reduced fat oxidation, and greater adaptation to the calorie deficit.

## 4. BE STRONG IN THE FACE OF PEER PRESSURE, AND CHOOSE FRIENDS WISELY.

If peer pressure is a problem, get tough and reaffirm your commitment to your goal. Decide in advance that you won't give in. If social temptation is a major problem, reconsider who you've chosen as friends. Most people don't care that you're working on self-improvement. In fact, some people resent it if you improve and they don't. It's easier for an average person to reach up and pull you down than to climb up and improve themselves.

People who aren't on the same path won't always support you if you tell them you're "on a diet" or "in training." It might make you a bigger target. Say, "No, thanks" and nothing else, or invent a good excuse, real or imaginary: "I have a stomach disorder, liver problem, etc.," works nicely. Instead of being in a tense peer-pressure situation, you could make a game out of it. "I'm the designated driver" is always a good way out that your friends may appreciate.

### 5. WHEN FAT LOSS IS YOUR GOAL, CONSIDER NOT DRINKING ALCOHOL AT ALL.

If your goal is fat loss, you must stay in a calorie deficit, so you have fewer calories to work with. (This is true for females especially.) This means that to include alcoholic drinks, which are calorie dense and nutrient sparse, you must displace other foods that are packed with nutrients and more filling. Even if you know you can fit in a drink or two and stay within your deficit, you may want to ask yourself if those calories are worth it. If you're stuck on a progress plateau, the answer is obvious.

## HYDRATE LIKE AN ATHLETE AND BURN MORE FAT!

The next time you're in a bar (hopefully not very often), take a look around. You won't find many successful fitness or bodybuilding champions hanging out there at 1:00 or 2:00 a.m. And the next time you go to the gym, check out the bodybuilders and fitness models. You'll notice that they all lug around a bottle of water or even a gallon (3.8-litre) jug – all the time. Then look at how lean and muscular they are. Coincidence? Or do they know something that you don't? Drink up! Your $H_2O$, that is!

CHAPTER 13

# Nutrient Timing

"From a muscle-development standpoint, when you eat is arguably as important as what you eat. This concept, called nutrient timing, has been extensively investigated by researchers, and studies show that consuming nutrients around your training session has a greater effect on anabolism than consuming them at other times of the day."

– Brad Schoenfeld, author of *The MAX Muscle Plan*

## WHY WHEN YOU EAT MATTERS

So far, you've learned that if you want to burn fat and achieve great health at the same time, the quantity and the quality of your food are both vitally important. But improving your body composition is not entirely about what you eat and how much you eat, it's also about when you eat.

Food quantity, quality, *and* timing all work together with exercise to increase your ability to train hard, recover from your workouts, gain lean muscle, and burn more fat. *Burn the Fat, Feed the Muscle* is not about nutrition or exercise alone – it's about the synergy you get from putting both together – and these principles apply to every man and woman who trains hard.

To maximize that synergy, you must provide fuel and building materials to your body when it needs them most, otherwise your nutrition plan won't work as well and even a well-designed training programme becomes less effective. By using the nutrient timing strategies you'll learn in this chapter, you can transform your body in a way you could never achieve with dieting alone or eating haphazardly.

## NUTRIENT TIMING TACTICS OF THE LEANEST PEOPLE IN THE WORLD

Fitness models, bodybuilders, and other super-lean people do things differently to the average dieter. Their meal plans are highly structured, they eat on time, they don't skip meals, they eat special pre- and post-workout meals, and they almost always eat breakfast. They typically eat four to six smaller meals per day rather than three big ones.

For the average person, breakfast, lunch, and dinner is the most common and traditional meal schedule. As long you hit your goals for calories, macronutrients, and you eat healthy foods that give you all the nutrients you need, this programme will still work well for you if you prefer only three "squares" a day. However, on *Burn the Fat, Feed the Muscle*, five or six meals a day is the standard best practice for men. Because women have lower calorie needs, four or five meals are more typical. That's an average of five feedings per day, and all our sample meal plans fit this schedule.

Why do so many athletes eat like this and swear by it? Many reasons have been proposed over the years, including more energy, less hunger, better muscle growth, increased fat loss, and psychological advantages. Not all the benefits once cited for eating often (such as increasing metabolism) have been scientifically verified, and meal frequency is a subject of great debate.

However, one thing we do know is that this is how the leanest, most muscular people in the world have been eating for years. The success record in the fitness world goes back more than three decades, and this is the most tested, proven, and widely used meal plan in physique sports today for accomplishing both goals, getting leaner and building muscle. Here are some of the most common reasons in favour of eating often and on a regular schedule:

### 1. It gives you the amount of fuel you need for great workouts when you need it.

Couch potatoes don't burn many calories, so they don't need to eat as much, nor do they have to worry about pre- and post-workout nutrition. On the *Burn the Fat, Feed the Muscle* programme, you do two types of workouts: cardio training and weight training. When you train like an athlete, you burn more calories and you have to feed your body like an athlete. The more often and more intensely you train, the more calories you need and the more important nutrient timing becomes. With more frequent meals, it's also easy for an athlete to fuel and refuel optimally and do it without feeling stuffed and bloated.

### 2. It provides a steady flow of fuel and helps maintain high energy levels.

Almost everyone who switches to a *Burn the Fat*–style meal plan says they have more energy. No more mid-morning crashes, no more late-afternoon drowsy spells, no more brain fog, no more ups and downs; just steady, high energy all day long – and more energy for workouts. Many people who have problems regulating blood sugar find it especially valuable to spread out their food intake. Eating regular meals with natural, slow-releasing carbs, fibre, lean proteins, and healthy fats stabilizes your blood sugar and prevents the energy ups and downs.

### 3. It helps reduce appetite, control cravings, and prevent binges.

When you go a long time without food, hunger becomes a problem. Mid-afternoon crashes or nighttime cravings that send you running for a junk food fix are often the result of skipping breakfast, leaving long gaps between meals or eating randomly without a schedule at all. If you eat more often, hunger is rarely a concern. You feel psychologically satisfied as well and the impact on your eating behaviour can be profound. Even if you get hungry, you can say to yourself, "I can wait, because the next meal is just an hour or two away," and when you do eat, there's no need to binge.

### 4. It makes it easy to hit your protein quota.

You need more protein when you're weight training. Getting the optimal daily amount is easy when it's spread over at least four or five servings compared to cramming it into two or three. Eating protein at each of those meals adds to the appetite control benefits as well.

### 5. It supports muscle growth.

Most bodybuilders believe that they get better muscle growth with more frequent meals. Getting the proper amount of daily calories and protein is most important, but research also supports the idea that spreading your protein intake throughout the day helps improve your muscular development.

### 6. It builds discipline.

Putting emphasis on structure, numbers, and timing develops discipline and attention to detail. I believe these are major factors that separate people with average bodies from people with the best bodies in the world. Quite simply, people with highly structured plans (they know what, when, how much, and even where they're going to eat) follow their plans better, reduce their risk of impulsive eating, and get better results. This discipline is transferable. When you're disciplined about eating, you become disciplined about training and other areas of life as well.

### 7. It promotes healthy attitudes and behaviours toward food and fat loss.

I also believe that eating often on a regular schedule is far healthier psychologically than typical deprivation diets or going entire days at a time eating nothing. Athletes think of food as fuel and the building blocks of health and muscle, not something to fear. In a world where many dieters are starving themselves and afraid to eat, looking at each meal as an opportunity to nourish, build and, energize your body makes you realize that food is your solution, not your problem.

## SHOULD YOU EAT LIKE A BODYBUILDER?

Everyone is different, so I'm not suggesting you must do what I did strictly because it worked for me. What I am saying is that bodybuilders and physique athletes are the exemplars in this field: They're the leanest people in the world. If you isolate the common denominators of success from a large group of high performers like this one, you have a success blueprint that you can copy with great confidence.

If more muscle and less fat are your goals, try this type of meal schedule. I think you'll be amazed with the results. You can always customize your plan later so it suits your preferences and, most importantly, so it fits into your schedule and is easy to follow every day. For long-term success, you have to pick a plan that you can stick with as a lifestyle.

So, if eating four to six times a day is good, then seven or eight times must be better, right? Not necessarily. Bodybuilders are famous for constantly eating. Some have been known to set their alarms to eat in the middle of the night! That might work for the pros, but it's unnecessary and probably impractical for most people.

If you eat too often, you'll simply pile food on top of undigested food. For people with low-calorie needs, such as short or petite women, splitting the day's intake into too many meals could make each meal too small to be satisfying. If you're the nibbler type of personality, you can certainly eat more than six times per day, but do that only if it suits you. There's no evidence that you can force your body to gain more muscle or burn more fat by trying to "drip feed" protein and other nutrients into your system.

## WHAT IS THE IDEAL MEAL SCHEDULE?

Traditional mealtimes on *Burn the Fat, Feed the Muscle* are early morning breakfast, mid-morning snack, lunch, mid-afternoon snack, dinner, and evening snack, but you should customize eating times to fit your schedule. For example, if you work nights, you can simply eat your first meal whenever you wake up (even if that's in the afternoon) and arrange your meals so you eat every three or four waking hours after that.

If you have an unusual work schedule that doesn't allow breaks for long stretches of time, if your meals are unevenly spaced, or your day has fewer meals – don't panic. The important thing is to set up a regular meal plan you can stick with, hit your calorie and protein targets by the end of your day (every 24 hours), and follow the other programme guidelines to the best of your ability.

Whatever meal schedule you choose, follow it consistently every day. Missing a meal occasionally won't make your metabolism crash or your muscles waste away, but missing *planned* meals or eating unplanned calories are major mistakes to avoid.

A study from the University of Nottingham in the UK found that irregular meal patterns can lower the thermic effect of food, disrupt glucose metabolism, increase insulin resistance, and create other types of metabolic disarray. The study also said that irregular eaters have trouble properly adjusting their calorie intake as the day goes on, which can lead to weight gain over the long term.

I've discovered something similar: People who eat without structure find it almost impossible to troubleshoot fat-loss plateaus because they've never established a baseline. Haphazard eating patterns lead to fat-loss failure.

## WHAT IS THE PERFECT MEAL SIZE?

The size of your meals can vary a lot. It depends on your total calorie needs and how many meals you eat, but if you follow the *Burn the Fat, Feed the Muscle* guidelines, meal size is easy to figure out.

The average fat-loss meal plan has about 2,100 to 2,500 calories per day for men and 1,400 to 1,800 for women. If you're a serious athlete or fitness enthusiast with high activity levels, your calorie needs will be higher. To get your ideal intake per meal, simply choose how many meals you want and then divide your total daily calories by the number of meals:

MEN:
**Average optimal calorie intake for fat loss = 2,300**
**Desired number of meals = 5 or 6**
**Target calorie intake per meal = 380 to 460 calories**

WOMEN:

**Average optimal calorie intake for fat loss = 1,600**

**Desired number of meals = 4 or 5**

**Target calorie intake per meal = 320 to 400 calories**

As you can see, these are fairly small meals. Just for fun, let's compare this with the calories in some meals you might see on some US restaurant menus:

**Spaghetti with tomato sauce, restaurant serving (490 g = 17 oz) = 850 calories**

**Big Mac and large fries = 980 calories**

**IHOP hearty ham and cheese omelette = 1,000 calories**

**Denny's Grand Slam breakfast = 1,100 calories**

**Cinema popcorn (medium-size) with butter = 1,100 calories**

**Porterhouse steak, restaurant-size serving (450 grams /1 pound) = 1,150 calories**

**Five Guys large French fries = 1,314 calories**

**Kung Pao chicken with rice (one order) = 1,620 calories**

**Uno Chicago Grill deep dish macaroni & 3-cheese = 1,980 calories**

**Cheesecake Factory bistro prawn pasta = 2,290 calories**

The problem is obvious: Most people, especially in America, have no awareness of calories per portion and they're massively overeating. A typical restaurant meal, whether we're talking about steakhouse, fry-up breakfast, Italian, Chinese, or fast food, can easily top 1,000 calories. If you count starters, drinks, and/or desserts, it's not hard to blow past your entire day's calorie quota in one sitting! If you want to get leaner, you must choose your meals wisely and control your portion sizes, especially at restaurants.

The simplest and easiest way to split up your daily calories is to divide them evenly between each meal. However, there are some adjustments you could make to your meal sizes that might help improve your results even more.

## BREAKFAST … STILL FIT FOR KINGS!

A typical pattern for most dieters is nothing in the morning or a skimpy breakfast like a bagel or doughnut, a big lunch like fast-food burgers or cafeteria food, concluding with a huge dinner and, of course, the ubiquitous late-night snack. By contrast, we usually see most athletes and lean people – including long-term weight-loss maintainers – consistently eating a hearty breakfast.

In one study of breakfast eaters, Dr. Holly R. Wyatt of the University of Colorado examined a group of formerly overweight subjects in the US National Weight Control

Registry (NWCR). The NWCR was established in 1994 to investigate what makes people successful not just at losing weight but at keeping it off. Today the NWCR is the largest ongoing study of successful weight-loss maintainers. The average registry member has lost 66 pounds (30 kg) and kept it off for five-and-a-half years.

The NWCR research identified some fascinating characteristics associated with successful weight maintenance. One of those success behaviours is eating breakfast: 78 per cent of registry members reported eating breakfast seven days a week, and 90 per cent reported eating breakfast on most days of the week. Only 3.9 per cent of subjects reported never eating breakfast. Breakfast eaters also reported higher levels of physical activity. Wyatt and her research team said they found it "striking" that breakfast eating was such a frequent behaviour among successful maintainers.

Most of the research on breakfast shows correlations, not cause and effect, and obviously breakfast is not an absolute necessity to lose weight. However, research like this does reveal what happens to the majority of people who skip breakfast: Hunger and cravings kick in and they're more likely to eat impulsively later in the day. Breakfast skippers also tend to make poor food choices, which lower the nutritional quality for the entire day. "I don't have time" is the usual justification, but it's an unpardonable sin when all you have to do is set your alarm 15 to 20 minutes earlier.

If the thought of becoming a morning person makes you groan, consider this: In his studies of successful people over several decades, personal achievement expert Brian Tracy said, "I've never found any highly successful person who was a late riser." To increase the odds of putting yourself among the achievers, get up early, review your goals, prep your meals, and have a nutritious breakfast so you're well fuelled and mentally sharp for the day.

## THE TRUTH ABOUT NIGHTTIME EATING

Circadian rhythms can affect your hormones, including insulin, cortisol, leptin, growth hormone, and thyroid-stimulating hormone, so all kinds of theories have been proposed for eating (or not eating) at certain times based on the hormonal response it creates. The real question is: Do any of these short-term hormone fluctuations affect fat loss in a significant way over time? We don't know for sure, but if they do, it's probably not much compared to the bigger priorities like getting your calories and protein right.

If you stay in a 24-hour calorie deficit, you'll lose weight regardless of what time of day you eat. It's a myth that eating at night makes you fat. It's true, however, that night-eating syndrome is a clinically significant problem for some people and heavy eating at night is more likely to push the average person into a calorie surplus, especially if they're not tracking food intake.

Psychologist John de Castro's research at the University of Texas shows that food eaten late at night lacks satiating value, which increases intake late in the day, while food eaten in the morning is particularly satiating, which reduces calorie intake later in the day. His study concluded: "A dietary regimen that encourages the ingestion of relatively large amounts of food in the morning and restricts intake during the evening might reduce overall intake and serve as a treatment or preventative measure for obesity."

Some people eat less at night hoping it will help them control calories and burn more fat. This is known as calorie tapering. Recent research has suggested that nighttime protein is beneficial for protein synthesis, which has prompted some people to avoid carbs at night, but they still go for a protein meal or a bedtime protein shake (casein protein is popular for this purpose). Pulling back on the carbs in the evening is appropriately known as carb tapering.

Calorie or carb tapering has been recommended for years by countless physique athletes and coaches and it can be a good strategy for calorie control. However, strict rules such as "Never eat carbs after 7:00 p.m." or "Don't eat within three hours of bedtime," though well-intentioned, are not mandatory. Front-loading the calories early in the day probably works best for people who train early in the day (with my mid- to late morning workouts, that's how I've done it for years). If you train at night, you may want to do it the opposite way.

The basic concept of nutrient timing is to provide more fuel and nutrients when you need them most. Good nutrition is a 24-7 discipline and the muscle growth process takes place for many hours after training, but you need the most nutritional support around your workouts. Moving some of your carb calories to support your training is known as carb targeting, and it's the most modern and scientifically supported technique. If you train late in the day, you might experiment with moving *more* carb calories to your post-workout meal, even if it's in the evening.

## POST-WORKOUT NUTRIENT TIMING

It's important to have one of your protein-containing meals fairly soon after resistance training, because this is an important time for muscle recovery and growth.

Many experts have created formulas to help you calculate the exact calorie, protein, and carbohydrate amounts for your post-workout meal. In the *Journal of the International Society of Sports Nutrition*, Alan Aragon and Brad Schoenfeld analysed all the scientific literature and recommended a "simple, relatively fail-safe general guideline" of 0.4 to 0.5 grams of high-quality protein per kilogram of lean body mass (LBM) both before and after exercise.

With this formula, someone with 70 kilograms of LBM would have between 28 and 35 grams of protein in both the pre- and post-exercise meal. If you had more protein than this, there's no downside, but if you neglected these protein feedings or fell below the recommended amount, you would not maximize the anabolic response.

The amount of carbs in your post-workout meal can vary but should probably be at least equal to the protein. The US National Strength and Conditioning Association's *Guide to Sport and Exercise Nutrition* suggests a minimum of 30 to 40 grams of carbs after weight training, but this number could be much higher, depending on your calorie budget, the intensity of your workouts and whether your goal is fat loss, maintenance, or muscle gain. For intensively training athletes pursuing muscle gain, the carb amounts could be twice that. For strict fat-loss programmes in a calorie deficit, the carbs would stay on the lower end of the range.

## Five Post-Workout Nutrition Strategies to Boost Muscle Growth and Improve Recovery

Post-workout nutrition is important, but many people overcomplicate it by micromanaging macronutrients and obsessing over the timing. *Burn the Fat, Feed the Muscle* makes it simple with five easy guidelines:

1.  **Eat soon after resistance training.** The 45 to 60 minutes immediately after intense training is an important window when proper nutrition makes the biggest difference. If you ate a pre-workout meal, there's less urgency to eat your post-workout meal immediately, but it's a no-brainer, number one strategy to eat within an hour or sooner after you train.

2.  **Eat protein and carbs in the post-workout meal.** Protein is an important part of your post-workout meal. Scientists are still debating the optimal amounts, especially carbs, but carbs and protein together is ideal.

3.  **Eat some of your carb calories in your post-workout meal.** Eating carbs after training helps restore blood sugar, suppresses cortisol, causes a beneficial spike in insulin (which helps amino acids into your muscles when insulin sensitivity is high), and stimulates protein synthesis. The carbs you eat after training are used to replenish muscle glycogen and rarely get stored as body fat.

4. **Drink your protein and carbs post-workout if you prefer.** Liquids are often recommended for post-workout nutrition because they're absorbed more quickly than whole foods. If you opt for a liquid "meal," you can use a commercial post-workout drink or make your own. Several studies found that milk makes an excellent post-workout drink (add chocolate protein powder for "healthy chocolate milk").

5. **Eat simple carbs or high glycaemic carbs if you prefer.** The post-workout period is a time when quickly absorbing carbs are acceptable. Normally, you'll keep simple sugars low, but if you're going to eat them, right after intense and exhaustive workouts is a good time to do it.

If your primary goal is fat loss and you have the endomorphic body type or carb-intolerant metabolic type, you may want to be more cautious about high-sugar post-workout drinks and stick with natural food. Whole food gives you micronutrients and fibre, not just calories and carbs while satisfying your appetite better, and these are decided advantages over liquids.

## WHAT ABOUT INTRA-WORKOUT NUTRITION?

Serious athletes and sophisticated dieters may want to keep their eyes on research regarding intra-workout (during workout) nutrition, which often comes in liquid form and sometimes includes additional amino acids or other nutrients. For most everyday fat-loss seekers, however, it's best to avoid over-analysing these details.

In fact, if someone tries to sell you on the necessity of a special drink during your workout, remember that if you have a proper pre-workout meal, you'll still be digesting it and releasing the nutrients into your system during the workout. This makes nutrition during the workout optional.

## THE PRE-WORKOUT MEAL

Most people eat their pre-workout meal an hour or two before training. The most recent research suggests that pre- and post-workout meals should not be separated by more than 3 to 4 hours, assuming the weight training workout doesn't go longer than 45 to 90 minutes.

For many people, pre-workout meal timing also depends on stomach comfort. If you get nauseated working out right after a meal, simply push back your pre-workout meal far enough to let your food digest comfortably before training.

It's a common belief that the ideal pre-workout meal should be high-carb and high-sugar for quick energy. Like the post-workout meal, however, protein is most important before resistance training. For carbs, it's best to stick with your usual natural, slow-burning carbs plus lean protein meal combination. Pre-workout sugar gives you a short-lived energy boost, but you may crash later, right in the middle of your workout.

If you train at the crack of dawn and can't work out comfortably with a big meal sloshing around in your stomach, have a light meal, snack, or protein shake as your pre-workout feeding (meal one) and then eat your big breakfast (meal two) afterward. Doing weight lifting or intense training totally fasted, without even providing amino acids, is not optimal.

## THE BRACKET TECHNIQUE FOR
## PRE- AND POST-WORKOUT NUTRITION

Many people report fantastic results using the bracketing technique: They handle pre- and post-workout nutrition in one fell swoop by surrounding (bracketing) their workouts with two of their meals, which are often the largest meals of the day. Even if you prefer lower-carb nutrition, shifting your limited amount of daily carbs around (or at least right after) your weight training sessions is one of the biggest bang-for-your-buck nutrient timing strategies you can use.

---

*QUICKSTART*

"Bracket" your workout in between two of your daily meals and make sure each meal contains a protein. If it's easier, use a protein drink. This is one of the simplest and easiest nutrient timing strategies to help you burn more fat and build more muscle.

---

## SEVEN PLANNING AND PREPARATION TIPS
## TO MAKE FAT-BURNING MEAL PLANS EASY

Eating like a physique athlete or fitness champion does require some discipline until you get used to it and it becomes habitual. But with a little planning, preparation, and scheduling, it's not as hard as you might think. Here are seven tips to help make it easier.

## 1. Think of where you'll be tomorrow and plan your day in advance.

American motivational speaker Jim Rohn once said, "Never start your day until you've finished it." This is simple but profound advice about time and life management. Always think ahead to the next day and schedule your entire day in advance. If you put your ideal day on paper before you start it, you'll always have a plan and you'll never be caught off guard without healthy food.

## 2. Schedule a time for each meal and stick to it.

When you customize your daily meal plans, choose a start time for each meal. Once you establish it, make this your permanent time to make habit work for you. If you stay with the same schedule long enough, eating at the prescribed time will become an ingrained habit that requires little or no thought. Your body will thrive on the regularity and even cue your hunger when mealtime arrives.

## 3. Use the meal-splitting technique.

Dr. Dan Benardot of Georgia State University is a dietician and sports nutritionist to national and Olympic champions. As one way to make an athlete's eating plan easier, Dr. Benardot recommends meal splitting. This allows you to cook just three meals and spread them across six feedings. "Eat half of what you normally have for breakfast, and eat the other half three hours later," says Benardot. "Do the same for lunch and dinner. This will spread out the calories and ensure that you don't eat more than you're currently eating."

## 4. Prepare an entire day's worth of meals every morning or the night before.

Spontaneity may be nice in some areas of life, but your meal plan shouldn't be left to chance. Early every morning or each evening (the night before), cook your food and pack it in plastic containers, bag it, or wrap it in foil so that it's ready to take with you wherever you go. If you eat at restaurants or cafeterias, decide in advance exactly where you're going and what you'll eat when you get there.

## 5. Cook in bulk.

A huge time-saving strategy is to cook large quantities of food for several days or even a week in advance and keep it refrigerated or frozen until you need it. Some people cook a whole turkey on Sunday, then slice off portions as needed every day. You can easily prepare large batches of lean meats on a George Foreman grill, a large stovetop grill pan, or an outdoor barbecue. Boil eggs in quantity and refrigerate them (they make a great portable protein snack!). Many of your carbohydrate sources, such as potatoes, sweet potatoes, beans, and brown rice, can also be cooked in bulk. Crock-Pots or slow-cookers and rice cookers are standard features in many *Burn the Fat* kitchens.

## 6. Keep your kitchen and refrigerator well stocked with healthy foods.

If your kitchen isn't well stocked with healthy food, you'll be more likely to call for fast food or buy convenience foods on impulse. Plan your food shopping in advance, preferably setting aside the same day every week. (Many people choose Sunday so they're prepared for the busy work week ahead.) Better still, and especially if you're a busy executive or professional, hire a personal assistant to shop for you, order groceries online, or use a home delivery service. Never stockpile junk in anticipation of cheat meals. When it comes time for a cheat meal, make sure you have to go out of your way to get it. If it's not in your house every day, you won't eat it every day.

## 7. Plan ahead when travelling.

Being in hotels, on the road, or in a plane is no excuse to let your nutrition plan fall apart. All it takes is a little planning. If you book yourself into a hotel with a full kitchen and hit the grocery store, then your food preparation is business as usual. Road trip? No problem. Cook in advance and get a small, portable cooler. It also makes life easier when you think in terms of "portable foods." You can make tuna or turkey sandwiches or wraps using 100 per cent wholemeal bread that don't need to be refrigerated and are easy to eat on the go. Or try this amazing recipe, one of the all-time *Burn the Fat, Feed the Muscle* favourites:

**APPLE-CINNAMON HIGH-PROTEIN OAT PANCAKES**

INGREDIENTS:

**65 g (2¼ oz) rolled oats**
**1 whole egg**

**3 egg whites**
**1 scoop vanilla protein powder**
**half an apple, chopped**
**dash of cinnamon**
**no-calorie sweetener (optional)**

Mix the ingredients in a bowl until they are a thick pancake-batter-like consistency. Lightly coat a frying pan with nonstick cooking spray. Pour the mixture into the pan and cook on medium until one side is lightly browned. Flip the pancake over until the other side is done. Presto! Eat it hot or wrap it in foil and take it with you for a super-convenient, fully portable 400-calorie travel meal.

## HOW SNACKING FITS IN

Most people's snacks of choice are refined carbs and fatty foods such as crackers, biscuits, sweets, muffins, pastries, crisps, and pretzels. This is mainly because packaged convenience foods and "carb snacks" are so readily available. (It's not like you can grab a chicken breast or salmon steak at the checkout counter of every corner shop.)

When you follow the *Burn the Fat, Feed the Muscle* meal plan, you won't need snacks because you'll be eating every few hours, so serious hunger and cravings between meals will be a thing of the past. However, if you choose a traditional three-meal schedule of breakfast, lunch, and dinner, I recommend planning healthy snacks for between meals: for example, one mid-morning, one mid-afternoon, and an optional evening snack (or bedtime protein shake). This way, you're still getting four to six feedings per day, but only three of them are sit-down meals that require cooking or food preparation. Even busy people can manage this with ease.

A man with a 2,300-calorie-per-day target might split that into three meals of 550 to 600 calories each and three snacks of about 200 to 225 calories each. A woman with a daily calorie goal of 1,600 calories might go with three meals of about 425 to 450 calories each and two snacks of about 125 to 150 calories each. Post-workout drinks, meal replacements, and protein shakes can be counted as snacks or as "liquid meals," depending on how many calories they have.

Some snack ideas include raw vegetables (carrots, broccoli, celery, cherry tomatoes, cauliflower, etc.), fruit (all kinds, but beware of the high calories in dried fruits), nuts and seeds (in small quantities, within your calorie limits), fat-free or low-fat cottage cheese, fat-free or low-fat cheese, fat-free or low-fat yogurt, hard-boiled eggs, sardines and other canned fish, and protein shakes.

## SHOULD YOU USE MEAL REPLACEMENTS AND PROTEIN DRINKS?

Work, school, or family commitments can make it hard for some people to fit in all their meals. In some business or personal situations, it's not appropriate to open up a plastic container and take a 20-minute break for sweet potato, vegetables, and salmon in the middle of the afternoon just because it's time for meal four. Whole foods should be your first choice, but in a time crunch, a meal replacement product (MRP) can be the difference between following your plan or not.

MRPs are usually high in protein and come as powder in tubs, cans, or individual packets. You simply shake or stir it in water (or milk if you have the calories to spare) or blend it up into a smoothie. Don't go overboard with shakes, however. These products are supplements, not a replacement for good eating habits. The primary advantage of meal replacement shakes over whole food is convenience.

## WHAT TO EAT WHEN YOU DON'T HAVE A MEAL READY

In a pinch, most people reach for carbohydrate snacks, usually high in refined sugars. By contrast, if you look at the habits of bodybuilders and fitness pros, you'll notice something very interesting: They reach for protein. Eating protein by itself (without the carbs) may leave you short on calories, but at least you'll be taking advantage of what is arguably the most important macronutrient during a fat-loss programme.

That's why it's a good idea to keep some protein powder or a high-protein MRP handy in case of a "nutritional emergency." Keep some in your desk, in your car, and in your backpack, briefcase, or handbag. Get a shaker bottle and fill it with two or three scoops of protein powder. Bring along a bottle of water and then you're ready to mix yourself a protein shake anytime, any place. Add a piece of fruit if you need the carbs. Two minutes and you're done.

What about protein bars? Many so-called nutrition bars are a compromise at best and sweets in disguise at worst. Read labels carefully. You're likely to find refined sugars, corn syrup, trans-fatty acids, and other artificial ingredients. Some are also very calorie dense for their small size and not very filling. If you can find bars high in protein and made with mostly natural ingredients (or make your own protein bars), they can make good snacks for travel and convenience.

If there's a health food café nearby, you could pop in for a quick protein drink to tide you over until you get home for your next food meal. What if there's nothing but fast-food restaurants around? No problem: Grab a grilled chicken salad. A corner shop? Grab a can of tuna or salmon; they make them now in foil bags and pop-top lids. Many stores these days carry ready-to-drink protein shakes and even hard-boiled eggs. Greek yogurt is a popular quick high-protein snack. There's always a way when you're committed. If getting caught without food happens to you a lot, you need to spend more time planning your schedule and preparing food in advance.

If you miss a meal completely, don't stress out. As long as you follow your schedule most of the time, you'll get great results. Don't use missing one meal as an excuse to abandon your schedule for the rest of the day. Get back on track with your next meal. That's all there is to it.

## ONE UNIVERSAL TRAIT OF ALL PEOPLE
## WHO GET LEAN AND STAY LEAN

Whatever meal schedule you choose, establish a regular daily pattern, seven days a week. Because most people work Monday through Friday, some find it easier to follow their programme on weekdays. On the weekends, it's tempting to sleep in, miss meals, eat at restaurants, stay out late for drinks, have an entire cheat day, or fall off your regular schedule. Habits are a powerful force if you harness them to your advantage. Whatever behaviour you repeat on a daily basis, week after week, will become habitual. If you eat haphazardly, apply these principles inconsistently or follow the programme five days a week and let it fall apart on weekends, you'll never establish good habit patterns and you'll never get optimal results. One trait shared by every person who gets lean and stays lean is consistency.

## BECOME DISCIPLINED AND CONSISTENT
## AND YOU WILL SUCCEED!

For many experienced fitness enthusiasts, the information in this chapter is not new because nutrient timing is common knowledge among the fitness savvy and frequent eating has been the traditional approach in bodybuilding for decades. However, it's talked about more often than it's practised, because it takes discipline to do it!

When starting *Burn the Fat, Feed the Muscle*, most people love it because they have more energy, they get to eat more, and they never go hungry. But some say that eating five times a day is a pain in the gluteus maximus. Like any new lifestyle change, the longer you do it, the easier it gets. Eventually, "feeding the machine" like clockwork becomes such a deeply ingrained habit, you won't be able to imagine doing it any other way.

Of course, you might think that all this nutrient timing stuff sounds like too much trouble and you'd rather just eat like the average person: coffee for breakfast, whatever lunch is available, a king-size dinner, and then late night munchies. Then again, if you look around and see what kind of shape the average person is in, you may find that thought passes – quickly!

# CHAPTER 14

# The *Burn the Fat, Feed the Muscle* Meal Planning System

"Have a plan. Follow the plan, and you'll be surprised how successful you can be. Most people don't have a plan. That's why it's easy to beat most folks."

– Paul "Bear" Bryant, University of Alabama American football coach

## PUTTING IT ALL TOGETHER: FROM FOODS TO MEALS TO MEAL PLANS

This is where we take all the nutrition knowledge you've learned so far and put it together into a practical, actionable plan that you can follow every day. In this chapter, you'll learn which foods are best for burning fat and which are worst. You'll discover a simple formula for combining individual foods into fat-burning meals and you'll see how to turn individual meals into a daily meal plan. You'll find out why generic meal plans don't work and customized meal plans do. Most important of all, you'll understand why starting your day without a meal plan is the worst mistake you could make.

## THE SIMPLE CURE FOR EVERY DIET PROBLEM

I must have heard every reason for why people eat poorly or fall off the diet wagon:

"I had to eat airline food."
"I was in the car driving all day."
"I didn't have anything else with me."
"The only place to eat was McDonald's."
"I was a guest – it would have been rude to turn down dinner."
"It was the only thing on the menu."

"I couldn't help myself – I had a major craving."

"I was starving – I had to eat something."

The truth is there are no good reasons for poor food choices, only excuses, because planning is the simple cure that solves every diet problem.

A meal plan is your eating goal for the day. Without goals, you wander aimlessly or float wherever the current of life takes you, and in the case of eating, for most people, that's right to the nearest fast-food joint. Without planning, you leave yourself at the mercy of impulse and circumstance. Even worse, eating haphazardly makes it impossible to establish a baseline, so you can't track your weekly progress or troubleshoot problems.

As simple as it seems, having a meal plan on paper is one of the most powerful fat-burning strategies you can use. It's a core principle of *Burn the Fat, Feed the Muscle*.

## GRADING YOUR FOOD CHOICES

Meal plans start on the individual food level, but it can get confusing to know what to eat every day, so let's start there first.

We often use the words "good foods" and "bad foods" as figures of speech, but in reality food doesn't fall neatly into these two categories. Although some foods may deserve their bad reputations, a better way to rate whether a food is good or bad is based on dose and context. A small, infrequent dose of ice cream never made anyone fat. A large dose every night has. It's also helpful to think of food quality like temperature or colour, with good and bad as simply two ends of a spectrum, not an either/or distinction.

An easy way to start making better decisions is to give your food a grade. Simply ask yourself, "How processed is this? How calorie dense is this?" The more a food is processed and the more calorie dense a processed food is, the lower the grade. The less a food is processed (the closer it is to its natural state), the higher the grade. Salmon, broccoli, and a sweet potato are A+ foods, making an A+ meal. A cheeseburger, fries, and milk shake get an F.

You don't need straight As to pass. As long as you choose mostly A and B foods – even an occasional C – and you're conscious of portion sizes, you can feel confident that your meal plan is healthy as well as effective for fat loss. There are, however, some danger foods (the Ds and Fs) to avoid. No foods or food groups are completely forbidden in this programme. But if you want the best results possible – better body composition and better health – highly processed and fattening foods should not become staples in your daily meal plan.

# ARE SOME FOODS REALLY MORE FATTENING THAN OTHERS?

You could argue that foods aren't fattening, excess calories are. But you're far more likely to overeat some foods than others. These are foods with more calories per unit of volume (high calorie density). Certain foods are also more palatable. Did you ever notice how some snack foods make it almost impossible to eat just one? How easily does ice cream go down? (If it weren't for the "brain freeze," most people would probably stuff it down even faster.) So if we're talking about calorie density or ease of consumption, then fattening foods definitely exist.

Certain food *combinations* are doubly disastrous. Fat and sugar is one of the worst. Common examples include cheesecake, peanut butter cups, and ice cream. Starchy carbs plus fat is another dangerous combo. A prime example is white pasta with a cheesy, creamy, or buttery sauce (think spaghetti carbonara). A typical restaurant serving is about 800 calories. Cheesy chips are notorious in this category: potatoes (starchy carb) fried in oil (fat), topped with full-fat cheese rocket the calories in a large portion to a stratospheric 2,000 or more per plate.

Even healthy, unprocessed foods can become calorie bombs, depending on what you put on them. Salads can be a great starter or even a complete meal (if you include some lean protein), but when they're topped with full-fat cheeses, croutons, bacon bits, and high-fat dressings, they pack a caloric wallop. Dry baked potatoes are a good, natural starchy carb choice, but when loaded with bacon bits, cheese, or sour cream, the calories can double.

Frequent or unrestrained eating of fat-storing foods, especially combined with calorific drinks, can stuff you with thousands of surplus calories. Have you ever seen the mathematical equation for a weekend binge? It's $5 - 2 = 0$. That's five days of perfect eating minus two nights at the bars and restaurants equals zero results for the entire week. Back to square one on Monday.

## THE 12 WORST FAT-STORING FOODS

One of the best ways to start the meal planning process is to learn which foods to keep out of your daily meal plans. Then your odds of choosing the most nutritious foods are automatically higher.

### The Terrible 12

- ✘  Chips and other deep-fried foods
- ✘  Ice cream and milk shakes
- ✘  Doughnuts and pastries

✘   Sweets and confections
✘   Sugar-sweetened soft drinks
✘   Sugar-sweetened juice drinks, energy drinks, teas, and dessert coffees
✘   White bread and white flour products
✘   Crisps, and fried tortilla chips
✘   Bacon, sausage, and processed meats
✘   Hot dogs and fast-food burgers
✘   Pizza with thick crusts and fatty meat toppings
✘   Sugary breakfast cereals

If you're in tears right now because I just took away all of your favourite foods, don't worry. No foods are totally forbidden. For cheat meals – which you can work right into your plan – eat anything you want. In fact, cheat meals and re-feeds can have positive effects in physical and psychological ways – if they're used strategically and kept under control. What you eat occasionally has little impact on your health or body composition. What you eat every day is what matters the most. Take it seriously.

By eating as many of your daily calories as possible from natural, nutrient-dense food, you're doing more than losing weight: You're building health. You're also building self-discipline and gaining momentum. Every time you eat a healthy meal, you get the same good feeling you get after a great workout; it's like an endorphin rush. You pat yourself on the back and say, "Job well done." You build the confidence of a person who has a goal and is going after it, who has a plan and follows it.

Eating the same healthy foods every day also taps into the power of habit. Any behaviour you repeat daily becomes habitual and eventually effortless. Willpower can only take you so far. The best way to harness the power of positive habits is to follow a well-structured meal plan until it becomes second nature. Building meal plans starts with choosing healthy, fat-burning foods.

## THE 12 BEST FAT-BURNING FOODS

Like "fattening foods," the term, "fat-burning foods" may be a misnomer because all foods add calories to your energy balance sheet; they don't subtract them. Some foods have a very low calorie density, but there's no such thing as negative-calorie foods that take more calories to digest than they contain. Clearly, however, certain foods are better for fat loss than others, for a variety of reasons.

Lean protein foods have the highest thermic effect and suppress your appetite better than any other macronutrient. This is one of the many reasons you include a lean protein with every meal. Fibrous vegetables are always a superb choice because they're high in fibre and low in calories. The most "fat burning" of all meals is lean protein plus fibrous carbs (fish and broccoli or chicken and a green salad, for example).

Whole fruits and natural, high-fibre starchy carbs are also good choices, although you must control the starchy carb quantities to keep your calorie deficit. The amount of starchy carbs in a meal plan can vary a lot, depending on your goals. Accelerated fat loss or competition-level diets usually include fewer starchy carbs. But overall, these are the staple foods that make up the foundation of the programme for most people.

### The Terrific 12

✓  Whole fresh fruit
✓  Vegetables (any fibrous carb or nonstarchy vegetable)
✓  Yams (or sweet potatoes)
✓  Potatoes
✓  Oats, rolled or steel-cut (unsweetened)
✓  Brown rice
✓  Beans and pulses
✓  100% whole wheat or whole grains*
✓  Low or fat-free dairy products*
✓  Chicken and turkey breast
✓  Eggs and egg whites
✓  Lean cuts of red meat, game meats

*If you have allergies or intolerances, you may need to avoid certain foods, such as dairy or grains.

---

**QUICKSTART**

Many *Burn the Fat, Feed the Muscle* readers who lost over 100 pounds (45 kg) started their body transformation journey simply by eating the foods recommended on the 12 best fat-burning foods list and avoiding the 12 worst fat-storing foods.

---

This short and simple food list might be one of the most valuable resources in the book, so you'll want to keep it handy. Brian, a *Burn the Fat* reader who shed 127 pounds (58 kg) of fat, told me, "At first I just wanted to know what to eat. I figured, if eating these foods worked that well for bodybuilders, then I wanted to try it myself. Following the 12 fat-burning foods list alone is what got me started." Many other readers have shared similar stories: Kick-starting your fat loss can be as simple as following a list of foods to eat every day.

By the way, this is the same list of foods you'd use for gaining muscle as well. The difference is in the amounts. As you learned in chapter 7 when we talked about calories, to gain muscle, you have to eat in a surplus: same foods, but more of them.

## THE SIX EXCHANGE GROUPS AND
## *BURN THE FAT, FEED THE MUSCLE* FOOD LIST

*Burn the Fat, Feed the Muscle* makes more precise distinctions about food groups than most diets. We subdivide carbs into starchy, fibrous, and simple. Proteins are narrowed down into lean proteins, because we usually don't want the extra fat calories (with some exceptions, such as fatty fish). Dairy products are narrowed down to non- or low-fat (to save calories), and fats have their own category. That makes six food groups, and the foods within each group can be exchanged.

| CARBS | | |
|---|---|---|
| **Starchy Complex Carbs (Starchy Vegetables and Whole Grains)** | **Fibrous Complex Carbs (Nonstarchy Vegetables and Leafy Greens)** | **Natural Simple Carbs (Fruit)** |
| Potatoes | Broccoli | Apples, apple sauce |
| Sweet potatoes | Spinach | Bananas |
| Yams | Asparagus | Blueberries |
| Oats | Cucumber | Raspberries |
| Beans | Tomatoes | Strawberries |
| Brown rice | Cauliflower | Blackberries |
| Lentils | Brussels sprouts | Nectarines |
| Chickpeas | Celery | Plums |
| Black-eyed beans | Onions, spring onions, leeks | Peaches |
| Green peas | Pepper (green or red) | Pears |
| Sweetcorn | Bok choy, cabbage | Grapefruit |
| Pumpkin | Kale | Oranges |
| Barley | Mushrooms | Watermelon |
| Winter squash | Aubergines | Pineapple |
| Quinoa | Courgette (summer squash) | Cherries |
| Millet | Carrots | Mango |
| Whole wheat | Runner beans, green beans | Kiwi fruit |
| 100% whole grain bread, cereal, and pasta | Lettuce and all leafy salad leaves | Melon/cantaloupe |
| All other whole grains and starchy vegetables | All other nonstarchy vegetables and greens | All other whole fruits (dried fruits in limited quantities) |

## LEAN PROTEIN, HEALTHY FATS, AND DAIRY

| Lean Proteins | Healthy Fats | Dairy (Fat-free or Low-Fat) |
|---|---|---|
| Chicken breast | Fish oil (supplement) | Milk |
| Turkey breast | Flax oil (supplement) | Cheese |
| Lean beef | Olive oil, extra virgin | Cottage cheese |
| Fish | Nuts | Yogurt |
| Shellfish | Nut butters | Greek yogurt |
| Eggs and egg whites | Seeds | |
| Lean pork | Avocado | |
| Venison and other game meats | Coconut | |
| Protein powder (supplements) | | |

## THE BURN THE FAT, FEED THE MUSCLE MEAL BUILDER: A SIMPLE TEMPLATE FOR CREATING FAT-BURNING MEALS

Once you're familiar with the highest-quality foods and you understand the different food groups, the next step is to pick the foods you like and put them together into your own customized meals. The classic bodybuilder's meal is a lean protein, a starchy carb, and a fibrous carb. Here's the template:

**STEP 1: Choose a lean protein for every meal.**
**STEP 2: Choose a starchy carb for every meal.**
**STEP 3: Choose a fibrous carb for every meal.**
**STEP 4: Add healthy fats into some meals as needed to reach your daily goal.**

It doesn't get much simpler. As long as you understand which foods are lean proteins, starchy carbs, and fibrous carbs, it's as easy as one, two, three. Even if you don't track your macronutrients by the numbers, if you follow this template for most of your meals, your numbers will be in the ballpark.

Think of all our templates for meals and daily meal plans as easy starting points and guidelines, not as commandments carved in stone. Later in the chapter, I'll show you some alternative templates and ways to customize daily meal plans. For now, here are a few ways you can modify the meal template to suit your preferences.

1.  **Swap fruit for fibrous carbs.** Some people eat vegetables for breakfast (veggie omelettes, for example), but fruit is a popular breakfast food, so in the *Burn the*

*Fat, Feed the Muscle* meal template, you can swap fibrous carbs for fruit if you choose. Fruit doesn't have its own slot in this template, but I encourage you to include fruit in your meal plans.

2. **Swap fruit for starchy carbs.** Although fruits have fibre, most fruits also have a substantial amount of metabolizable carbohydrate calories, so fruits make a suitable exchange for starchy carbs at times. For example, in a meal of eggs, spinach, and oats, you could drop the oats and have fruit instead. If you need to keep your calories low or you want a very simple meal, another option is a lean protein and fruit (for example, hard-boiled eggs and a banana).

3. **Dairy products are optional.** Lactose intolerance is common and some people don't want to use dairy for other reasons. An advantage of including dairy foods is that they're a source of high-quality protein. There's not as much protein in most servings of dairy as there is in lean meat, fish, or eggs. But foods such as Greek yogurt and fat-free cottage cheese give you enough to count it as a lean protein in our meal template.

4. **For variety, eat more than one fibrous or starchy carb per meal.** As long as you stay within your calorie and macronutrient target ranges, you can have more than one of each natural carb if you choose. For example, broccoli and cauliflower (two fibrous carbs), or rice and beans (two starchy carbs).

### *Burn the Fat, Feed The Muscle* Meal Ideas: Breakfast

The first step in creating a breakfast is to select a lean protein; eggs are the classic choice. Using egg whites can help you get more protein while controlling the calories. But including at least one whole egg in your egg meals provides valuable nutrients from the yolk, and the whole egg is more filling than the whites alone. The second step is to choose a starchy carb such as porridge or a 100 per cent whole grain bread or cereal. The third step is to choose a fibrous carb such as veggies for an omelette, or have fruit instead. Walnuts or ground flaxseed are also popular additions to porridge.

There's no reason you can't have vegetables and fish for breakfast if that's what you want. But a more traditional breakfast usually includes either hot cereal, cold cereal, or whole grain bread for complex carbs; a piece of fruit for simple carbs; and eggs, protein powder, or a dairy product for protein. Be careful with cold cereals: Most of them are processed and filled with sugar, which is one reason why hot old-fashioned porridge made from rolled or steel-cut oats is so popular on this plan. If you want it sweeter, try it with berries or natural apple sauce.

If you're looking for easy ways to eat more vegetables, put them into your omelettes and scrambles. Spinach and mushroom omelettes are a low-carb favourite. Peppers, onions, and tomatoes are also great for egg recipes. Potatoes go well with eggs when you have room for more starchy carbs. For Mexican eggs, add salsa (and low-fat cheese if you have room for the calories). For a Greek omelette, try spinach, feta cheese, and olives.

Yogurt or cottage cheese and fruit is a popular light, quick breakfast or mid-morning snack. Protein smoothies with fruit are also great in the morning or anytime you're in a hurry. Rolled oats can also be added as a whole food ingredient in a protein drink; that's been a hotel room breakfast for me many times (cheaper than the restaurant too).

Here's a week of sample breakfasts:

|  | Lean Protein | Starchy Carb | Fibrous Carb (or Fruit) |
|---|---|---|---|
| **Breakfast 1** | Scrambled eggs | 4-grain hot cereal with flax | Blueberries |
| **Breakfast 2** | Vanilla whey protein | Old-fashioned porridge with cinnamon | Apple sauce or chopped apples |
| **Breakfast 3** | Hard-boiled eggs | Sprouted grain bread | Mixed fruit bowl |
| **Breakfast 4** | Egg omelette (with veggies) | Steel cut oats (with chopped walnuts) | Spinach and mushrooms |
| **Breakfast 5** | Egg scramble | Potato | Peppers, onion, salsa |
| **Breakfast 6** | Skimmed milk | Shredded Wheat | Grapefruit |
| **Breakfast 7** | Greek yogurt | None (light meal or snack) | Banana |

### *Burn the Fat, Feed the Muscle* Meal Ideas: Lunches and Dinners

As with all meals, for lunch or dinner, you begin by choosing a lean protein such as chicken breast, lean beef, or fish. Second, you choose a starchy carb such as brown rice, yam, or potato. Third, choose a fibrous carb such as broccoli or salad.

Here's a week of sample lunch or dinner meals:

|  | Lean Protein | Starchy Carb | Fibrous Carb (or Fruit) |
|---|---|---|---|
| **Lunch/Dinner 1** | Chicken breast | Brown rice | Broccoli |
| **Lunch/Dinner 2** | Salmon | Yam | Asparagus |

| Lunch/Dinner 3 | Lean beef, topside | Baked potato | Green and veggie salad with olive oil balsamic dressing |
|---|---|---|---|
| Lunch/Dinner 4 | Tilapia fish | Lentils | Mixed vegetables |
| Lunch/Dinner 5 | Lean minced turkey | Rice and beans | Salsa |
| Lunch/Dinner 6 | Extra-lean minced beef | Whole grain pasta | Tomato sauce, salad |
| Lunch/Dinner 7 | Sliced turkey breast | Wholemeal bread | Lettuce and tomato, apple |

## *BURN THE FAT, FEED THE MUSCLE* TEMPLATE FOR CREATING DAILY MEAL PLANS

You can use a template for daily meal plans just as you did for individual meals. Using templates makes everything "plug-and-play" easy and allows unlimited variety. All you have to do is choose the foods and plug them into the slots. The baseline nutrition template is where most people start. The accelerated fat-loss ("competition diet") templates, which have fewer starchy carbs and more protein, are the next level; we'll cover that in the final chapter.

### The *Burn the Fat, Feed the Muscle* Daily Meal Plan Template

First, let's take a look at a blank template:

| Meal 1 Time: | Lean protein Starchy carb Fibrous carb |
|---|---|
| Meal 2 Time: | Lean protein Starchy carb Fibrous carb |
| Meal 3 Time: | Lean protein Starchy carb Fibrous carb |
| Meal 4 Time: | Lean protein Starchy carb Fibrous carb |
| Meal 5: Time: | Lean protein Starchy carb Fibrous carb |

Here's an example of a *Burn the Fat, Feed the Muscle* daily meal plan for men, based on the previous template:

| Meal 1 | Scrambled eggs/omelette (2 whole, 3 whites) | 5 |
| Time: 6:00 a.m. | 1 slice wholemeal toast | 1 slice |
| | Spinach | 30 g (1 oz) |
| | Mushrooms | 30 g (1 oz) |
| | Orange | 1 medium |
| Meal 2 | Vanilla whey protein | 1.5 scoop |
| Time: 9:00 a.m. | Old-fashioned rolled oats | 65 g (2¼ oz) |
| | Banana | 1 large |
| Meal 3 | Chicken breast | 175 g (6 oz) |
| Time: 12:30 p.m. | Baked potato | 225 g (8 oz) |
| | Green salad with cucumber and tomato | 135 g (4¾ oz) |
| | Olive oil and balsamic dressing | 2 tbsp |
| Meal 4 | Salmon | 150 g (5 oz) |
| Time: 3:30 p.m. | Yam | 175 g (6 oz) |
| | Asparagus | 175 g (6 oz) |
| Meal 5 | Lean beef, topside | 175 g (6 oz) |
| Time: 7:30 p.m. | Brown rice | 200 g (7 oz) |
| | Broccoli | 100 g (3½ oz) |

Total: 2,344 calories; 195 grams protein, 278 grams carbs, 47 grams fat

Here's an example of a *Burn the Fat, Feed the Muscle* daily meal plan for women calories), based on the previous template:

| Meal 1 | Scrambled eggs/omelette (1 whole, 3 whites) | 4 |
| Time: 6:00 a.m. | 1 slice light wholemeal toast | 1 slice |
| | Spinach | 30 g (1 oz) |
| | Mushrooms | 60 g (2 oz) |
| Meal 2 | Greek yogurt, vanilla | 175 g (6 oz) |
| Time: 9:00 a.m. | Banana | 1 medium |
| Meal 3 | Chicken breast | 115 g (4 oz) |
| Time: 12:30 p.m. | Baked potato | 175 g (6 oz) |
| | Green salad with cucumber and tomato | 135 g (4¾ oz) |
| | Olive oil and balsamic dressing | 2 tbsp |
| Meal 4 | Salmon | 150 g (5 oz) |
| Time: 3:30 p.m. | Yam | 150 g (5 oz) |
| | Asparagus | 75 g (2¾ oz) |

| Meal 5 | Lean beef, topside | 115 g (4 oz) |
| Time: 7:30 p.m. | Brown rice | 150 g (5 oz) |
| | Broccoli | 70 g (2½ oz) |

Total: 1,690 calories; 144 grams protein, 195 grams carbs, 34 grams fat

An alternative schedule with a later morning start might be: meal 1 – 8:00 a.m.; meal 2 – 12:00 p.m.; meal 3 – 3:30 p.m.; meal 4 – 6:30 p.m.; meal 5 – 9:30 p.m.

Women who are short and small framed, who don't have a large calorie budget, might opt for the four-meal plan or the three-meals-with-snacks plan.

To make sure your calorie and macro numbers are on target, add up your meal subtotals and your daily meal plan totals. Then increase or decrease the serving sizes so you're close to your calorie and macronutrient goals. If you want the most precision, use a spreadsheet, app, or nutrition software. You can download a free interactive meal planner Excel sheet at www.BurnTheFatFeedTheMuscle.com.

Some people find making daily meal plans challenging at first, but usually only because they're trying too hard to micromanage their macronutrients. Remember, macronutrient ratios don't have to be perfect. If you stick close to this template, the macros will fall right into the ballpark. After your initial setup, you'll simply need to adjust the serving sizes to get close to your calorie target.

Schedule a time for each meal, because those mealtimes will become habitual. If you have an unorthodox schedule, don't worry that you're not eating when most other people are eating; eat at your own times, but make it a regular schedule. Your body thrives on regularity, so avoid random or haphazard eating.

The old rule was that you must eat six times per day, or every three hours. This is the approach that I use and that helped me win more than two dozen trophies in natural bodybuilding championships. There's no question about how well it works, especially for building muscle. But nowhere is this carved in stone. Many people adopted it simply because it has been the most popular meal plan in the physique world.

There has, however, been a shift in recent years toward greater flexibility in meal schedules to accommodate goals, personal preference, and metabolic individuality. Even among fitness athletes, today you'll see some choose fewer meals if they are small bodied, less active, and pursing weight loss, while others spread their calories into more meals if they are large, active, and pursuing muscle gains. This customized approach makes more sense than any rigid, prescribed plan, which leans in one direction or the other.

## CUSTOMIZING YOUR DAILY MEAL PLANS

The modern style of bodybuilding nutrition we use in *Burn the Fat, Feed the Muscle* is so flexible that anyone can do it. Eating anywhere from four to six times per day fits into our basic template, and every meal doesn't need to be a formal sit-down affair that requires food prep and cooking. There are many solutions for customizing your meal plan to make it fast, easy, and convenient. Here are three of them:

1.   **Include snacks in your daily meal plan.** Most people already eat at least four or five times per day, they're simply not eating the right foods and they don't have any structure; they grab snacks at random between meals or on impulse at night. Instead of snacking carelessly on junk food, build snacks strategically into your schedule and, if possible, include protein in most of them. If you eat breakfast, lunch, and dinner and include two or three snacks in between, you're eating five or six times. There you have it: You're feeding the muscle and eating like the leanest, fittest people in the world.

2.   **Make a shake or smoothie for one of your meals.** Protein drinks and meal replacement shakes are a big help to many people – and I'm not saying that because I sell them. I have no affiliations with the protein supplement industry. I recommend getting the majority of your calories and nutrients from whole foods. I mention shakes simply because they solve the convenience problem for many people while simultaneously helping you reach that important protein goal. When you're in a hurry, drink a meal instead of eating it. If you get creative with smoothie recipes, you can also boost the nutritional value of your drinks by adding whole food ingredients such as fruits, vegetables, oats, flaxseeds, nut butters, and so on. If your shakes taste good, it makes compliance easier too.

3.   **Try a four-meal schedule.** Another option for the busy person is the four-meal-a-day plan: breakfast in the morning, lunch in the afternoon, dinner in the early evening, and one more meal (or a snack/shake) later in the evening. Many people avoided this type of schedule in the past because they thought eating at night was not allowed if you want to burn fat. We cleared up that misconception in a previous chapter. If you want a nighttime meal, you can, but you must plan for it and keep it inside your daily calorie budget. If you train at night, then a big night meal may be a great option because it gives you the proper post-workout nutrition.

If I wrote one set of meal plans and said you had to follow them to the letter, it might create some problems. What if you were allergic or intolerant to half the foods? What if you don't like some of the foods? The fact is I don't know what you like to eat. No other diet expert knows, either, without consulting you personally.

There are nutrition principles that everyone must follow, but if you want the best results and the most enjoyable experience, the ultimate solution is to customize your meal plans rather than follow someone else's. Suggested food lists, sample meals, and sample daily meal plans are helpful as idea starters, but you should be able to fill in the blanks and make swaps easily. The best news is that all it takes to get started is one good meal plan that you enjoy.

## MEAL PLAN VARIETY:
## WHAT THE LEANEST PEOPLE IN THE WORLD DO

When it comes to the need for variety, everyone is different. But among the leanest people in the world, they usually share a unique trait: When they're pursuing an important physique goal, most of them follow the same meal plan every day. People who've had the greatest success on *Burn the Fat, Feed the Muscle* eat mostly the same thing during the early phases. As time goes by, they swap out foods and try new meals whenever they get bored. Most have two or three favourite meal plans – a total of 10 to 15 different favourite meals – and they rotate those over and over again.

Contrary to what many people have been taught, eating the same thing every day or following the same meal plan each day can help you automatically eat less and maintain long-term fat loss. Behavioural studies have shown that when you're given too many choices, you not only become confused about what to eat, you also tend to eat more. Eating more or less the same every day also turns new behaviours into habits quickly, makes it easy to track calories, and helps you establish a baseline sooner, making it a snap to troubleshoot plateaus. One caveat: If you're like me and you eat mostly the same foods every day, it's a good idea to get as much within-day variety as possible (make each meal different). There are more than 40 essential nutrients you must consume to maintain good health and no food contains all of them. It's also a good idea to take a multivitamin/mineral supplement for nutritional insurance, especially when you're in a calorie deficit.

If you're the gets-bored-easily type of eater who demands more variety, exchanging foods is simple when you have a template. From your original meal plan, swap the old food for a new food *from the same category*: fibrous carbs for fibrous carbs; lean proteins for lean proteins; and so on. This will keep your macronutrient numbers approximately the same.

For example, if you want to exchange rice, look on the food list for other types of natural starchy carbs. You'll find yams, baked potatoes, beans, pulses, whole grains, and many other options. The possible meal combinations are endless. You're not limited to the foods listed in this book, but our *Burn the Fat, Feed the Muscle* food lists will give you a lot of good ideas.

## HOW TO MEASURE AND TRACK YOUR CALORIES AND MACRONUTRIENTS

Weighing food is the most accurate way to track calories and macros, and that's why a set of kitchen scales are a prominent appliance in every *Burn the Fat, Feed the Muscle* kitchen. A set of scales are helpful for weighing meat, fish, vegetables, potatoes, and many other foods. If the weight is listed on a package, you can eyeball the serving size from that alone. For example, a typical bag of frozen vegetables is 450 grams (1 pound), so if you want 225-grams (8-ounce) serving, then use half of the bag. If a package of chicken is 500 grams (18 ounces) and you need a 170-gram (6-ounce) serving, simply divide the package into thirds. You can also use measuring cups for tracking calories and nutrient values by volume. Oats and cereals are typically measured dry and uncooked. Rice and pastas are generally measured after cooking. Keep in mind that some calorie counter guides include cooked and uncooked food values. The important thing is to not confuse the two.

With enough repetition of positive habits, making healthy choices and getting your numbers in the right ballpark becomes second nature. You won't need to count, weigh, and measure everything for the rest of your life, unless you want to. But in the early stages, think of counting and tracking as vital parts of the learning process. The precision is also helpful when you're going after big goals. For example, I don't weigh and measure my food all year round. After eating this way for years, it's totally habitual and unconscious for me. But if I want to prep for a competition, you'd better believe I'll go back to doing it by the numbers.

If you never count, weigh, or measure, you'll never go through the learning process that allows you to become unconsciously competent. You'll always be guessing, running blind, and probably underestimating your calorie intake badly more often than you think. Give counting and tracking at least 28 days, and by then you'll already have new habits developing. Give it a few months and you'll have a real knack for portion sizes, and then, just by estimating, you'll have a better idea of approximately how many ounces or grams are in any food item.

## HOW TO MAKE NUTRITIOUS FOOD DELICIOUS FOOD

There's a persistent myth about fat-burning nutrition that if it's health food, it must taste bad – or the flip side, that if something tastes good, you shouldn't eat it. Even the fitness legend Jack LaLanne said it (one of my idols, so God bless him, even if his well-meaning advice wasn't quite accurate). This myth was probably perpetuated because many athletes choose to eat very plain and simple diets, which makes it easy to prepare the food, follow the plan, and track the numbers.

The truth is, as long as you hit your calorie and macronutrient goals, you can do as much cooking as you want and as much spicing as your taste buds desire. You can enjoy delicious meals every day if that's important to you. If not, you can keep your meal plans plain and simple.

Starting with basic, plain meals is simply another part of the learning process. Unless you're already a food-savvy master chef, the learning curve usually goes like this:

1.  Familiarize yourself with the best foods and work off a food list.
2.  Learn how to put together individual foods into meals.
3.  Move on to fancier, multi-ingredient, multi-step recipes.

Step three could easily fill up another book (if enough people bug me for a *Burn the Fat, Feed the Muscle* cookbook, we'll see about that). For now, I'll give you a few tasters (below) that are so easy to make, they don't require explanation. Also, you should know that you can freely use herbs, spices, and seasonings such as black pepper, garlic powder, chilli powder, oregano, parsley, tarragon, thyme, dill, ginger, cinnamon, nutmeg, chopped onion, cumin, paprika, and, yes, even a pinch of salt here and there.

You can also add any low- or no calorie condiments, sauces, lemon juice, light dressings, low-calorie marinades, rubs, salsa, or sweeteners (if you wish to avoid artificial sweeteners, stevia is popular and now widely available). If you use any condiments that have calories, be sure to add those into your meal plan totals because little things forgotten can add up to an "unexplainable" plateau over time.

Sometimes extra virgin olive oil is an essential ingredient in some recipes, but you'll save a lot of calories by getting away from butter and oil in general. On fat-loss programmes, most people don't have the extra calories to spend. Instead, a light coat of nonstick cooking spray does the trick.

## SAMPLE BREAKFAST RECIPES

| Meal Template | Portable Apple-Cinnamon High-Protein Oat Pancake | Healthy Greek Omelette | Lazy Person's Mexican Eggs | Pumpkin Spice Porridge |
|---|---|---|---|---|
| Lean Protein | 1 whole egg 3 egg whites | 1 whole egg 3 egg whites | 1 whole egg 5 egg whites | 1 scoop vanilla whey protein |
| Starchy Carb | 65 g (2¼ oz) rolled oats | | | 55 g (2 oz) oats |
| Fibrous Carb | | 30 g (1 oz) spinach | 30 g (1 oz) low-fat grated cheese | ½ can pumpkin |
| Extra (Spices, etc.) | 1 scoop vanilla whey protein; ½ apple, finely chopped; cinnamon | 8 olives, pitted; 120 g (4 oz) feta cheese | 65 g (2¼ oz) salsa, chilli powder | cinnamon, nutmeg, sweetener |

## LUNCH AND DINNER RECIPES

| Meal Template | Muscle-Making Teriyaki Chicken Stir-fry | Simple Salmon Salad Sandwich | Tom's Baked Tilapia | Beefy Spanish Rice |
|---|---|---|---|---|
| Lean Protein | 150 g (5 oz) chicken breast | 1 x 175 g (6 oz) can salmon 1 tablespoon light mayo | Tilapia | 350 g (12 oz) lean minced beef |
| Starchy Carb | 150 g (5 oz) brown rice | 2 100% whole grain pittas (makes 2) | Sweet potato | 350 g (12 oz) long-grain brown rice (cooked) |
| Fibrous Carb | 90 g (3¼ oz) each chopped carrots, green pepper, mushrooms, onions | 25 g (1 oz) finely chopped celery; 80 g (3 oz) finely chopped onion | Broccoli | 425 g (15 oz) can diced tomatoes; 2 tbsp tomato purée; 1 green pepper; 1 large yellow onion |
| Extra (Spices, etc.) | Low-calorie teriyaki sauce | 2 tbsp lemon juice; 1 tsp ground black pepper; 2 tsp dill | Season tilapia with olive oil, lemon juice, paprika, parsley, oregano, pinch of salt | Worcestershire sauce, thyme, garlic powder, black pepper |
| | (serves 1) | (serves 2) | (serves 1) | (serves 2–3) |

## WHY YOU SHOULD "CHEAT" AND MAKE
## FREE MEALS A PART OF YOUR PLAN

To an athlete, food is fuel, food is building material, and at times great nutritional discipline is required to achieve big goals. But food is also one of life's great pleasures and an important part of our social lives. When you deprive yourself completely, it can make you more likely to binge, crave missed foods, and give up. It's simply human nature to want what you can't have. That's why, for most people, it's better to allow cheat meals. But there's a right and wrong way to do it.

Many diet programmes recommend an anything-goes cheat day once a week. That might work for some people some of the time, especially when a big cheat day follows a week or more of very strict dieting. But while I do recommend strategic re-feed days, I don't recommend free-for-all cheat days. The former are planned and measured parts of your programme. The latter are more like gluttony and can easily go too far, break your momentum, and backfire. If you care about your physical and mental health, stay away from anything remotely resembling bingeing or a starve-binge cycle.

Even with cheat meals, the key is planning. The most effective strategy I've used is to stay on a meal schedule seven days a week, but enjoy one or two weekly cheat meals as part of the plan. A good rule of thumb for most people is the 90 per cent compliance rule. That means follow the *Burn the Fat, Feed the Muscle* food lists and eat healthy, natural, nutrient-dense foods 90 per cent of the time (90 per cent of your weekly calories or weekly meals). For your cheat meals, eat anything you want and lose the "forbidden foods" mentality.

Consistency is another key. Honouring your compliance rules and staying on a meal schedule are hallmarks of all the fittest and leanest people. If you're inconsistent, you don't allow good habits to form and you stay stuck in that horrible cycle of cheat/guilt, binge/starve, and "start-over Mondays." If it's a part of your plan, it's not really cheating, and if it's not cheating, there's no reason to feel guilty. That's why many followers of *Burn the Fat, Feed the Muscle* prefer to call them "free meals," not "cheat meals."

Most people track the calories in their free meals carefully, but either way, remember that there are two kinds of compliance. First, there's compliance to a calorie deficit, which is mandatory for weight loss. There's also compliance to a food list, which is actually more flexible than you might think. I know some people who comply with their clean foods list only about 80 per cent of the time, but as long as they hit their calorie deficit and macronutrient goals, they still get great results. But be careful not to get too lax. The lower you drop compliance to your healthy food list, the easier it is to start forming bad habits, the lower the nutrient density of your meals, and the unhealthier it gets.

## WHAT TO DO WHEN YOUR BEST-LAID PLANS GO AWRY

Life isn't always predictable and sometimes things happen that interfere with even the best of plans. But there's a solution for unexpected events: plan B, the plan for when you can't follow your plan.

First, remind yourself that there's no reason to get upset or frustrated just because you miss a meal or can't have an ideal meal. Most people beat themselves up mentally and emotionally after a single slipup (perfectionist thinking). Even worse, some equate a single mistake with absolute failure, as if one bad meal ruins an entire day or one bad day ruins an entire month (all-or-nothing thinking). One meal doesn't make or break you. Your habits make or break you. It's what you do every day, over and over, week after week, that matters the most.

Second, remind yourself that you *always* have choices. Then make the best choice possible in every situation. Even at a fast-food restaurant, you have choices. You can have a grilled chicken and water instead of the double bacon cheeseburger and fizzy drink. Even when only one type of food is being served, you *still* have a choice. You can choose *how much* food you eat. The calorie *quality* might be poor, but if you choose a smaller serving and get the calorie *quantity* right, at least you're obeying the law of energy balance and you won't get fatter.

## NOW CREATE A PLAN AND COMMIT TO IT!

*Burn the Fat, Feed the Muscle* is the next generation of fat-burning and muscle-building nutrition programmes – structured, by-the-numbers, but also more flexible than any conventional diet. Whether you're as disciplined as an athlete or you customize your plan to suit a more relaxed lifestyle, you must have a plan. Don't try to wing it. You can't "intuitively" eat properly from day one without educating yourself about food and developing a meal plan. The opposite is true: Proper eating gets turned over to your subconscious (i.e., becomes habit) only after you do the work and go through the conscious stages of the learning process first.

In our modern obesogenic environment – with social pressure, food marketing, eating cues tempting us at every turn, and technology making us more and more sedentary – being able to successfully guesstimate your nutrition or trust your innate feelings of hunger and satiety are not things that come naturally or easily. The surefire way to make eating well become second nature is by going through a learning process, and that includes setting goals, crunching numbers, planning meals, tracking food, and measuring progress. Then repeat. That is how you achieve unconscious competence and mastery.

It takes time to make changes in your daily eating habits and make those changes stick. There's no quick fix, but this chapter was loaded with little tips and tricks that you can start implementing not next week, not tomorrow, but today. As General George S. Patton said, "A good plan … executed now, is better than a perfect plan next week." So create your first meal plan, keep it where you can see it – as you do with all your goals – and get to it!

# *A*CTIVATE:

## CARDIO TRAINING (The 3rd Element)

Did you ever wonder why so many people fail to burn the fat off and keep it off by dieting? It's because that's all they do – diet! Eating less without moving isn't going to cut it. You must get active!

Good nutrition alone can get weight loss started and improve your health, but there's one thing eating right can't do: it won't make you fitter. Why settle for leaner and healthier when you can get leaner, healthier and fitter? How would you like more endurance, more energy, and a natural endorphin "high" as bonuses? You get all that when you add cardio training into the mix.

The benefits don't end there. Why settle for getting leaner when you can get leaner faster? That's what else cardio training does for you. You can only cut calories so far. Why work on only one side of the fat-burning equation when you can work on both sides – with cardio – and burn fat faster?

Wait, it gets even better. Burning fat off is only half the battle. Keeping fat off is the other half, and for most people it's the toughest fight to win. That's the one solution that all the experts agree on: getting active and staying active is the key to lifelong maintenance.

Before you jump to it, here's a piece of advice to help you be absolutely sure you get permanent results. As you read through the chapter on cardio training, you'll see that there's no single best type of cardio. There's no one exercise that I force you to do. You get to customize your own plan, and your choices are endless.

The real key to success is to find an exercise you enjoy – then it won't even seem like work. You'll start to look forward to training, and when that happens, you've got it made: you're on your way to getting healthier, leaner, and fitter – for life!

# CHAPTER 15

# Maximize Your Fat Loss with Cardio Training

"To lose fat, you need to create a calorie deficit. This can be done using high- or low-intensity exercise. In other words, the best exercise for weight loss is to burn as many calories as you can in the time you have available."

– Christian Finn, MS, founder of muscleevo.net

## THE AMAZING BENEFITS OF CARDIO

If you know the secrets, cardio can be the number one key to accelerating your fat loss beyond what you could achieve with diet alone. If you do cardio right, you could double or even triple your rate of fat loss, boost your metabolism, increase your conditioning to an athlete's level, and get healthier than you've ever been. If you do it wrong, you will waste time and suffer consequences such as muscle loss, metabolic adaptation, joint pain, boredom, and burnout.

Enjoying the positives of cardio without the negatives is all about intelligently integrating cardio with nutrition, fine-tuning the balance between intensity, duration and frequency, and choosing the right cardio programme for your goals, your body type, and your lifestyle. This chapter will show you how.

## EXERCISE OR NUTRITION: WHICH IS MORE IMPORTANT FOR FAT LOSS?

Even if you ask top personal trainers, whose entire careers are devoted to preaching the benefits of exercise, almost all will concede that the priority for fat-loss success is nutrition, not training. There are two major reasons for this.

First, it's easier to create the initial calorie deficit by decreasing your food intake. If you are maintaining your weight and you eat 500 fewer calories every day – even if you did nothing else – you'll start losing weight. Yes, without the slightest physical exertion. If you are smart, however, you won't stop there, because as important as it is, nutrition is only one piece of a complete fitness programme.

Second, it's not only possible, it's easy to out-eat any amount of exercise if you're not watching your balance between calories burned and calories consumed. Trainers are constantly frustrated when their clients leave the gym and proceed to destroy all the hard work they did … with a fork and a knife! Sometimes they cancel an entire workout's calorie burn with one visit to the coffee and doughnut shop.

If you think, "There's no way I could eat so much that it would undo all my training," think again. Lean endurance athletes are a perfect example. They might burn as many as 5,000 calories a day biking, swimming, or running, but they don't lose weight. How is that possible? Simple: They put all those calories back – on purpose – to match their training demand. People who want to lose weight often do the same thing: They train like crazy, but they put all the calories back. The difference is they do it accidentally. They don't lose weight either. Oops!

This is why so many so-called experts believe that exercise doesn't work for weight loss. They claim that people compensate by eating too much after starting an exercise programme, replacing the extra calories they burned. "Well, no kidding!" I yell at them. "Don't put all the calories back! It's called dietary restraint!" Working out isn't a free pass to eat as much as you want.

## THE ULTIMATE SECRET TO FAT LOSS

The secret to fat loss is so simple, it's a tragedy that it hasn't clicked yet for the millions of people struggling with excess body fat. Read the following paragraph as many times as you need to until you get it. Understanding this distinction is the key to it all.

The secret to fat loss is not exercise. It's not what foods you eat either. *The ultimate secret to fat loss is achieving a calorie deficit, and consistently staying in that deficit until you reach your goal.* Nutrition is only one way to achieve the deficit: You decrease calories in. Training is the other way: You increase calories out.

Your gut reaction on reading this may be "It can't that simple: We've heard 'Eat less and exercise more' for years and it hasn't solved the problem." I agree. I didn't say *eating less and exercising* more is the secret. I said *maintaining a calorie deficit* is the secret. Exercising more is a poor crutch for a bad diet or ignorance of calorie maths. Training more to increase a deficit, on the other hand, accelerates fat loss every time.

Focus on the deficit. It's a simple concept on paper, but not easy to manage in the real world. It takes knowledge, awareness, diligence, discipline, honesty, and consistency. The good news is, when you get it intellectually and then you apply it, you'll gain total control of your body and you'll never have to worry about body fat again.

## THE FINAL NAILS IN THE COFFIN
## FOR DIET WITHOUT EXERCISE

If nutrition gets ranked as the most important element for fat loss and you can lose weight with diet alone, then why bother training? Why not just cut calories and save yourself a lot of time and sweat? This is not an unreasonable question. My answer is: If you burn the fat with training, you get better body composition, better health, and better fitness than if you starve the fat with diet alone. You can also get results faster.

If you have a 500-calorie daily deficit, and you want to accelerate fat loss, increase it to 750 or 1,000. One way to do this is by decreasing your food intake more, but you can cut only so many calories until you're starving and bad stuff starts to happen. That leaves cardio training – on the "burn more" side of the equation – as the prime method for increasing your deficit.

If there are two sides to the energy balance equation – food in versus calories burned – then working only on the food intake side is like going into a fistfight with one hand tied behind your back. You could fight one-handed, but why would you want to? You'll be at a disadvantage. You can lose weight without training, but without some type of vigorous physical work, you'll never burn fat at the maximum possible rate.

Exercise is also crucial for keeping the fat off. There's so much research backing up this point, even experts who promote only dieting for weight loss admit that exercise is vital for weight maintenance.

Simply eating less does nothing to make you stronger, fitter, or more athletic. Diets can actually make you a smaller version of your old self – weighing less, but still flabby and weak. If you want only a smaller trousers size, you can achieve it by dieting. If you want a new body that's lean, muscular, and looks as good out of clothes as it does in clothes, training is mandatory.

## THE DIFFERENCE BETWEEN ACTIVITY AND TRAINING

All physical activity counts. Even gardening, walking around town doing errands, and vacuuming the house burns calories. But obviously some activities don't burn much or have much effect on carving out a muscular body, so we don't count them as formal training.

Your miscellaneous activity is part of NEAT, which, if you recall, is the acronym for non-exercise activity thermogenesis. The more you walk and the more activity you get throughout the day, the better. It all adds up, and it can nudge along your fat loss nicely over time. But it's the formal type of training we'll focus on, because that's what really transforms your body quickly and dramatically.

In *Burn the Fat, Feed the Muscle*, there are two types of formal training, resistance and cardio. Both can burn large amounts of calories and help you lose fat, but we'll consider them as two separate endeavours, with distinctly different purposes. You'll focus on weight training for gaining strength, building muscle, and reshaping your body. You'll focus on cardio training for heart health, conditioning, and fat burning.

## WHAT TYPES OF EXERCISE ARE BEST FOR CARDIO TRAINING?

Our definition of "cardio" is any exercise that's rhythmic in nature, involves large muscle groups (namely your legs), and raises your heart rate and breathing, and which you can sustain for extended periods of time. The idea here is to pick an activity that has the potential to burn a lot of calories. You have plenty of choices.

### Running or Jogging Outdoors

On the pro side, running is an outstanding cardio workout, the fat-burning potential is very high, it's free, and it doesn't require equipment. On the con side, running outdoors may not be possible, depending on the weather and where you live. If you're a beginner, running may be too intense, and if you're overweight, have orthopaedic problems, or are injured it may not be feasible. High-volume endurance training, especially running, can also interfere with muscle size and strength gains. If you enjoy running, ignore naysayers and go for it, but keep the risks and benefits in mind.

### Walking

Walking is ideal if you're overweight, a beginner, or you don't have the disposition for intense types of training. If you enjoy being outdoors and you have open space, parks, trails, or long stretches of beach near your home, walking or hiking can be a real joy and your cardio won't feel like work at all. There are few downsides except that the intensity is low, so you don't burn many calories per minute. Push the pace if you want to burn more. Walk at least 40 to 60 minutes a day for best results. Do it all at once or split it into shorter sessions. A pedometer is a great gadget for tracking your steps. The Fitbit is a popular one with *Burn the Fat, Feed the Muscle* readers.

### Treadmills

Many people prefer the outdoors, but treadmills do have advantages. They're nice when the weather is bad, and you can't beat the convenience of having cardio equipment at home. Good treadmill decks are designed to flex, which reduces impact forces. Treadmills also give you continuous feedback on their electronic consoles, including time, speed, distance, and heart rate. The calorie readouts on cardio machines are not always accurate, but if they let you input your body weight, it's a decent estimate. Most treadmills elevate to at least 10 per cent to 12 per cent. Walking uphill can increase the fat-burning potential and is a type of cardio almost anyone can do. Wearing a weighted vest can bump the calorie burn even more.

### Stationary Upright Bicycle

Stationary cycling has moderate to high fat-burning potential, it's superb for cardiovascular conditioning, and it's a killer leg workout. Cycling is also preferred by many bodybuilders because it doesn't compromise leg muscle size the way distance running does. Cycling is nonimpact, so injury potential is low, but you must pedal vigorously or turn up the resistance to maximize the calorie burn. A client once complained he wasn't losing much weight even though he was riding the bike an hour several times a week. I chuckled as I told him, "Turn on the power – you're pedalling at level zero." If you get bored easily, then crank up the tunes on your iPod or park your bike in front of a TV.

### Stationary Recumbent Bicycle

Recumbent bikes give you all the benefits of upright bikes, plus one more: The seats are ergonomically designed to be more comfortable, to support your lower back, and to reduce fatigue. This makes recumbent cycling a good option if you have lower back problems (or a bony butt!). Don't get too comfortable: Turn up the resistance and crank up the rpms if you want to maximize your calorie burn.

## Outdoor Cycling

Outdoor cycling can be a great fat burner, especially if you ride hills or push the pace and coast less. One long weekend ride can really boost your weekly calorie burn. Many people who prefer the outdoors find mountain biking or cross-country cycling not only excellent cardio but a great hobby or sport. If you dedicate yourself to a physically challenging sport you love – recreational or competitive – that can go a long way toward ending the struggle with body fat.

## Stair-climbers

Stair-climbing machines give you an intense cardio workout and they're excellent calorie burners, making them ideal for fat loss. Avoid leaning on the handlebars or side rails because it lowers your heart rate and reduces the calorie burn. Stair-climbing machines provide a nonimpact workout, although the repetitive motion can aggravate knee pain in people with pre-existing problems. The StairMaster StepMill is a favourite of mine: it looks like a mini-escalator with a rotating flight of steps to simulate real stair stepping. Killer!

## Cross-Trainer

Cross-trainers are similar to stair-climbers except they use a circular stride instead of an up-and-down stride. This circular, no-impact motion may be helpful for people working around certain knee injuries. Cross-trainers have increasing levels of resistance and ramps that let you change the angle, similar to a treadmill's incline. Some machines let you stride forward or backward or pump your arms. The fat-burning potential is moderate and may be high, but it's self-paced, so you must make a constant effort to maintain your speed.

## Rowing

Rowing machines give you a superb cardio workout with very high fat-burning potential. Rowing is a complete exercise, working all the lower body muscles as well as the upper-body pulling muscles. Rowing is a non-jarring, impact-free activity, so it's a good option for people seeking relief from lower body joint pain. Always use perfect form, and if you've ever had low back pain, use rowers with caution.

## Cross-country Skiing

Cross-country skiing has a very high calorie- and fat-burning potential because, like rowing, it also involves the upper and lower body. Being a no-impact activity is another advantage. Cross-country skiing machines are not found in many gyms, but they have a cult following. The machine does involve a certain degree of skill and coordination, but if you stick with it through the learning curve until the awkwardness is gone, you'll be well rewarded.

## Swimming

Swimming is a full-body exercise that puts your heart and lungs to the test. A great appeal for many people is the zero-impact nature of swimming: It's as friendly to your joints as cardio can get. The calorie burn can be very high, but to translate into significant fat loss, you have to be able to swim long enough for the calorie burn to add up.

An interesting debate raged for years because research and observation kept suggesting that swimming wasn't very good for reducing body fat. It was later discovered that exercising in water, especially cold water, can increase your appetite. This resolved the swimmer's body fat paradox and was another great example of how exercising more does not guarantee weight loss if you're not careful about your food intake.

## Classes and Boot Camps

Group exercise and aerobic dance classes have been around for ages, but in the last decade, boot camps, kickboxing, and circuit-training have taken off in popularity. Typically, body weight exercises and conditioning drills are done nonstop or in circuits, which is what makes the workouts cardiovascular in nature. Depending on the programming, the calorie burn can be extremely high. People who don't want to use cardio machines often find a happy home in these classes. But keep in mind that they usually can't replace traditional progressive resistance weight training. Cardio training and resistance training each stand alone as important elements of this programme.

## PICK THE CARDIO YOU ENJOY AND MIX IT UP IF YOU CHOOSE

You're not limited to this list or only one type of cardio; there are advantages to mixing it up. Constantly changing cardio programmes can make it difficult to calibrate and track the source of your results, but on the other hand, a change in cardio has been known to help break plateaus. Variety saves many people from boredom too. That goes for within the workout as well: There's no reason you can't pick three machines (or activities) and do 15 minutes of each instead of 45 minutes of one. If you do a lot of cardio, it's wise to alternate days of high-impact activities with days of days of low-impact activities, or alternate high-intensity cardio with low-intensity cardio. This simple trick saves a lot of people from chronic joint pain and burnout.

Workout styles come and go, but you don't have to do things by the book or follow the crowd. Sometimes it's the trendiest workouts that have the highest dropout rates. I believe that if you keep your options open and pursue the training you enjoy the most, you'll get the best results in the long run.

## FREQUENCY OF CARDIO TRAINING: HOW OFTEN?

How often you should train depends on your goals, your schedule and your desired rate of progress. Three days per week is a good starting point for almost everyone, because it's enough to enjoy health benefits, improve your conditioning, and increase fat loss. I like to call three cardio workouts a week a baseline. You may do more at times, but when you're committed to the fitness lifestyle, you usually won't do less.

If you're not highly active already, it's easy to increase your fat loss simply by increasing your training frequency. Suppose you burn 400 calories per workout, three times a week. That's a total of 1,200 calories a week. If you increased that to six days per week at 400 calories per workout, you would burn 2,400 calories per week. If all else remained equal, you've doubled your fat loss! That was a no-brainer, wasn't it?

What would happen if, in addition to increasing your cardio from three to six days per week, you increased the intensity so you were burning 600 calories per workout? With six workouts at 600 calories per workout, you'd be up to 3,600 calories per week. You just tripled your fat loss!

Could speeding up fat loss really be that simple? Well, your body is deviously complex in the ways it can adapt or trigger compensation, and there's a point where doing more brings diminishing returns or get impractical. But if all else remains equal, then yes: The more often you do cardio, the more calories you'll burn and the more fat you'll lose. You don't even need to know how many calories every workout burns; just realize that there's a direct dose-response relationship. When you multiply frequency with duration and intensity, you can accelerate your fat loss exponentially.

Let me put it this way: If I were overweight and I knew what I know now about fat loss, I would be doing cardio every day, possibly even twice a day, seven days a week, until I was happy with my weight. Only then would I taper down to a maintenance programme.

That said, it's usually better to build up gradually. Many beginners try to do too much too soon, then they find themselves burned out or injured, especially if the cardio was intense or high-impact. Start with at least three sessions per week, and if your goal is maximum fat loss, progressively build up to five, six, or seven days per week as your weekly results dictate.

---

***BURN THE FAT, FEED THE MUSCLE* FREQUENCY GUIDELINES FOR CARDIO TRAINING**

| For Maintenance, Health, and Fitness: | For Maximum Fat Loss: |
| --- | --- |
| 3–4 days per week | 5–7 days per week |

---

## DURATION OF CARDIO TRAINING: HOW LONG?

If your cardio is high in intensity, the sessions will be shorter and you'll still burn a lot of calories. If your cardio is low-intensity, you need to exercise longer for the calorie burn to accumulate. If your goal is fat loss, 30 to 45 minutes at a moderate intensity is usually more than enough time to achieve the type of calorie burn you need. In some cases, like interval training, where the intensity is very high, as little as 15 to 20 minutes can do it.

You could build up to 60 minutes a day, but you might consider splitting it up. For example, 30 minutes in the morning and 30 minutes in the evening is more doable for many people, and multiple sessions might stimulate your metabolism more. Keep in mind the possibility of diminishing returns. At some point it's better to tighten up your nutrition and train more efficiently. If you're doing an hour or more of cardio every day but you're not losing fat, you almost always have a nutrition problem. Double-check your food intake first, because throwing more cardio at this kind of "plateau" is like bailing water faster when there's a gaping hole in your boat. Fix the hole first, then bail!

Busy people need the most efficient workouts possible, and no one wants to waste time, so short, high-intensity workouts are popular for good reasons. Unfortunately, another reason that minimalist workouts are popular is because they sell better. The body of your dreams in "just minutes a day, a few days a week" is a powerful sales pitch.

There's a big difference between efficient training and fitness marketing hype. If you can't tell them apart, you're in trouble. I'm not sure whether to laugh, cry, or scream when I see other trainers advertising their "super-intense" four- or eight–minute workouts as ideal for fat loss. Claims like these are ridiculous. No matter how hard you train, you can burn only so many calories per minute.

Granted, don't fall into the trap of mindlessly punching the cardio time clock either. Logging a certain number of minutes doesn't necessarily guarantee the fat loss you want. If the intensity is too low, your progress will be slow.

Your mission is to find that "sweet spot" in the middle where intensity times duration yields the highest calorie burn. I believe that sweet spot – which provides both efficiency and effectiveness – is around 20 to 30 minutes of high-intensity cardio or 40 to 45 minutes of moderate-intensity cardio.

If you're a beginner, it's okay to increase the duration gradually. Many of our members said that walking to their mailbox was a "workout" when they were obese. They didn't get discouraged. They did what they could and added a little bit more each time. Today, some of them run marathons or ride in 100-mile bike races.

---

**BURN THE FAT, FEED THE MUSCLE DURATION GUIDELINES FOR CARDIO TRAINING**

| For Maintenance, Health, and Fitness: | For Maximum Fat Loss: |
|---|---|
| 20–30 minutes per session (moderate to intense) | 30–60 minutes per session (moderate) |
| | 20–30 minutes per session (intense) |

---

## INTENSITY OF CARDIO TRAINING: HOW HARD?

You can always burn more calories by working harder in the time you have, but there is a catch. If you sprint, you burn an enormous amount of calories per minute, but you won't last long. If you pace yourself leisurely, you could keep going for hours, but you won't burn many calories per minute. If you want maximum fat loss, the trick is to work hard enough so you hit that sweet spot for maximum calorie burn.

One way to find your ideal training intensity is by heart rate. The "age-predicted" method has been recommended in fitness books for decades. You estimate your maximum heart rate (MHR) with this formula: 220 minus your age. Then multiply your MHR by a target intensity range of 70 per cent to 85 per cent. Choose 70 per cent to 75 per cent for moderate; 75 per cent to 80 per cent for moderately hard; or 80 per cent to 85 per cent for hard.

Here's an example: If you're 30 years old, your estimated MHR is 190. For a moderately intense workout, multiply the 70 per cent to 75 per cent intensity range by 190 and you get a target heart rate zone of 133 to 143 beats per minute (bpm).

During each cardio session, periodically check your pulse at your wrist or neck. The easy way is with 10-second counts: Simply divide your 60-second target heart rate by 6. If your target zone is 133 to 143 bpm, your 10-second count is 22 to 24. If you're below your target zone, raise the intensity by increasing resistance, speed, or incline. Many people invest in a heart rate monitor. A chest strap transmits your heart rate to a wristwatch or cardio machine, letting you check your heart rate easily without interrupting your training rhythm.

The classic 220-minus-age formula can underestimate MHR in older adults and overestimate it in young people by as much as +/−10 bpm. A new equation (the Seals formula) was published in the *Journal of the American College of Cardiology*: 208 −(0.7 × age). This decreases the margin for error at the age extremes. If you really wanted to know your actual MHR, you'd need to do a maximal exercise test, in which an exercise physiologist hooks you up to a bunch of monitors and runs you faster and steeper until you cry uncle.

All heart rate formulas are only estimates, so use common sense about how your exertion level feels. If it feels ridiculously easy, then don't be afraid to increase the intensity. If it feels incredibly difficult, don't hesitate to decrease the intensity.

**BURN THE FAT, FEED THE MUSCLE INTENSITY GUIDELINES FOR CARDIO TRAINING**

| Moderate | Moderately Hard | Hard | Very Hard (Sprints) |
|---|---|---|---|
| 70%–75% of MHR | 75%–80% of MHR | 80%–85% of MHR | 85%+ of MHR |

## HOW TO ESTIMATE TRAINING INTENSITY WITH PERCEIVED EXERTION

The rating of perceived exertion (RPE) is a simple shortcut method for estimating the intensity of your workout. You simply rate how hard your workout feels on a scale from 1 to 10. Even though it appears simplistic and is completely subjective, perceived exertion is surprisingly reliable. Basically, if you think your workout is "very hard," like an 8 out of 10, it probably is.

Based on the 1 to 10 RPE scale, a 4 to 8 would be the ideal target zone for steady state cardio and also for hitting that fat-burning sweet spot – not too easy, not too hard.

**RATING OF PERCEIVED EXERTION (RPE)**
0   Nothing (no work: sitting or lying)
1   Very, very light
2   Very light
3   Light

4   Moderate
5   Somewhat hard
6   Moderately hard
7   Hard
8   Very hard
9   Very, very hard
10  Maximal (all-out)

## BREATHING AND SWEATING AS MEASURES OF EXERCISE INTENSITY

Breathing rate is another way to estimate training intensity. If you're not breathing heavily, you're not working hard. If you're so out of breath that you can't finish a sentence or hold a conversation (the "talk test"), your intensity is probably too high for steady-state training.

Sweating, on the other hand, is not a good gauge for training intensity or calories burned. Sweat is simply your body's cooling mechanism, which gets turned on when your body temperature rises. Heavy sweating will lead to weight loss but not fat loss. Water weight comes right back as soon as you rehydrate.

## HIGH-INTENSITY INTERVAL TRAINING (HIIT) FOR TIME-EFFICIENT FITNESS AND FAT LOSS

If you want to burn the most calories possible, the way to do it would be through high intensity and long duration. The problem is that intensity and duration are inversely related; or, as they say, you can't sprint through a marathon. You can't even sprint for 10 minutes. An all-out sprint will last only seconds, and a near-maximum sprint may last only a minute or two. There is a way, however, to combine higher intensity with longer duration and it's called high-intensity interval training (HIIT).

HIIT allows you to accumulate a larger volume of high-intensity work in a single session by alternating between short high-intensity work intervals and short lower-intensity recovery intervals. During the high-intensity interval, you push yourself above your normal training zone to the point where you start getting out of breath. During the recovery interval, you reduce the intensity enough so you reclaim the oxygen debt just in time to do another intense burst.

You can adjust the number of intervals, length of intervals, and the work-to-recovery ratio based on your goals and fitness level. Beginners might start with

6 rounds and work up to 8 to 12 rounds. The interval length can vary from 10- to 20-second all-out sprints to submaximal but intense 60- to 90-second bursts. You could make work intervals longer, but you'd be sacrificing intensity. Longer recovery intervals make it easier; shorter recovery intervals make it harder. For example, 60 seconds of work followed by 120 seconds of recovery (a 1:2 ratio) is easier; 60 seconds of work followed by 60 seconds of recovery (a 1:1 ratio) is harder.

For fat-loss goals, the duration needs to be long enough so the calorie burn adds up, but with interval training, you can get an effective fat-loss workout in as little as 20 minutes. That makes HIIT one of the most time-efficient types of cardio and a favourite for busy people. For cardiovascular conditioning, some types of HIIT are amazingly effective, even when the workouts are shorter.

You can do HIIT training on any type of cardio machine. You can also do HIIT running outdoors or with various body weight exercises or conditioning drills. There's no single best way, so be open-minded, experiment, and see what works best for you.

### Classic *Burn the Fat, Feed the Muscle* Fat-Loss HIIT Workout

The classic HIIT workout for fat loss is 8 to 12 rounds with 60-second high-intensity intervals and a 1:1 work to recovery ratio.

**Warm up for 3 to 5 minutes steady state at a low RPE.**
**High-intensity interval: Perform one minute of very hard work at 8 to 9 RPE.**
**Recovery interval: Perform one minute of light to moderate work at 3 to 4 RPE.**
**Repeat for 10 intervals (rounds).**
**Cool down for 3 to 5 minutes at a low RPE.**
**Total workout time: 26 to 30 minutes**

### Hill Running, Stadium Stepping, and Sprint Intervals

When you're ready for a real challenge, try running stairs. This is a form of sprint interval training in which you work all out, or close to it, for about 10 to 20 seconds, then recover. The work to rest ratio is usually 2:1 or 3:1. Here's how I do it:

I have access to a university stadium with a straight flight of 52 steps. Sprinting up takes about 10 seconds; walking down about 30 seconds. I warm up first, usually starting with walking, a slow jog, and then a run up before sprinting, usually 10 to 12 rounds. Some athletes do a lot more, but your intensity drops as your legs get fatigued, so go for quality, not just quantity.

If you want to top off the calorie burn to stimulate more fat loss, you could finish with a walk or jog around the track. Running stairs is also an amazing leg workout. Bodybuilders and figure athletes love it because they say it brings out the muscularity in their legs. Jogging up flights of stairs in a high-rise is another option if you don't have access to stadium steps.

No stairs? Hills get the job done, too, and may give you even more flexibility in the duration of your intervals because hills come in all sizes. Grassy hills are nice when available, as they spare you some of the impact from running on pavement. Running hills has a built-in safety factor too. Strength coach Steven Morris says, "Even an athlete with horrendous running form will be safe running hills. This is simply because the hill does NOT allow the athlete to over-stride nor does it allow them to reach top speed, both major factors in hamstring injuries."

No stairs or hills? Sprinting intervals on a level track, field, or beach are popular too. On these, be sure to warm up fully and play it safe, as pulled hamstrings are no fun. Because all types of sprint interval training are so intense, once to three times a week is all it takes. If you're also weight training, any more is overkill.

Running stairs, hills, or flat sprints are advanced workouts. Beginners need to slowly build up to it. If you're overweight, it may be a challenge just to walk up stairs, let alone run, not to mention that it might be too stressful on your joints. But as you get lighter and fitter, it's a challenge you might work toward. I know a man named Jon from Chicago who was at one time morbidly obese – 340 pounds (24 st 4 lb/154 kg), with a 60-inch (152-cm) waist. He lost 150 pounds (68 kg) and then started running the Willis Tower (formerly Sears Tower) and other skyscraper races. If he can do it, you can.

## HOW HIGH-INTENSITY TRAINING ACTIVATES THE "AFTERBURN EFFECT"

Here's another benefit of doing some of your cardio workouts with high intensity: It can boost your metabolism for hours after the workout is over. This is commonly known as the afterburn effect. The scientific term is excess post-exercise oxygen consumption (EPOC). This means you could literally burn extra fat all day long as you sit at your desk.

Low-intensity training doesn't stimulate much EPOC. The higher the intensity and the longer an intense workout is sustained, the higher the EPOC. According to Jack H. Wilmore, and David L. Costill in *Physiology of Sport and Exercise*, the EPOC after moderately hard training (75 per cent to 80 per cent of MHR) is approximately 0.25 kilocalories per minute. If the afterburn lasted for five hours, that would be an extra 75 calories burned after the workout is over. That's not earth-shattering, but if all else remained equal, that would burn an extra pound of fat every ten weeks.

When training intensity is high, that's when it gets really interesting. In a recent study from Appalachian State University, researchers had subjects cycle for 45 minutes nonstop. The intensity was about as high as it could go for steady state training: around 85 per cent of MHR. They measured an increase in metabolism that lasted 14 hours after the workout ended, including while the subjects were sleeping. The EPOC accounted for an extra 190 calories burned.

## IS THERE A BEST TIME OF DAY TO DO CARDIO?

The best time of day for cardio or any other type of training is the time you feel most physically energetic, most mentally focused, most motivated, and most likely to make it a habit and stick with it. The way I see it, all other considerations are secondary, even if there are physiological advantages from training at specific times. Your daily training schedule is one of those personal things where it's best to listen to your body and keep practical considerations in mind.

Many people have had great success training in the morning. Some of the benefits may be behavioural or psychological. Taking positive action in the morning starts your day on the right foot and makes you feel good all day long. This may help you stick with your plan the rest of the day because you'll want to stay consistent and keep your momentum going.

It's easy to blow off evening workouts when you're exhausted from work. When you train at the beginning of your day, your workout is out of the way. And remember, no matter how busy you are, you can always make time for training by getting up earlier in the morning.

## CARDIO FED OR FASTED?

Many bodybuilders believe that cardio on an empty stomach helps them get leaner. Their preferred time is first thing in the morning after the overnight fast. This practice has been controversial for as long as it's been popular. Downsides for fasted cardio include concerns about muscle loss and low training energy. The upside, say proponents, is that it should allow fat to be more easily released from fat cells into circulation and then burned for energy. Whether doing cardio fasted improves body composition from week to week is the question still being debated. We would need more long-term research on people with different body fat levels to know for sure.

Bodybuilders have low body fat to begin with. When you're already lean and you want to get even leaner, every little nutrition and training detail counts, so that might explain their preference for and apparent success with fasted cardio.

If you're debating whether to eat before a morning workout, there are a few factors to consider. One is intensity. Most people have more energy, feel better mentally, and perform better physically when they have some fuel in them. If you're lifting weights or doing intense cardio in the morning, it's probably ideal to have one of your meals beforehand, including protein. If you must train immediately at daybreak and don't want a full meal churning around in your stomach, you could at least have a light meal, a snack, or a protein drink and then eat your first full meal after training.

If your morning workout is only cardio, most people have no problem doing it fasted before breakfast (a cup of coffee helps!) as long as the intensity is not too high. Low or moderate intensity cardio isn't that stressful and doesn't require that much energy, so the risk of muscle loss is low. Who knows, you might see better fat loss too. In the bigger scheme of things, it probably doesn't matter much whether you do your cardio fed or fasted. If you do it consistently and maintain your calorie deficit you'll get leaner either way.

## CARDIO BEFORE WEIGHTS, AFTER WEIGHTS, OR IN A COMPLETELY SEPARATE SESSION?

When you schedule your training is completely up to you. Timing is secondary to training consistently and achieving your calorie deficit consistently. In a perfect scenario, there are advantages of doing cardio and weight training in separate sessions or at least doing cardio after weights in the same session.

Research at the University of Victoria in British Columbia found that weight-lifting performance suffered right after doing intense cardio and up to eight hours afterward, especially for the legs. It's tough to do cardio after an intense leg workout and even tougher to do a leg workout after intense cardio. If you separate cardio and weights, fatigue won't get in the way as much. The fresher you are at the start of each workout, the stronger you'll be and the harder you can train.

Sometimes, however, what's optimal on paper is trumped by personal preference and practical considerations. Many people feel fine doing cardio right after weights, not to mention that schlepping to the gym twice is inconvenient. So if you do cardio and weights in the same session, which should come first? The answer is: whichever is the higher priority. On *Burn the Fat, Feed the Muscle*, maintaining muscle is the top training priority, so weight training goes first and cardio second.

## DOES CARDIO MAKE YOU LOSE MUSCLE OR STRENGTH?

There's been a lot of research about the interference effects between strength training and endurance training. It's clear that your body can't achieve maximum results in both endeavours concurrently because many strength and endurance adaptations in muscle fibres, organelles, hormones, enzymes, and capillaries are antagonistic to one another. It's unlikely that you'll see an active marathoner win a bodybuilding contest. To excel at a sport, the training demands must be specific to that sport's goals. This is why so many strength athletes are conservative about cardio and some even shun it. But does cardio always interfere with weight training? Will cardio make you lose muscle? What about people whose primary goal is fat loss?

Research plus real-world results from competitive bodybuilders suggest there's plenty of room for both. Weights are the first priority, but most bodybuilders integrate cardio in small amounts year round and in larger amounts before contests. The cardio is instrumental in helping them achieve peak condition, and they have no problem maintaining their muscle mass as they get ripped.

In moderation, cardio might even enhance muscle development. Cardio helps increase nutrient clearance from the blood and uptake into the cells. It can increase capillary density, which enhances delivery of oxygen, nutrients, and hormones to the muscles. It also helps remove waste products from working muscle tissue. As your cardiovascular fitness improves, you can recover faster from weight training. And of course, if you've sucked wind after a set of squats, you can appreciate the role of good cardio in a strength training workout.

With moderate amounts of cardio, muscle loss shouldn't be a concern. If your cardio volume is so high it looks more like an endurance athlete's regime, you may be compromising some strength and it will pay to monitor your lean body mass closely. High-volume endurance training while on a very low-calorie diet can be catabolic, and has been known to cause metabolic adaptations even more severe than starvation dieting alone.

## CARDIO PERIODIZATION: THE FAT LOSS SECRET OF THE LEANEST PEOPLE IN THE WORLD

Despite the promise of getting leaner faster, there seems to be, if not a loathing of cardio due to the time, effort, or boredom involved, then certainly an irrational fear that too much cardio will do bad things to you. The fact is the human body is a remarkable machine, and at least for short periods can perform a lot more work than most people give it credit for. Almost all of the negatives you hear about cardio are related to long periods of high-volume training, without proper recovery periods in between, or from doing large amounts of cardio in an aggressive calorie deficit.

Getting all the positives that cardio has to offer, without the negatives, is mostly a matter of doing more cardio when you need it and less when you don't. In weight-lifting and other strength sports, periodization is a strategy used by all the top athletes. Instead of constantly pounding their bodies with long, hard, heavy workouts, they vary their intensity, volume, weight and other training variables in weekly, monthly and yearly cycles. This allows them to achieve peak performance without burnout or injury. Why more people don't apply this concept to cardio training is a mystery to me. Doing hard cardio for hours every day or seven days a week, month after month, year after year, is unnecessary and may lead to overuse injury, suppressed immunity, overtraining, mental burnout, or aerobic adaption.

To a certain degree, adaptation is a normal part of getting in shape. The more you train, the more efficient you get at doing the workouts until you eventually need a more challenging workout to keep improving. But the smart way to make improvements and reach new peaks is through cycles and seasons of varying workloads, not putting your body through ever-increasing and never-ending stress.

Competitive bodybuilders are the true masters of peaking their physiques for a deadline and getting better and better, year after year, throughout their careers. Cardio periodization is one of their secrets. There's a maintenance phase (athletes sometimes call it an off season) and a peaking phase (the pre-contest season). During the maintenance phase, you do less cardio and during the fat loss or peaking phase you do more. Your body fat level will go up a bit when you cycle back to the off-season phase, but with each successive phase you shoot for a new all-time best condition.

This isn't just for bodybuilders; it's a smart strategy for everyone. Once you've achieved your target weight and body fat level, don't stop doing cardio, but don't keep blasting away for hours either. Slowly downshift into a maintenance phase. Once or twice a year, if you want a challenge, ramp up the cardio again and go for a personal best.

## BURN MORE! BUT MORE IS NOT ALWAYS BETTER

When being introduced to *Burn the Fat, Feed the Muscle* and the burn-more philosophy for the first time, it's not uncommon for readers to misinterpret my enthusiasm for training as implying that more is always better. Considering the magnitude of the obesity problem and how profoundly sedentary most people are, more probably is better! But this is only true as far as it remains safe, practical, effective, and in alignment with your goals. For strength and power athletes, the best amount of cardio might be the least you can get away with. Physique athletes know they need more cardio before contests, but not so much in the off season. Endomorphs usually understand that they do better with more cardio all around.

What I'm really recommending is being willing to do what it takes to get the results you want at the speed you want them – and, most importantly, to customize your own plan.

---

### QUICKSTART

**Not sure how much cardio you should do for maximum benefit and minimum risk? Here's a simple shortcut formula, backed by research and experience: A fool-proof starting point is three to four days per week of the cardio of your choice, for 20–40 minutes at a moderate to high intensity. If you're already fit and your time is limited, do up to three sessions of high-intensity interval training (HIIT) per week. When you need to accelerate fat loss, simply increase the duration and frequency a little bit each week until you get the rate of fat loss you want.**

---

## YOUR PERSONAL CARDIO PLAN

The ultimate cardio programme is the one you design for yourself. This chapter has given you everything you need to create your own programme, so that's exactly how we're going to wrap it up. All you have to do is choose the following cardio training variables and write them down in the 28-day-plan calendar:

1. Frequency (how many days per week)
2. Type of cardio (you can mix it up or stick with the same type every session)
3. Duration (how many minutes)
4. Intensity level (% of MHR or RPE)
5. Mode/resistance/speed (steady state or intervals; incline, resistance level, or speed)

Let me give you three examples for one week and then you can map out your plan for all four weeks:

## Beginner Cardio Plan

| Mon. | Tues. | Wed. | Thurs. | Fri. | Sat. | Sun. |
|---|---|---|---|---|---|---|
| Treadmill walking | No cardio | Cross-trainer | No cardio | Treadmill walking | No cardio | No cardio |
| 30 min | | 30 min | | 30 min | | |
| RPE 5 | | RPE 5 | | RPE 5 | | |
| Steady state | | Steady state | | Steady state | | |
| 5% incline | | Level 5 | | 5% incline | | |

## Tom's Year-Round Fitness and Maintenance Plan

| Mon. | Tues. | Wed. | Thurs. | Fri. | Sat. | Sun. |
|---|---|---|---|---|---|---|
| Stationary cycle | No cardio | StepMill | No cardio | Lifecycle | No cardio | Hiking/walk |
| 24 min | | 30 min | | 24 min | | 60+ min |
| RPE 4/9 | | RPE 7 | | RPE 4/9 | | RPE 3 |
| 10 intervals | | Steady state | | 10 intervals | | Steady state |
| 1 min/ 1 min | | | | 1 min/ 1 min | | |

## Tom's Competition Fat-Loss Plan

| Mon. | Tues. | Wed. | Thurs. | Fri. | Sat. | Sun. |
|---|---|---|---|---|---|---|
| Stationary cycle | StepMill | Stairclimber | Stationary cycle | StepMill | Stairclimber | No cardio |
| 24 min | 30 min | 45 min | 24 min | 30 min | 45 min | |
| RPE 4/9 | RPE 8 | RPE 7 | RPE 4/9 | RPE 8 | RPE 7 | |
| 10 intervals | Steady state | Steady state | 10 intervals | Steady state | Steady state | |
| 1 min/ 1 min | | | 1 min/ 1 min | | | |

Now it's your turn: Go ahead and create your first plan. You can download additional free copies of the personal cardio planner at www.BurnTheFatFeedTheMuscle.com.

## Personal Cardio Planner

|  | Mon. | Tues. | Wed. | Thurs. | Fri. | Sat. | Sun. |
|---|---|---|---|---|---|---|---|
| **Week 1** | | | | | | | |
| **Week 2** | | | | | | | |
| **Week 3** | | | | | | | |
| **Week 4** | | | | | | | |

Remember to do a progress check at the end of every week, including weight, body composition, and a visual assessment. Cardio programmes are meant to be changeable and progressive. If you're not making the progress you want, then increase the intensity, duration, or frequency.

Ultimately, you can always depend on the feedback loop method; let your results dictate your approach. If your fat loss is too slow, crank up the cardio. If you're hitting your weekly goals with only a few sessions a week, no increase is needed. In fact, unless you have a deadline looming, it's best to do the minimum necessary and save the extra cardio for the peaking cycle or for breaking plateaus later down the road. It's always good to have an ace in the hole, and cardio should be one of yours.

# NEW BODY:

## WEIGHT TRAINING (The 4th Element)

What could be better than getting leaner, healthier, and fitter? How about getting leaner, healthier, fitter and stronger – and completely changing your shape into the body you've always dreamed of? Now we're talking! You can have all of that – if you'll commit to making this fourth and final element a part of your plan – and your lifestyle.

This is the part almost everyone misses when pursuing a weight-loss goal. And missing this element is why most weight-loss programmes fail. Including this fourth element – weight training – is what makes Burn the Fat, Feed the Muscle unique among fat-loss programmes, and why it succeeds so brilliantly.

In the two weight training chapters ahead, you'll learn all the reasons why weight training is so important, not only for fat loss, but to strengthen and shape your body. If you're a beginner who feels intimidated or scared by the weights, you can relax knowing that I've designed an entry-level "primer" programme just for you.

If you're experienced, don't worry about this programme being too easy. Even if you're a master's level lifter, I've designed a plan for your needs – it's called The New Body 28 (TNB-28). You can scale the difficulty level to where even athletes and bodybuilders will feel challenged.

When you think about how much effort you're going to put into this training programme, how diligently you'll follow the plan, and whether you'll merely do it for a month or two or, like the most successful physique athletes, you can make it a part of your lifestyle, remember this most of all: you can lose weight with a diet, but only weight training can increase your strength and literally give you a new body.

# CHAPTER 16

# Burn the Fat, Feed the Muscle Weight Training: The Principles

"There is nothing as good as bodybuilding to get your body tuned up and totally in shape."

– Arnold Schwarzenegger

## LIFT WEIGHTS, DROP FAT

It would be far beyond the scope of one chapter to teach you everything there is to know about weight training. A great example is Arnold Schwarzenegger's *Encyclopedia of Modern Bodybuilding*. It's 736 pages long, with 850 photographs! As an exercise science major in college, I spent an entire semester on weight training, and even that didn't scratch the surface. Weight training is an art, a science, and a discipline that you can study and practise your whole life, and it would take another book to do justice to the details.

However, no fat-loss programme is complete without resistance training because it plays such a crucial role in getting leaner. This surprises many people, who only think of diet and aerobics when they think of fat loss. A bodybuilder or strength athlete doesn't need convincing to make weight training priority number one. But most people with weight-loss goals think this doesn't apply to them. It's time to change that.

In this chapter, you'll learn the most important weight training fundamentals they teach you in school, as well as secrets from the trenches, known only by the best physique champions. You'll hear the truth about common muscle myths that might be holding you back and discover not only how to burn more fat but how to transform your body shape completely. You'll then be ready for my step-by-step 28-day training plan, The New Body 28 (TNB-28 for short), in the next chapter, which will get you started the right way and keep the results coming.

## SYNERGY: THE SECRET TO EXPONENTIALLY FASTER FAT LOSS

"It's 80 per cent diet!" is a common weight loss cliché. Even if this isn't literally accurate, it's fair to say that nutrition is the most important element for fat loss. That's because even if you have a perfect training programme, you won't lose weight without a calorie deficit. The success of any weight-loss goal hinges on getting this one nutrition detail right. But if you're smart and your goals go beyond weight loss to better body composition and permanent fat loss, then weight training is an equally vital part of the formula.

The secret to achieving your best body is in how well you implement all four elements of the programme at the same time. The combination of nutrition, cardio training, resistance training, and mental training together becomes greater than the sum of its parts. This is known as synergy, and it means that 1 + 1 + 1 + 1 might not equal 4, it might equal 40 or 400! When balanced properly, each element complements and enhances the others. The best example is the powerful phenomenon called partitioning, which is what happens when you put proper nutrition and weight training together.

The law of energy balance says that if you're in a surplus, excess calories will be sent into fat stores. That's more or less true for a couch potato. The law of energy partitioning says that if you're in a surplus, but you're weight training, some of those excess calories will be sent to your muscles for repair and growth. Imagine two people following the same meal plan with a calorie surplus. One lifts weights and the other doesn't. The one not lifting weights gets fatter. The one lifting weights not only doesn't get fatter, he gets more muscular by eating more!

This partitioning of calories and nutrients is even more interesting in the other direction. Two people go on the same meal plan in a calorie deficit. One person is lifting weights and the other isn't. Since the laws of thermodynamics can't be violated, you know they're both going to lose weight. The real question is: What kind of weight will they lose? The person not lifting weights loses lean body mass. The person lifting weights loses fat and keeps his lean body mass; he might even gain a little.

Two people. Same diet. Totally different results. This is more proof that weight loss and body transformation are not the same and that transformation goes far beyond calories in versus calories out. It's what your body does with the calories that counts.

Weight loss is a matter of energy balance. Body composition is a matter of energy partitioning. Your food choices, genetics, lifestyle, and hormones can all affect partitioning. But the biggest influence is weight training. Wouldn't you love to see the food you eat get delivered to your muscle cells for growth and recovery instead of being stuffed into your fat cells? Combine good nutrition with weight training and that's exactly what happens.

## HOW WEIGHT TRAINING HELPS YOU GET LEANER

One reason that weight training increases fat loss is obvious but is almost always overlooked: It burns a lot of calories. It's entirely possible for your weight training to burn more calories than your cardio, especially if you do a lot of energy-demanding exercises like squats, lunges, rows, presses, dead lifts, and other compound lifts.

An even bigger surprise is the metabolic boost. This afterburn effect is becoming mainstream knowledge, often written about in fitness magazines, but most people think it only comes from interval training. The truth is weight training can produce an equal if not greater metabolic boost than cardio. There's also a high-energy cost required for repairing muscle damage from training and for building new muscle. And these are only the short-term effects. There's also the long-term boost in metabolism you get from increasing your lean body mass. The higher your lean body mass, the higher your metabolic rate.

## WHY WEIGHTS SHOULD BE PRIORITY NUMBER ONE
## IN EVERY FAT-LOSS TRAINING PROGRAMME

For years, weight training was like the American comedian and actor Rodney Dangerfield: It got no respect. Weight lifters were viewed as weirdos or freaks. Athletes were encouraged not to lift weights. Just one generation ago, people thought that weight training made you slow and muscle-bound and raised your blood pressure. At one time even the medical establishment said to avoid weight training in favour of aerobics.

Today, all world-class athletes do serious weight training. Every pro sports team has a strength and conditioning coach. Doctors prescribe weight training for cardiovascular health, better bone density, and stopping sarcopenia as you get older. Psychologists recommend it for building self-confidence and even overcoming depression. In 1990 the American College of Sports Medicine released an updated position stand stating that weight training decreases cardiovascular risk factors and was good for your health all along.

It was great news when the scientific, medical, and athletic communities started supporting weight training, except for one thing. In perfect character with the notoriously fickle fitness industry, many strength-training gurus started flipping to the other extreme, saying that weight training is the only kind of training you need and that cardio is worthless or actually bad for you.

There's no question: You'll improve body composition far more with weights than you will with cardio alone. If you go overboard, cardio can interfere with strength, power, and muscle gains. However, in the right amounts, cardio and weights not only get along well together, they're great companions, producing the most rapid fat loss and dramatic physique transformations possible.

---

**QUICKSTART**

**Progressive resistance training – namely weight lifting – is the single most powerful body transformation tool you can use. A weight training programme combined with proper nutrition will burn fat and re-shape your body faster than any other single form of exercise. If you're ever in doubt about how to start working out, start with resistance training. Add cardio and other types of training from there.**

---

## THE TEN BIGGEST WEIGHT TRAINING MYTHS THAT HOLD YOU BACK FROM ACHIEVING YOUR BEST BODY

Weight training can seem intimidating at first because there's so much conflicting information about what it will and won't do for you. The misconceptions about training are endless, but these ten big ones are insidious because they prevent so many people from taking the first step. Let's bust these myths once and for all.

### MYTH #1: If fat loss is your goal and you don't have time for weights and cardio, you should just do cardio.

Resistance training is such a powerful health, fitness, and anti-ageing tool, it's the one type of training you never compromise. Weight training can burn fat, increase your strength, and maintain or build your lean body mass. Cardio alone can't do that. Weight training makes the difference between the person with an ideal weight but an average-looking body and the person who looks cut and chiselled like a fitness model. When you have time, do weights and cardio. When your time is limited, always prioritize the weights. With that said, please allow me to step on my soapbox for a minute to talk about time.

"I don't have time" is not a valid reason, it's an excuse. It's not that some people have more time; some people are simply better at prioritizing. You're being honest if you say, "Other things are higher priorities right now," but you can't honestly say, "I don't have time to work out." Many get up at five in the morning because it's the only time they can train. The rest of their day is full with work and family commitments. Paradoxically, it's often the busiest people who get more done than anyone else, because their schedule forces them to become masters of productivity. If they can do it, you can do it.

### MYTH #2: You should lose all the fat first, then start weight training later.

People who are extremely overweight may need to focus on nutrition at first if they're not very mobile yet. But if you're physically able to exercise safely, you'll get amazing benefits from starting a weight training programme, even if you still have a lot of fat to lose. Almost anyone can start with walking for cardio and basic lifts for strength, and it's never too soon to start developing good habits.

Yes, you can lose weight with diet and cardio or even diet alone, but many people who do that find they're not as happy with their bodies as they thought they'd be. They fit into smaller clothes, but they still don't want to be seen out of clothes. They look soft and unathletic. It's never too late to pick up the weights, but wouldn't it be better to start training from day one and finish with a stronger, harder and more athletic body?

### MYTH #3: You have to join a gym to get good results.

The best place to train is wherever you'll get the best workouts and do them consistently. I started working out in my parent's garage when I was 14 with nothing more than barbells, dumbbells, an adjustable Joe Weider bench, a squat rack, and an Arnold Schwarzenegger book to guide me. I did that for six months, then I joined a gym. I've been training in gyms ever since because I like having access to all the equipment and I enjoy the motivating atmosphere.

Gold's Gym, the original "bodybuilder's gym," where Arnold got his start, has been my favourite chain for decades (I even did a brief stint as a trainer for Gold's). It's my kind of place. Your kind of place may be different, but if you find the right one, your gym can become a second home and a great source of friends and partners who support your new goals.

The benefits of home training are convenience, privacy, and saving money you would have spent on gym memberships every year. If training at home helps you stick to your programme better, and you prefer the privacy, then train at home. Some of the exercises in the *Burn the Fat, Feed the Muscle* training programmes require machines, but it's easy to substitute other exercises.

Basic free weights are all you need to start at home. You can do hundreds of exercises with nothing more than dumbbells. Add a barbell set and a bench that's fully adjustable (from flat to inclined to vertical) and you can do hundreds more. If you have the space, the next equipment you want in your home gym would be a power (squat) rack with a pull-up bar, dipping bars, and a cable machine with a low and high pulley. You'll get more mileage from this simple setup than all the fancy machines they sell on shopping channels.

### MYTH #4: If you lift weights, you'll get bulky or look like a bodybuilder.

Most natural bodybuilders, myself included, would love to have more muscle size, but we're still working on it after years because gaining muscle is a slow and difficult process. Beginners can gain muscle easily at first, but the rate of progress levels off quickly. Only the most genetically gifted mesomorphs can gain muscle with ease. Putting on muscle size is even harder for women, who have less testosterone.

Despite my reassurance that every ounce of muscle gained is a hard-fought victory, most women (and some men) are still worried about getting too big. I think a major source of this fear is from misconceptions about pro bodybuilders. It's easy to look at the bulk on those guys and say, "If that's what lifting weights will make me look like, forget it!" What they don't realize is that they're looking at a mesomorph on steroids whose full-time job for the last ten years has been eating and training. Even if you do have Olympian genetics, you're not going to wake up one morning and notice that you've sprouted new muscle overnight. The process occurs very slowly and it doesn't happen by accident.

When you master the art of training, you're in total control of how your body looks. You're the artist and your body is your masterpiece. Cardio chisels away the excess you don't want. Lifting adds muscle like clay – right where you do want it. You can sculpt your body into the exact figure you want. You may not be a bodybuilder, but if you lift weights, you are a body sculptor. And remember, you can't sculpt anything with diet alone.

### MYTH #5: If you stop lifting weights, the muscles will turn into fat.

If you stop lifting, your muscles will eventually shrink, and if you eat too much, your body fat will increase. This may appear as if your "muscles have turned to fat," but muscle can't change into fat because fat and muscle are two different types of tissue.

This myth probably comes from the retired-athlete syndrome. Elite athletes practise, train, or compete for hours every day, burning huge amounts of fuel. When their athletic careers end, their activity levels drop, but if they keep eating the same amount of food, they instantly create a calorie surplus and start gaining fat. This makes it look like their muscles "turned to fat" purely because they stopped working out.

This programme is all about helping you develop long-lasting habits and a long-term outlook. If you make training a part of your new lifestyle, you'll never have to worry about shrinking muscles and rising body fat. If your activity level ever drops suddenly due to an injury or lifestyle change, all you have to do is recalculate your calories based on your new activity level and adjust your food intake.

### MYTH #6: If you lift weights, you'll lose flexibility and get muscle-bound.

The surest way to decrease your flexibility is to sit on your butt all day long doing nothing. Weight training can actually increase your flexibility if you perform the exercises through the full range of motion. I've seen male bodybuilders weighing 230 pounds (16 st 6 lb/104 kg) of solid muscle do full splits as part of their posing routines. As for the women, watch a professional fitness show like the Fitness Olympia. You'll see some of the most flexible athletes in the world, even though they train with weights every bit as hard as the men.

If increasing flexibility is one of your fitness goals, then devote some time for stretching at the end of your lifting sessions and emphasize the tightest areas. An easy way to fit stretching into your routine with no extra time commitment is to stretch in between sets. Some people add yoga into their weekly plan to gain more flexibility. Just remember that yoga is a good adjunct to weight training, it's not a substitute for it.

### MYTH #7: Women must train differently from men.

Most women who say they want to be "toned" mean that they want to get fitter and firmer without getting bigger. Guess what? The best and fastest way to achieve the "fitter and firmer" look women want is the same way that men achieve the "muscular" look they want: with weight training. And without it, a woman will never get much stronger.

A muscle either gets stronger and more developed or it doesn't. There's no such thing as "toning" or gender-specific exercise; these are just the perceptions created by the fitness industry. I don't think that's a bad thing if it gets more women involved. What I'm saying is that if women squat, lunge, row, press, and deadlift, just like men, they'll be rewarded with many times greater results than if they pursue some kind of dainty "toning" exercises with 3-pound (1-kg) pink dumbbells or follow exercise programmes that don't use resistance at all.

### MYTH #8: You have to lift for hours every day to get a great body.

You can finish an effective and thorough weight training workout in 60 minutes or less. While some people train longer for various reasons, and competitive athletes put in more hours a week than recreational lifters, more is not always better when it comes to resistance training. Short but intense workouts always produce great results, but intense training done too long or too often is counterproductive. Even if you could squeeze out more results by putting in more time, long workouts aren't practical for most people.

If your time is limited, avoid the all-or-nothing mind-set and make the most of the time you have by working as hard and efficiently as possible. The obvious way is to reduce the number of exercises while maintaining or increasing the intensity. You can also use supersets, where you do two exercises in a row nonstop, or decrease rest intervals between sets. These techniques can help busy people get great results in as little as 30 to 45 minutes.

### MYTH #9: Weight lifting will make you slow and unathletic.

Weight training makes you a faster and better athlete. Stronger muscles can contract more quickly and produce more power. Athletes in almost every sport depend on weight training to improve their performance. Look at sprinters: They're the fastest people in the world, and heavy lifting is a major part of their training.

Some strength coaches and athletes strongly endorse weight training but say that doing the wrong workouts will make you "nonfunctional." Outside of sport-specific training, "functional" has become a buzzword in the fitness world, but the definition is fuzzy. Usually it means that you should train in a way that improves your ability to function well in daily life or perform better in your sport.

If you're an athlete, you may need a specialized training programme designed specifically for your sport, so consult your coach for advice. Strength and performance are top motivations for athletes, but looking great and getting healthier are the top motivations for everyone. The good news is it's not an either/or choice: With my programme, you can have it all! You can get stronger, healthier, more functional – and get a killer body too.

### MYTH #10: You're the only one who feels overwhelmed, uncomfortable, confused, or not sure where to start.

You have the knowledge of all the world's experts at your fingertips today on the Internet, but more than ever you're also drowning in a sea of conflicting opinions and information overload. It's normal to feel a little confused or overwhelmed at first. The good news is you can relax, because what would take months or even years to find online and pull together, you have right between the covers of this book. You can also trust that the information here is backed by science and experience.

Even with a coach you trust and a plan you put faith in, most people feel a little intimidated when they first pick up the weights, especially in front of other people. I've lost track of how many times I heard this: "I would join a gym, but I have to get in shape first." The irony there might make some people chuckle, but maybe you can relate. The important thing to remember is that discomfort is normal, not just in training, but in every new endeavour. You're uncomfortable the first time you do anything, but you must step outside your comfort zone to grow.

## THE NINE *BURN THE FAT, FEED THE MUSCLE* RESISTANCE TRAINING SUCCESS PRINCIPLES

Now that you understand the importance of weight training in the fat-loss equation and we have all those pesky myths out of the way, we're ready to dive into the *Burn the Fat, Feed the Muscle* training plan.

First, you'll learn the training principles. Fads come and go every year, but core principles never change. If you build your training plans on a foundation of principles, you will never go wrong.

After the principles, we'll go on to the training plans. Start with the "primer programme" if you've never lifted weights before. After that, I'll give you the new flagship training programme of *Burn the Fat, Feed the Muscle*: the TNB-28 plan.

### Principle #1: Progressive overload

Progressive overload is the number one principle of all successful training programmes. Progression means that, whenever it's possible, lift more weight, do more reps, do the same workout in less time, or increase the workload in some other way that your body is not accustomed to doing. Stated differently, overload means that you're going on a mission to continuously aim for personal improvement and new personal records (PRs).

Any type of progressive overload can cause a positive adaptation – but progressive resistance, where you lift more weight than you have before, is the Holy Grail of building muscle and strength. It's not uncommon for beginners to add weight to the bar almost every week if not every workout. As you get more advanced, your improvements will naturally slow down to the point where progress must be coaxed slowly, in small increments every workout or even each week. PRs come even less often. Still, your goal remains the same: Keep challenging yourself. Keep improving.

Using a repetition range (such as 8 to 12) is helpful for guiding progression. When you reach the upper end of your rep range, then it's time to increase the weight.

Increasing reps, then weight, is known as the double progressive system. Here's an example of what slow progression on an exercise like the squat might look like:

| Weight in Pounds (kg) | Reps | Progression Stage |
|---|---|---|
| 225 (102) | 8 | Start at low end of rep range. |
| 225 (102) | 9 | Increase by one rep. |
| 225 (102) | 10 | Increase by one rep. |
| 225 (102) | 11 | Increase by one rep. |
| 225 (102) | 12 | Achieved rep goal; increase weight. |
| 235 (107) | 8 | Drop back to low end of rep range. |
| 235 (107) | 9 | Increase by one rep. |
| 235 (107) | 10 | Increase by one rep. |
| 235 (107) | 11 | Increase by one rep. |
| 235 (107) | 12 | Achieved rep goal; increase weight. |
| 245 (111) | 8 | Drop back to low end of rep range. |

This is a simplified example. Your progress usually isn't this linear. More often, progress comes in spurts and then plateaus. You might jump three steps forward and then one step sideways (or back). Sometimes you'll make fast strength gains and increase the weight every workout. At other times, you must be patient and move up one rep at a time. If you add even one more rep with the same weight each workout, that's progress.

When the honeymoon period of fast newbie gains is over, most people get frustrated at how long it takes to add even the smallest amounts of muscle or strength. But slow and steady is the secret to winning this race. Keep after it and be sure to track your progress using a written training journal. Each year, when you review your journal, you'll be amazed when you look at your PRs and see how far you've come.

The antithesis of progression is to go through the motions and repeat the same workout at the same workload over and over again. That might maintain your current condition, but it won't improve it. If you ever feel stuck, as if you're putting time into your workouts but not getting results, ask yourself how well you've been applying this principle of progression.

Write this on Post-it notes and add it to your affirmations list: "*I don't go to the gym to maintain; I go to the gym to improve. And if I want to improve, then today I must aim to beat my previous workouts and do something I've never done before.*"

Not every workout should be 100 per cent and you can't always increase the weight, but you can develop a constant improvement mind-set and a low tolerance for standing still. That makes training much more exciting, challenging, and motivating.

## Principle #2: Intensity

Training intensity is the amount of effort you exert – or, if you prefer, hard work! If you've selected the right amount of weight, the last two or three reps in a set should be difficult. You'll feel fatigue, the burn intensifies, the weight feels heavier, and it gets harder and harder to finish each rep. If your rep range goal is 8 to 12 and you hit the upper rep number – 12 – and it feels easy, the weight is too light and the set was not intense. If you stop when you still have three, four, or more reps left in you, then you're not challenging yourself. If you push yourself through the "good pain" of burn and fatigue to squeeze out those last reps, it can make the difference between a great body and an average body.

If you continue a set to complete fatigue, you'll hit a point where you momentarily can't do another rep. In lifter's lingo, that's known as reaching "failure." Whether you should push yourself this hard is a topic of great controversy. The science tells us that training to failure can increase muscle fibre recruitment, muscle tension, metabolic stress, and anabolic hormone release, which can all contribute to better muscle gains. However, training to failure all the time could lead to overtraining and mental burnout. As long as you keep using the progressive overload principle, you'll keep making progress whether you reach failure or not.

The ideal method is to include intense training (to failure) during some but not all of your workouts as part of a training cycle. This gives you the benefits of failure training without the overuse problems. When you train to failure, be sure to do it safely and intelligently. If you train alone, don't train to failure on exercises where you could get stuck under the bar. Use a spotter when you need one and *never, ever* push through the "bad pain" of injury.

## Principle #3: Optimal resistance

"Resistance training" is the general term used for lifting any kind of weight or working against any form of resistance, including your body (as in pull-ups or push-ups), elastic bands, and so on. An advantage of weight training is being able to measure and monitor the load down to the pound. Choosing the right amount of weight is important for getting the results you want.

The traditional way to calculate your optimal training load is the one-rep maximum test. It's exactly what it sounds like: You build up to the heaviest weight you can lift one time and that's your one-rep max. When you know your one-rep max, then you choose your training load based on a percentage of it. The traditional prescription is:

**70 per cent or less = light**
**70 per cent to 85 per cent = moderate**
**85 per cent or higher = heavy**

The one-rep max and percentage method are still widely used in strength sports, but to simplify this programme and avoid the need for heavy one-rep max testing, the loads in this workout are simply dictated by a rep max range or bracket:

**The 4 to 7 rep max range is considered heavy and is associated with the strength workouts.**
**The 8 to 12 rep max range is considered medium and is associated with the muscle workouts.**
**The 13 to 20 rep max range is light and associated with endurance workouts.**

What separates this programme from many others is that we use a combination of rep ranges instead of one prescription such as 3 sets of 10 or 5 sets of 5. Working in more than one rep range gives you the best overall results because it develops greater strength as well as greater muscle development.

Adding in some occasional lighter sets can be helpful for giving your joints a break, building endurance, and inducing circulation, but it's a mistake to drop all your heavy work. Doing high reps with light weights will not develop muscle definition or burn more fat; you can add that to the lifting-myths column.


### Principle #4: Optimal rep range

Choose a repetition bracket based on your goals or the effect you want to produce. To get stronger, athletes do a lot of training in the 4 to 7 rep range with heavy weights. Training in the 8 to 12 rep range with moderate weights is ideal for muscle growth. If you want muscular endurance or pump (increased blood flushing into the muscle), work in the 13 to 20 rep range.

Most people want both strength and muscle and that's one reason why it makes sense to train in multiple rep ranges, either in the same workout (concurrent) or alternating (undulating). I recommend doing both; that's why there are strength days and "muscle" (hypertrophy) days in this programme.

The simplest and easiest way to get started is to choose one rep range such as 3 × 8–12 (three sets of 8 to 12 reps) or, in the case of our muscle primer programme, 10–15 reps. Giving yourself a range lets you know when it's time to increase the weight and helps you use the progressive resistance principle.

| Rep Category | Rep Range | Weight | Benefit |
|---|---|---|---|
| **Low** | 4–7 | Heavy | Maximum strength |
| **Medium** | 8–12 | Moderate | Maximum muscle development, some strength |
| **High** | 13–20 | Light | Muscular endurance, metabolic conditioning, little strength |

## Principle #5: Optimal volume

There's no question that one set per exercise can produce results if the intensity is high enough. But as more studies have been done over the years, research has validated what I and other athletes have discovered through experience: The optimal approach is to do multiple sets of each exercise. In a review published in the *Journal of Strength and Conditioning Research*, author James Krieger concluded that multiple sets are associated with a 40 per cent greater increase in muscle growth as compared to the single-set approach.

Three sets per exercise has been a best practice for decades, but there's no reason you can't do two sets or four sets per exercise. Five sets of five is actually one of the most popular strength workouts. For strength workouts, when the reps are low, the number of sets per exercise is sometimes increased to keep the total training volume up. The total number of sets in a workout can also vary based on the body part. Larger muscle groups like your back can handle more volume than smaller muscle groups like your biceps.

## Principle #6: Optimal rest intervals

As a generalization, rest intervals can be described as very short (30 seconds), short (1 minute), medium (2 minutes), or long (3 minutes). If you're training for muscle, resting 60 to 90 seconds between sets is a good rule of thumb. That gives you enough time to recoup your energy and work capacity just enough to perform the next set without too much residual fatigue from the last set. If you're training for strength, it's ideal to extend rest intervals between sets to two or three minutes. This lets you recover more fully so you can do each subsequent set with maximum strength, but it's not so long that you start cooling off. You can use a wristwatch or timer if you want, but don't have to time your rest periods exactly; just get as close as you can and remember the general rule.

In some cases, there are advantages to reducing your rest intervals to as little as 30 seconds. Obviously, short rest periods between sets are a time-saver. Doing more work in less time is known as increasing training density. It burns more calories in less time and it's a way to use progressive overload without having to increase weight. The disadvantage is that short rest intervals provide incomplete recovery between sets and dramatically reduce the amount of weight you can use, which is not as conducive to strength gains.

Cutting all the rest between every set of every exercise would be circuit training, which is good for fitness conditioning and time efficiency, but then you're no longer doing true strength training; it's more like doing cardio with weights. On TNB-28, we keep cardio and strength training separate and distinct. A superset is where you perform two exercises in a row with no rest between them. You rest after the second exercise. In this programme we superset the arm exercises. For busy people who want to finish their workouts faster and don't mind the compromise, including more supersets and reducing rest intervals are great efficiency techniques.

### Principle #7: Optimal Tempo

Tempo is how fast or slow you do each repetition. We're going to keep it simple and use a two-point tempo prescription: lifting (concentric) and lowering (eccentric).

The concentric action is where you lift the weight and the muscle shortens or contracts. For example, when you curl a barbell up, that's the concentric part of the rep, where your bicep contracts and shortens. The concentric part of the rep should be done quickly but under control. It usually takes one to two seconds to lift the weight, depending on the exercise. As your muscles get fatigued toward the end of the set, it's normal for the movement to slow down as you struggle to finish the final reps.

The eccentric action is where you lower the weight back down and the muscle lengthens. If you go a little slower on the way down (eccentric emphasis), this may help increase your strength and muscle gains. A typical eccentric action is about two or three seconds, which simply means that you should lower the weight a little more slowly than you lift it. An easy way to remember this is to "fight gravity" on the way down instead of dropping the weight quickly.

Some trainers have taken this method to the extreme and promote "super-slow" reps, which may take 10 or 15 seconds to complete. It might sound like a good idea at first, but it's counterproductive to do your reps too slowly. Aside from being a tedious way to train, the biggest problem is that you have to use weights that are so light, you don't trigger the muscle response you want.

## Principle #8: Variation

Changing your overall workout structure and individual exercises regularly helps prevent you from getting bored and losing motivation. It lets you work your body from various angles with different training stimuli. It also helps you avoid plateaus from adaptation and keeps the progress coming.

Beginners can get results on the same workout for months before seeing the progress curve flatten. The more years you've been training (training age) and the more conditioned your body becomes, the faster your body adapts to each new stimulus and the more you'll benefit from frequent variation.

On the other hand, you don't want to change workouts too often. By constantly hopping from one programme to another, you don't establish continuity from one workout to the next, you don't allow time for progression on each exercise, you don't optimize your strength gains, and you really don't know what's working and what's not.

There are potential benefits to changing something in your workout every day, but don't change everything and don't change at random for no reason. Milk each routine for all its worth before switching to the next one. You can stay on the same programme as long as it keeps working for you, but as a best practice, every 12 weeks is a good time for an overhaul involving changing some of the exercises and trying new training tactics. Beginners should stick with their initial programme for at least three months. As your training age increases, you may want to make changes as often as every four weeks.

## Principle #9: Periodization

At its simplest level, periodization is planning. It means you never go into the gym without knowing what you'll be doing and what your goals are for the workout. Going deeper, periodization means a special type of planning where you structure your programme in blocks, phases, or cycles and you change the training variables regularly in a way that maximizes your strength and muscle gains while minimizing plateaus and injuries. A nice bonus: It keeps your workouts interesting and prevents boredom or burnout.

This typically means rotating or periodically changing loads, reps, exercises, and intensity. That might seem complicated, but the *Burn the Fat, Feed the Muscle* programme makes periodization easy. We use it in several simple but effective ways: We cycle intensity in 4-week (28-day) blocks, rotate exercises, change repetition ranges, and alternate heavy and moderate workouts, with a few lighter ones thrown in for good measure. Our way borrows techniques from both the strength training world and the physique world, so it's ideal for body transformation goals. What's most important to know is that a programme using periodization is always more effective than one that doesn't.

## PUTTING THE PRINCIPLES INTO PRACTICE

This may have seemed like a lot of details to take in, especially for a beginner. Anyone new to weight training might want to go back and review the information more than once before getting started on the workouts. Because these are foundational principles and not training fads that come and go like the latest fashion, it's well worth it for advanced trainees to review as well. No matter what your level of experience, in the next chapter you'll see how easy these principles are to follow and how they all come together seamlessly into a practical plan.

# CHAPTER 17

# *Burn the Fat, Feed the Muscle* Weight Training: The Programme

"If you could have only one reason to make strength training part of your fitness life, you might try this fact: It is the only way to reshape your body. Attempting to transform a body with cardio alone is futile."

– Shawn Phillips, author of *Strength for Life*

## FROM PRINCIPLES TO ACTION

In the last chapter, we dispelled the most common myths that prevent people from starting a weight training programme or from doing it most efficiently. We also listed the nine training principles that are most important to your fastest body transformation and continuous progress. That gives you all the background details and tools you need to start building, so in this chapter we are jumping right into the workout.

I first want to re-emphasize that this entire programme is built on principles. Change is a constant. You'll always need to change your workouts to prevent plateaus. You'll need new ideas to avoid boredom. You'll always be cycling the acute training variables such as choice of exercise, intensity, volume, and repetition ranges, just to keep progress coming. But those changes in methods take place on top of a bedrock-solid foundation of experience and science-based principles, not on the most fashionable current trends. The core concepts worked decades ago. They work today. They'll still work decades from now.

In this chapter, I'm going to give you the flagship training programme of *Burn the Fat, Feed the Muscle*: The New Body 28 (TNB-28) plan, which puts all these principles into action. The programme uses a template that's plug-and-play simple. The cycle lasts 28 days, but it doesn't end after 28 days: You can plug in new variables and continue on to your next level by repeating these 4-week cycles.

I'm thrilled to welcome men and women who are new to weight training to this programme and to our community. For the beginners, we'll start with a simple and easy but ultra-effective workout called the Muscle Primer Plan. Enjoy the beginner gains: It's the most exciting time to make quick progress! Combined with *Burn the Fat, Feed the Muscle* nutrition, mental training, and cardio training, even this basic starter programme can produce dramatic results in the first 28 days.

## THE MUSCLE PRIMER SCHEDULE

If you have at least three to six months of consistent training experience, then you can skip right ahead to the TNB-28 plan. If not, start with this Muscle Primer Plan, which is perfect for beginners or anyone who has been away from lifting for a long time.

You'll train your whole body at each workout, three days per week, on non-consecutive days, such as Monday, Wednesday, and Friday or Tuesday, Thursday, and Saturday. If you've never lifted weights before, you can break in slowly the first week and do one set your first day, two sets your second day, and three sets on your third day. This gives a beginner's body the first week to acclimatize to the new stress and prevent excessive muscle soreness. By week two, you'll be doing 3 sets of each exercise.

| Mon. | Tues. | Wed. | Thurs. | Fri. | Sat. | Sun. |
| --- | --- | --- | --- | --- | --- | --- |
| Full body weights | Off | Full body weights | Off | Full body weights | Off | Off |

### Equipment Required

I've chosen each exercise for a reason. They're not only the most effective and essential movements everyone needs to learn (squat, dead lift, press, row, etc.), I've chosen a variation of each exercise that's easy for a beginner to master and that can be done at home with minimal equipment. All you need is dumbbells.

Dumbbells (free weights that some people know as "hand weights") are a fantastic training tool on many levels. They encourage equal development on each side of the body, they allow natural, unrestricted range of movement, they require more activation in the stabilizer muscles, and they're great for every type of fitness goal. You can use them in a gym or at home, and if you lack space at home, you can get dumbbell handles that take weight plates of increasing sizes. You can also use adjustable dumbbell sets where one pair is the equivalent of an entire rack of solid dumbbells (examples: PowerBlock or Bowflex SelectTech).

Dumbbells will never go out of style: They are the first and best resistance training equipment investment you can make. You can buy dumbbells at any fitness or sporting goods shop or you can even shop for them online. You can buy a whole rack all at once, or you can add heavier sets one or two pairs at a time as you get stronger. If you plan to continue training at home, I recommend adding a fully adjustable bench, which will allow you to challenge yourself with a wider variety of weight training exercises when body weight exercises like push-ups get too easy. Add a soft mat for floor exercises, and you have everything you need.

### Warm-up and Stretching

It's important to warm up before each weight training session. Warming up raises your body temperature, increases joint mobility, stimulates blood flow, and increases your physical and mental readiness for the workout ahead.

The traditional way to warm up is to hop on a cardio machine for five to ten minutes. That's fine as a general warm-up, especially on lower-body day, but another option is joint mobility drills or dynamic flexibility exercises. Arm circles, trunk circles, leg swings, Spider-Man steps, squat to stand, body weight lunges, and so on not only warm you up, they also increase mobility and flexibility in the joints you're about to train. You can see these and other warm-ups in the free exercise demos at www.BurnTheFatFeedTheMuscle.com.

To increase your performance and decrease risk of injury, do at least one or two light, nonfatiguing sets of each exercise before moving on to your heavy work sets. It's not wise to jump right to your heaviest set or attempt a personal record if you're still cold.

It's important to remember that static stretching is for increasing flexibility, not for warming up. In fact, an ideal time to stretch is after you're already warm. That's why most athletes do warm-up and mobility exercises before lifting and do static stretching *after* the workout.

### Muscle Primer Plan Exercises

The exercises in the primer plan are so basic that they're self-explanatory or already familiar to people who have lifted weights before. However, any kind of free weights, even dumbbells, can be intimidating for a first timer, so I've listed the exercises below with a description of the form. I've put additional training information on the website for free. You can see photos of every exercise with more details and grab a quick-reference workout chart and log sheet at www.BurnTheFatFeedTheMuscle.com.

### 1. DUMBBELL SPLIT SQUAT (THIGHS): 3 SETS × 10–15 REPS

Holding a dumbbell in each hand, step forward into a lunge (split) position, with one leg in front and one leg in back. Squat down, lowering your back knee until it almost touches the floor. Stand back up, keeping a slight bend in your front leg so you maintain tension on your thighs.

### 2. ROMANIAN DEAD LIFT WITH DUMBBELLS (HAMSTRINGS/LOWER BACK): 3 SETS × 10–15 REPS

Hold a dumbbell in each hand, with your palms facing your body (pronated). Stand up tall with your feet no wider than shoulder width apart. Slowly bend forward, hinging at the waist. Keep your knees slightly bent and the dumbbells close to your body as you bend forward and lower the weights toward the floor. Keep your entire core tight and maintain a neutral back position, which means a flat back or slight arch in your lower back; do not round over your back. Return to the standing-straight-up starting position.

### 3. ONE-ARM DUMBBELL ROW (UPPER BACK): 3 SETS × 10–15 REPS

Grab one dumbbell with your right hand and place your left hand on a bench, chair, or ledge for support. Step back with your right leg so you have a stable support base. From arm's length, pull the dumbbell up to your waist. Keep your palm facing your body and keep your head up and back flat throughout the exercise. Slowly lower the dumbbell back down until your arm is straight and you feel a stretch. Switch arms and repeat.

### 4. DUMBBELL BENCH PRESS (CHEST): 3 SETS × 10–15 REPS

Grab a set of dumbbells and lie on your back on a bench. Begin with the dumbbells at arm's length over your chest, palms facing toward your feet. Lower the dumbbells to the sides of your chest, then press them back up to the starting position. If you train at home and don't have a bench, you can substitute push-ups for the bench press. Since it's a body weight exercise, you can keep increasing your reps beyond 15 each week instead of adding weight.

### 5. DUMBBELL OVERHEAD PRESS (SHOULDERS): 3 SETS × 10–15 REPS

Grab a set of dumbbells and sit on the edge of a bench or chair. Begin with the dumbbells at shoulder height with your palms facing away from your body. Press the dumbbells up until your arms are straight overhead. Slowly lower back to the starting position. You can also do this exercise standing.

#### 6. OVERHEAD DUMBBELL EXTENSION (TRICEPS): 3 SETS × 10–15 REPS

Standing, or sitting on the edge of a chair, hold a single dumbbell between both hands, cupping the weight so one side of the bell rests in the palms of your hand. Start with the weight over your head and your arms fully extended. Lower the dumbbell behind your head by bending at the elbows. Push the dumbbell back over your head (extend) until your arms are straight again.

#### 7. DUMBBELL CURL (BICEPS): 3 SETS × 10–15 REPS

Standing with your feet shoulder width apart, or seated on the edge of a bench or chair, hold a dumbbell in each hand with your palms facing up. Curl both dumbbells up together to shoulder height by bending at the elbows. At the top of the movement, your palms should be facing upward. Hold the contraction briefly and squeeze the biceps, then slowly return the dumbbells to the starting position. Keep your torso vertical and avoid leaning backward.

#### 8. SINGLE LEG CALF RAISE WITH DUMBBELL (CALVES): 3 SETS × 15–20 REPS

Stand on just the ball of your right foot at the edge of a step, a block of wood, or a thick book so your heel is off the edge. Holding a dumbbell in your right hand, rise up on the ball of your foot as high as you can go. Drop your heel below the edge until you feel a slight stretch in your calf. Repeat for the desired number of reps; then, without stopping, switch to the left leg and repeat.

#### 9. PLANK (ABS/CORE): 3 SETS X 30–60 SECONDS

Lie on your stomach on an exercise mat or carpeted surface. Prop your body up on your forearms and position your body in a straight line from head to feet. Hold the straight line position with your body several inches off the floor for 30 seconds. Increase your hold time by 10 seconds each week until you reach 1 minute per set (hold longer if you're an overachiever).

#### 10. CRUNCHES OR BICYCLE CRUNCHES (ABS): 3 SETS × 15–20 REPS

Lie flat on your back on a mat or soft surface with your knees bent and feet flat on the floor (or your heels on the edge of a bench or chair). Put your hands behind your head, touching your fingers to the back of your head. Raise your head, shoulders, and upper back off the floor in a curling motion, contracting your abdominals. To avoid neck strain, avoid pulling on the back of your head. To involve the oblique muscles on the side of the waist more heavily, perform the bicycle crunch variation, where you perform the crunch with a twist, touching your elbow to your opposite knee.

### Adjusting the Weight and Reps

In the last chapter I explained how to select the right amount of weight (principle #3). It's important to get this right because making progress is all about applying the proper resistance. Keep in mind that it may take a couple of sets or even a couple of workouts to adjust the initial weight.

An advantage of working in a rep range is that it helps you choose the right weight. If your target rep range is 10 to 15 reps, then you should be able to do at least the lower number (10). If you can only do 6 reps, for example, the weight is too heavy. If you can hit the upper number in the range (15) and it was easy, that's your signal that the weight was too light, so you should increase it.

In the primer phase, the reps for most of the exercises are a little higher (10–15) because that allows you more opportunity to practise proper form and ingrain the new movement patterns into your nervous system.

### When to Advance to the Next Workout

Follow this programme for the first three months. Some people find it tedious to continue with the same exercise for two or three months, so if you feel your progress is plateauing after the first or second month or you're losing motivation, then switch the exercises. Stick with the same exercises if you're enjoying the workouts and still progressing in weight and reps. After three months on the primer plan, you'll be ready for TNB-28.

There's nothing wrong with staying with a full-body workout for up to six months or longer if you continue to get great results from it and the simplicity of full-body training suits your style. What you'll need to do, however, is rotate your exercises every 4 to 12 weeks and continue to use the progressive overload, intensity, and variation principles. You'll also benefit from implementing the periodization principle, alternating heavy-rep-range and medium-rep-range workouts every other session or scheduling a heavy, medium, and light day for each of your three workouts.

## INTRODUCING TNB-28

Most people are not interested in building the mass of a heavyweight bodybuilder and they certainly aren't going to tan up, pump up, and flex in posing trunks or a teeny bikini onstage under a spotlight. But I've never met anyone who wasn't interested in staying lean and developing a more sculpted physique. I developed the TNB-28 plan with that in mind.

This programme borrows some of the most effective techniques from bodybuilding and physique sports, used by the leanest, most muscular people in the world, and combines them in a programme that fits the goals and lifestyle of the regular guy or girl. It's designed to work equally well for men and women, and to be done in a gym or at home (some equipment is required). You can easily modify it to fit busy schedules.

Follow it and you'll get stronger and leaner and completely transform your body shape. Guys will achieve the natural muscular look (think *Men's Fitness* cover model or all-natural bodybuilder if you want to take it further). Girls will sculpt a curvaceous "hard body" with feminine muscle in all the right places in just the right amount. (Have you seen what figure athletes look like?)

Wherever your body is now, this plan will take your physique to the next level. The TNB-28 programme will challenge you even if you're already in good shape, because you can increase the difficulty level and repeat the 28-day cycles more than once, each time hitting new personal records and new peaks in your condition. I'll give you tips to customize the programme so it fits your level of experience the best.

In all my years as a fitness pro, TNB-28 is the most popular, most effective, most talked-about type of resistance training programme I've ever created. It's been tested behind the scenes in our Inner Circle community for years, and what you're getting here is the newest evolution of the plan. TNB-28 is the lean-muscle training programme of the future.

### Equipment Needed

This programme uses a mix of barbells, dumbbells, and weight machines. You can do it in a gym or you can follow it at home with basic equipment. If you don't have access to all the machines, you can easily substitute an equivalent free-weight exercise. For example, if you don't have a cable pulley machine for triceps push-downs, you can do a barbell or dumbbell triceps extension. If you don't have a lat pull-down machine, you can do dumbbell rows, dumbbell pull-overs, or even inverted rows under a sturdy table. You can also go off the TNB-28 exercise list and pick any alternative exercise you want.

## Exercises

Changing exercises and other programme variables at least every few months gives your body new challenges and keeps training fun and interesting.

There are a handful of very important basic movement patterns including squats, lunges (split squats), dead lifts, rows, pull-ups, chest presses, and shoulder (overhead) presses. Master them. These exercises should always be a major part of your training plans. However, there are countless variations on each of these movements: barbell and dumbbell versions, different stance or grip positions, different bars, and so on. You can use these variations on the basics to mix things up without getting away from the primary movements.

The "big lifts" – multi-joint, compound exercises such as squats, dead lifts, rows, and presses – have the highest calorie burn and are the most effective muscle builders. They're also the most challenging. Single-joint isolation exercises like leg extensions and small-muscle exercises like concentration curls can be a part of any weight training programme and they're especially useful for bodybuilding and fine-tuning physique details. But avoiding the difficult exercises like squats in favour of the easier ones like leg extensions is a sure way to short-circuit your results.

Adding more exercises on top of a beginner routine is another method of progressive overload. But more isn't always better. For example, in workout one of the TNB-28 plan, there's only one exercise for biceps and one for triceps. In their eagerness to build arms like Mr. Olympia, many lifters add a second or even a third exercise for the arms or they double the number of sets. On a two-day split with four workouts per week, this is unnecessary. Between one direct exercise and all the pushing you do on shoulder and chest exercises and all the pulling for back exercises, your biceps and triceps get plenty of stimulation. If you add too many more exercises, your workouts take a lot longer and could lead to overtraining.

The following exercise menu includes all of the exercises listed in the primer workout and the TNB-28 workout. Underneath, you'll also find exercises that you can use as alternatives, based on your equipment availability and preferences. TNB-28 is a workout template. When it comes time for a new routine, you simply choose new exercises and plug them in. To see proper form for all the exercises, visit www.BurnTheFatFeedTheMuscle.com. Be sure to subscribe to the e-mail newsletter to get updates about new and advanced workouts.

## *BURN THE FAT, FEED THE MUSCLE* EXERCISE MENU

| Quads | Hamstrings | Back | Calves | Abs/Core |
|---|---|---|---|---|
| BB squats | BB Romanian dead lift | DB one-arm row | Standing calf raise | Plank/side plank |
| DB split squats | DB Romanian dead lift | Chin-ups | Seated calf raise | Reverse crunch |
| Leg press | Lying leg curl | Lat pull-downs | DB single leg calf raise | Cable crunch |
| | Low back extension | BB rows | | Hanging leg raise |
| | | | | Leg raise/toes to sky |

| Chest | Shoulders | Biceps | Triceps | Crunches |
|---|---|---|---|---|
| BB bench press | BB shoulder press | BB curl | Tricep push-down | Bicycle crunches |
| BD bench press | DB shoulder press | Incline DB curl | Lying triceps extension BB | |
| DB incline press | DB side laterals | DB curl | DB overhead extension | |
| DB incline flyes | DB bent-over laterals | | | |

*Key: BB = barbell, DB = dumbell*

## Alternative Exercises

**Quads:** front squats, dumbbell squats (two dumbbells or goblet squat), barbell lunge, dumbbell lunge, Bulgarian split squat, hack squat, leg extension

**Hamstrings:** seated leg curl machine, single leg curl machine, single leg Romanian dead lift, glute-ham raise, one-leg low back extension

**Back:** conventional dead lift, pull-ups, one-arm dumbbell row, inverted row, dumbbell pull-over

**Calves:** calf press, donkey calf machine

**Abs/core:** barbell rollout (or ab wheel), crunches, Swiss ball crunches, Swiss ball jackknife, cable woodchopper

**Chest:** incline barbell press, wide grip dips ("gironda" dips), cable crossover, flat dumbbell flyes, machine flyes, hammer strength chest press (any angle)

**Shoulders:** dumbbell upright rows, barbell upright rows, cable upright rows, cable pulls to face (rear delts), dumbbell front raise, barbell front raise, cable front raise, dumbbell shrugs, barbell shrugs

**Biceps:** preacher bench curl, dumbbell concentration curl, cable curl, hammer curl

**Triceps:** close-grip barbell bench press, dumbbell kickbacks, overhead cable extension, overhead barbell extension (French press), rope push-down, reverse bench dips

**Forearms:** dumbbell wrist curl (one or two dumbbells), barbell-behind-back wrist curl, gripper machine, cable wrist curl

## The Exercise Rotation System

One feature that sets TNB-28 apart from others is the exercise rotation technique. This means that the programme is actually two workouts, not one. Every other workout, you rotate between the two. For example, on workout one you do chin-ups, and on workout two you do lat pull-downs. There are huge benefits to this system.

First, it's a boredom killer. There is nothing wrong with working the same exercises for months as long as you can keep applying the progressive overload principle. The problem is many people get bored and lose motivation even if they're still getting results. Rotating between two workouts keeps it interesting a lot longer.

Rotating exercises also helps you avoid overuse injuries caused by repetitive pattern overload. If you do the same exercises week after week for months on end, especially if you train hard and heavy, eventually your joints take a beating. Joint pain from training is common, and rotating exercises (in addition to alternating heavy and lighter workouts) may help alleviate it.

By rotating some of the exercises you also all hit your muscles from a variety of angles and planes with different equipment (barbells, dumbbells, cables, and so on). This helps stimulate the maximum number of muscle fibres and develops every part of every muscle. The variety also helps slow down the adaptations that lead to plateaus, so you keep getting results longer.

In TNB-28, not all of the exercises are rotated, which keeps this plan a little simpler and easier. For example, you stay with basic movements like squats through the whole programme (you rotate the rep ranges), and only the second leg exercise is rotated. As you get more advanced, rotating two workouts that are 100 per cent different is an option.

## The Two-Day Split Routine

The TNB-28 programme uses a two-day split routine, in which you divide your workout into an upper-body day and a lower-body plus abs day. Why not stick with a full-body workout? You could, but beyond the beginner stage, your body will respond best when you accumulate a higher volume of work. Splitting your body in two gives you time in each workout to add those additional sets and exercises. As you advance, it's also important to use more variation in the training stimulus, both in rep ranges and exercises. These goals are difficult to achieve with full-body workouts, without turning them into marathon 90- to 120-minute sessions.

Split routines also allow you to focus your mental and physical energies more efficiently. Training your entire body in a single session can be exhausting. When you only have to work half your body, you can give more energy and intensity to each muscle group. There's a little more volume to be done on the upper-body days, but since leg training is so demanding, it's better that the volume is lower on leg day. It also leaves you plenty of time to do a thorough job on your abs.

## The Weekly Workout Schedule (frequency)

TNB-28 calls for four workouts per week:

**Day 1: upper-body strength and muscle**
**Day 2: lower-body strength and muscle**
**Day 3: upper-body muscle**
**Day 4: lower-body muscle**

| Mon. | Tues. | Wed. | Thurs. | Fri. | Sat. | Sun. |
|---|---|---|---|---|---|---|
| 1. Upper-body strength/ muscle | 2. Lower-body strength/ muscle | Off | 3. Upper-body muscle | 4. Lower-body muscle | Off | Off |

This is an ideal weekly schedule for most people because it gives you an extra day of total rest from resistance training between the third and fourth day, which enhances overall recovery. It also leaves weekends open. This schedule has some room for flexibility. If you prefer, you can change the days of the week you train, moving workouts to the weekend or inserting an off day in between two training days.

## Three-Days-per-Week Option

If you're pressed for time, or if you feel you don't recover completely from four workouts a week, you can reduce this schedule to three workouts every seven days. You would simply train on any three nonconsecutive days per week, such as Monday, Wednesday and Friday (or Tuesday, Thursday, Saturday). With a Monday-Wednesday-Friday schedule, you would do workout 1 on Monday, workout 2 on Wednesday, workout 3 on Friday, workout 4 on the following Monday, and then repeat the cycle.

| Mon. | Tues. | Wed. | Thurs. | Fri. | Sat. | Sun. |
|---|---|---|---|---|---|---|
| 1. Upper-body strength/ muscle | Off | 2. Lower-body strength/ muscle | Off | 3. Upper-body muscle | Off | Off |
| **Mon.** | **Tues.** | **Wed.** | **Thurs.** | **Fri.** | **Sat.** | **Sun.** |
| 4. Lower-body muscle | Off | 1. Upper-body strength/ muscle | Off | 2. Lower-body strength/ muscle | Off | Off |

### The Workout

**WORKOUT 1: MONDAY, UPPER-BODY, STRENGTH/MUSCLE**
**A.**  Barbell rows: 4 sets × 4–7 reps, 120–150 seconds rest
**B.**  Chin-ups: 3 sets × 8–12 reps, 90–120 seconds rest
**C.**  Barbell bench press: 4 sets × 4–7 reps, 120–150 seconds rest
**D.**  Dumbbell incline press: 3 × 8–12 reps, 90–120 seconds rest
**E.**  Dumbbell lateral raise, seated: 3 sets × 8–12 reps, 60–90 seconds rest
**F.**  Barbell shoulder press, seated: 3 sets × 4–7 reps, 90–120 seconds rest
**F1.** Lying triceps extension: 3 sets × 8–12 reps, 0 seconds rest (superset)
**F2.** Barbell curls: 3 sets × 8–12 reps, 60–90 seconds rest

**WORKOUT 2: TUESDAY, LOWER-BODY AND ABS, STRENGTH/MUSCLE**
**A.**  Barbell squat: 4 sets × 4–7 reps, 120–150 seconds rest
**B.**  Dumbbell split squat (static lunge): 3 sets × 8–12 reps, 90–120 seconds rest
**C.**  Barbell Romanian dead lift: 4 sets × 8–12 reps, 120–150 seconds rest
**D.**  Lying leg curl: 3 sets × 4–7 reps, 90–120 seconds rest
**E.**  Seated calf raise: 3 × 15–20 reps, 60–90 seconds rest
**F1.** Hanging leg raise: 2–3 × 10–15 reps, 0 seconds rest (superset)
**F2.** Reverse crunch: 3 sets × 15–20 reps, 60 seconds rest
**G.**  Plank: 3 sets × 30–60 seconds, 60 seconds rest

**WORKOUT 3: THURSDAY, UPPER-BODY, MUSCLE**

**A.** Barbell row: 3 sets × 8–12 reps, 1 set × 15–20 reps, 60–90 seconds rest

**B.** Lat pull-downs: 3 sets × 8–12 reps, 60–90 seconds

**C.** Barbell bench press: 3 sets × 8–12 reps, 60–90 seconds rest

**D.** Incline dumbbell flyes: 3 sets × 8–12 reps, 60–90 seconds rest

**E1.** Dumbbell shoulder press: 3 sets × 8–12 reps, 60–90 seconds rest

**E2.** Bent-over dumbbell lateral raises: 3 sets × 8–12 reps, 60–90 seconds rest

**F1.** Tricep push-down (cable): 3 sets × 8–12 reps, 0 seconds rest (superset)

**F1.** Incline dumbbell curls: 3 sets × 8–12 reps, 60–90 seconds rest


**WORKOUT 4: SATURDAY LOWER-BODY, ABS, HYPERTROPHY**

**A.** Barbell squat: 3 sets × 8–12 reps, 1 set × 15–20 reps, 90–120 seconds rest

**B.** Leg press: 3 sets × 8–12 reps, 1 set ×15–20 reps, 60–90 seconds rest

**C.** Lying leg curl: 3 sets × 8–12 reps, 60–90 seconds rest

**D.** Low back extension: 3 sets × 8–12 reps, 60–90 seconds rest

**E.** Standing calf raise: 3 sets × 15–20 reps, 60–90 seconds rest

**F1.** Kneeling cable crunch: 3 sets × 15–20 reps, 0 seconds rest (superset)

**F2.** Lying leg raise/toes to sky: 3 sets × 15–20 reps, 60 seconds rest

**G.** Side plank: 3 sets × 30–60 seconds, 60 seconds rest


## The Four-Week Periodization Cycle

This is a four-week programme that changes rep ranges within the week and progresses weekly in load and intensity. On strength and muscle days you'll do a mix of heavy sets for 4 to 7 reps and muscle sets for 8 to 12 reps. On muscle days, you'll do sets of mostly 8 to 12 reps and an occasional higher rep set. There are no low-rep-only (strength) days because this is a body transformation programme, not a powerlifting or strength sports programme. However, there's enough heavy work to guarantee you'll get a lot stronger. You'll progress through the following four one-week cycles:

**WEEK 1: INTRODUCTORY LOADING**

You'll be introduced to the new exercises and training techniques. The loads are submaximal. For example, if you estimate that you can do 10 reps with 100 pounds (45 kg), you would select only 90 pounds (41 kg). The intensity level is low, which means you won't take any sets to failure: You'll complete the entire set easily.

### WEEK 2: BASE LOADING

You'll increase the load in every exercise whenever possible. The intensity level will be moderate, which means you'll come close to failure on your hypertrophy sets and the final reps of each set will be hard.

### WEEK 3: OVERLOADING

You'll increase the loading again to above your previous max, whenever possible while maintaining good form. Your goal is to start beating your previous week's bests. The final reps of each set will be very hard, and this week, you'll probably hit failure on some of your sets.

### WEEK 4: SHOCK (PR) LOADING

You'll once again increase the load above the previous week's bests and aim to hit some personal records (PRs). Intensity is very high. This is where you push yourself. You'll take many of your sets to failure and you may miss some reps (for example, your goal is 8 to 12 reps but you barely got 7). If you have any favourite high-intensity techniques such as forced reps or drop sets, this is when to use them.

### WEEK 5: BEGIN NEW CYCLE

You can repeat the four-week cycle by starting over again with introductory loading (submaximal load and no sets taken to failure). At this point you'll be stronger, so your introductory phase will be at least equal to your previous base-loading phase. With each cycle, you continue to increase the weights used as your newfound strength allows.

## WHAT'S NEXT AFTER TNB-28?

Most people can keep getting amazing results on the TNB-28 plan for months – even years. The training template and weekly schedule never go bad. Simply continue focusing on progressive overload, and keep challenging yourself to hit new personal records.

I recommend you repeat the programme for at least three 4-week cycles (12 weeks). After 12 weeks, most people will start experiencing significant adaptation, so it's time for a change. Stick with the TNB-28 weekly schedule and set/rep guidelines, but change some (or all) of the exercises. Rinse and repeat as long as it's still working well for you.

Men and women who are interested in competition-level figure or bodybuilding training may want to move on to advanced three- and four-day body part split routines. You can learn more about these advanced physique programmes on the website at www.BurnTheFatFeedTheMuscle.com and at our private members-only support community at www.BurnTheFatInnerCircle.com

## WEIGHT TRAINING CUSTOMIZATION

You can follow these routines exactly as outlined or customize them to suit your situation better. If you prefer different exercises or training techniques, by all means, use them. *Burn the Fat, Feed the Muscle* nutrition works well with other weight training programmes and even body weight resistance programmes. The important thing is that you always include the resistance training element of our four-part fat-loss formula. If you're not doing some form of resistance training, you're not doing *Burn the Fat, Feed the Muscle.*

Consider this training programme as a great starting point. No training plan can remain the same and keep working forever. You may move to other weekly split routines or stay with this one, but no matter what schedule you follow, to prevent staleness or muscle adaptation, you must periodically change the other variables: exercises, exercise combinations, exercise order, intensity, sets, reps, rest intervals, poundage, and so on. The number of potential workouts you can create by mixing these training variables is infinite.

We've covered a lot of ground in this chapter, and you have everything you need to get started. Advanced programme design is a complex subject, and the more years you've been training, the more variation and sophistication you need to keep making progress. So I encourage you to become a serious student and keep testing different techniques. Become your own science project, and remember: The results of your own personal experiments are what matter more than anything else.

# THE NEXT LEVEL:

## ADVANCED STRATEGIES

# CHAPTER 18

# Breaking Plateaus

"If you do what you've always done, you'll get what you've always got. If what you are doing is not working, do something else."

– Joseph O'Connor and John Seymour,
*Introducing NLP [Neurolinguistic Programming]*

## UNDERSTANDING FAT-LOSS PLATEAUS

You've made progress for weeks or even months and things are going great: You're lighter, leaner, and already looking a lot fitter. Then, for no apparent reason, your fat loss slows down. The next thing you know, your progress stops completely, but you haven't reached your goal yet. You still have fat you want to get rid of. You don't understand what's going on because you're following the same programme that was working before.

To the best of your knowledge, you haven't fallen off track. You had some cheat meals each week, but you built those into your plan and never overdid it. You haven't skipped any workouts either. But there they are: the last stubborn pounds of fat, defiantly clinging to your lower abs, love handles, hips, or thighs – ironically, the places you want that fat gone the most. That's when it dawns on you: "I've hit a fat-loss plateau."

At that point, many people think there's something wrong with them. "Maybe it's my thyroid," they wonder. "Do I have a slow metabolism? Am I one of those extreme endomorphs that can't be helped? Maybe getting really lean just isn't in the cards for me." It's normal to feel frustration and have these types of doubts when progress stops coming. But getting through plateaus is as much psychological as it is physical. When you're stuck, that's when it's more important than ever to redouble your commitment, stay focused on your goal, and be positive. That's plateau-breaking strategy number one.

Discouragement and frustration cause many people to give up even though they're so close to the finish line. They would have easily broken through with a shift in attitude and an extra dose of persistence. Many people also quit when they stall because they don't understand the real reasons why plateaus happen and they don't know about all the strategies they can use to break through them and reach the next level. The good news is those strategies are now right at your fingertips in this chapter and the next.

The bad news about plateaus is that they're common. In fact, you should expect them. You're more likely to zigzag your way to your goal, with sticking points and good weeks and bad weeks, than you are to shoot to your goal in a straight line without a hiccup. Fortunately, if you understand how plateaus are a normal part of the way your body adapts, it won't bother you so much. You'll simply make the right adjustment, get back to work for another week, and be back on target.

Before we look at the specific techniques for breaking plateaus and keeping progress coming week after week, let's first look at why progress stalls in the first place.

## PSYCHOLOGICAL AND BEHAVIOURAL REASONS FOR PLATEAUS

In the majority of cases, a faulty thyroid gland or a slow metabolism is not the cause of stalled fat loss. Lack of compliance is the biggest reason for fat-loss plateaus and slower-than-expected weight loss. Stated differently, you didn't follow your plan closely enough – and you may not have realized it. Your goal is to see some kind of positive result every week. If you're getting no results after seven days, before considering a change, the first thing to do is check your compliance to your current plan.

Ask yourself honestly: "Have I been doing everything I need to do every day or am I missing something? Have I done my best or could I have given it more? Have I been consistent in my eating habits every day or eating well one day and poorly the next? Am I doing a great job all week, then blowing it on the weekends?" The cause of your plateau may be uncovered with the answers to these simple questions.

When you're rating yourself for compliance, remember to rate yourself in all four areas:

1.  **Mental training.** Do you have a current set of updated goals in writing, and have you been keeping your goals in front of you, reading them every day?

2.  **Nutrition.** Do you have a customized meal plan in writing and have you followed it every day to the best of your ability?

3.  **Cardio training.** Do you have a customized cardio schedule and have you been following it consistently?

4. **Resistance training.** Have you been following your weight training programme and applying progressive resistance consistently, week by week?

When you rate your compliance to your nutrition programme, be sure to rate yourself twice: once for compliance to your food quality and again for compliance to your food quantity.

When most people think about compliance, they only think about whether they followed their allowed-foods list (food quality). They pat themselves on their back for eating so cleanly and say, "I followed my plan!" But for fat loss, the real question is: How was your compliance to your calorie deficit (food quantity)? Too much healthy (a.k.a. "clean") food is the cause of many fat-loss plateaus.

You also should ask yourself whether it's possible you underestimated your calorie intake or overestimated your activity level. Almost everyone reports eating fewer calories than they really do; it's one of the most well-known facts in weight-loss research.

The landmark study on this was done at St. Luke's–Roosevelt Hospital Center in New York and published in the *New England Journal of Medicine*. Steven W. Lichtman and his research team hypothesized that many overweight people do not lose weight because their calorie intake was substantially higher than what they reported. The subjects were chosen specifically because they had a claimed history of "diet resistance." They had made at least eight attempts at weight loss in the past, they believed they were eating less than 1,200 calories a day, and many of them thought they had a metabolism or thyroid problem.

The results were a big surprise to the subjects but confirmed the hypothesis of the researchers: Under laboratory-controlled conditions, they found that the study participants underestimated their food intake by a whopping 47 per cent and overestimated their physical activity by 51 per cent! The authors concluded that "failure to lose weight despite a self-reported low-calorie intake can be explained by substantial misreporting of food intake and low physical activity."

Even health professionals are not immune to this error. In another study, a group of dieticians underreported their food intake by an average of 16 per cent. They self-corrected when confronted with the discrepancy, but you would think that dieticians would be among the people most likely to report food intake most accurately. The major lesson here is to be sure you rule out the most common and obvious cause of plateaus before you make any other assumptions: You may simply be eating more than you thought you were.

The plateau-breaking lesson that naturally follows is that if you've been guesstimating food portions, it's time to get serious about your calorie and macronutrient numbers. Measure, count, and track your food intake. When you do it the first time, you may be shocked at how easy it is to underestimate your calories. But you'll be glad you did it because you can then self-correct and start making progress again.

If you realize that compliance was your problem, don't beat yourself up; simply refocus and recommit to your original plan. Rewriting and rereading your goals will help. Map out your training and nutrition strategy for the next seven days in advance and schedule the workouts right in your daily planner with the rest of your appointments. Increase your accountability by sharing your goals with a friend. Then go back to work with renewed motivation and enthusiasm.

If you were tracking carefully and you know your compliance was spot-on, then it's time to consider the other possible causes of your plateau – the biological ones.

## PHYSIOLOGICAL REASONS FOR PLATEAUS

Your body doesn't like to change. Every system in your body is tightly regulated to maintain homeostasis. Blood sugar, body temperature, and acid-base balance are a few examples. When the delicate balance in your body is disturbed, your body sees that as a threat to your survival, so feedback mechanisms automatically kick in to bring you back to normal. Your weight is no different. You adapt hormonally and metabolically to dieting and weight loss. The more you restrict calories and the more weight you lose, the more your metabolism slows down.

If all else is equal and you've remained compliant to your original plan, a plateau means that your body has adapted. In chapter 2, you learned the six strategies to avoid as much of this adaptation as possible. By avoiding starvation diets, you reduce the frequency and severity of adaptation and the frequency of plateaus. However, metabolic adaptation is unavoidable: It's what your body does naturally when you lose weight and restrict calories.

This drop in metabolism is highly misunderstood. Most people don't realize that it occurs for two reasons. The first part of the metabolic slowdown is from the loss in total body weight. Smaller people burn fewer calories than larger people, so the more weight you lose and the lighter you get, the more your deficit shrinks, even at the same calorie intake. That's one reason why the more weight you lose, the harder it gets to continue losing weight.

Here's an example. Kevin is a 40-year-old active male, 5 feet 8 inches (172 cm) tall and 235 pounds (16 st 11 lb/107 kg). If you run his numbers through the calorie formulas, you'll see his maintenance level is about 3,200 calories per day. With a 20 per cent deficit, which is fairly conservative, he would want to eat 2,600 calories per day to lose weight.

Suppose Kevin successfully loses 50 pounds (23 kg) and becomes a lean 185 pounder (13 st 3 lb/84 kg). But then he wants to knock off that last 10 pounds

(4.5 kg) so he can be "ripped." Now that he weighs 185 pounds (13 st 3 lb/84 kg), if you run his calorie calculations again you see that *the mathematical equation has changed!*

Kevin is a smaller guy now, so he needs fewer calories. At 185 pounds (13 st 3 lb/ 84 kg), his maintenance level is now only 2,800 calories a day. He's burning 400 calories a day less than when he started! If he keeps eating the same way he did when he was a bigger guy, he will hardly lose any weight because he doesn't need that many calories to sustain his weight any more. Suppose Kevin also forgets to account for a measly 200 calories per day – now his deficit is gone and his plateau has been fully explained.

The second part of the metabolic slowdown is adaptive thermogenesis. This means that when you restrict calories and lose weight, your metabolism slows down even more than you'd predict from the weight loss alone. It happens through a complex weight-regulating mechanism, involving numerous hormones and body systems becoming more efficient.

It's similar to how the thermostat in your home turns on when the temperature drops. You have the temperature set at a nice, comfortable level, and when the temperature regulation system detects a drop below that set point, it automatically turns on the heat to bring the temperature back up. If your weight regulating system detects a change in body weight below its usual set point, the metabolic thermostat turns the calorie-burning hormones down and the hunger hormones up. Your body becomes more efficient, and burns fewer calories while simultaneously tricking you into eating more.

With fewer calories out and more calories coming in, your caloric deficit shrinks, your fat loss slows down, and eventually you reach a plateau. Although the weight regulating mechanism that causes metabolism to slow down and hunger to go up is extremely complex, you should see by now that the explanation for a fat-loss plateau is very simple: If you were losing weight but your weight loss has stopped completely, you had a calorie deficit, but now you've lost it.

## THREE TYPES OF PLATEAUS, THREE TYPES OF SOLUTIONS

When you finally understand the true nature of fat-loss plateaus, the solution seems clear: to start burning fat again, you must re-establish your calorie deficit. You can do that by eating less or burning more and I'll show you the progression variables you can use to do that in the last section of the chapter.

Depending on how long you've been dieting and training, and how severely, you can also use strategies designed to restimulate your metabolism and reverse the adaptive responses. This makes it easier to establish a significant calorie deficit or allow your body to recognize a deficit.

Before you start training harder or dieting stricter, you should consider that the condition your body is in might affect the type of strategy you use to kick-start your progress. Sometimes you need to push harder; sometimes your body needs a rest before pushing harder again will have much effect.

A dieted-down and depleted body doesn't respond the same way as a well-fed and well-rested body. Your metabolic, hormonal, and mental state are not the same. In fact, some of the strategies that work best in the early stages work the least in the late stages. Late-stage plateau-breaking strategies are often counterintuitive. Many people do the opposite of what they should and dig themselves into deeper metabolic holes.

### 1. Early-stage plateau: Break it with harder work and progression.

The early stage on the programme is the first and second month. When you hit a plateau in the early stages, it usually means you need to apply some type of progression. More of the same will only get your more of the same. You need to challenge yourself.

Many people underestimate how much effort it really takes to get lean. They've been sold on rapid weight-loss diets and minimalist training programmes, so their expectations get distorted. The truth is it takes dedication and hard work to get results, and even harder work to continue making progress. If the effort you're putting in isn't getting you the results you want, then quietly, and without complaining, accept that you may need to work longer, harder, more often, or all of the above.

You can try to hone in on the one area likely to make the biggest difference, because you've identified it's the area where you have the most room for improvement. Or you can completely smash a plateau by applying changes across all four areas: nutrition, mental training, cardio training, and resistance training. Remember the mental aspect. When you're stuck, you're most likely to slip there, yet it's the time you need proper focus and a positive attitude the most.

Overall, the mandate is clear: Tighten the diet belt, train harder. Be meticulous. Weigh, measure, and count your food more diligently. Get stricter about everything.

### 2. Mid-stage plateau: Break it with cycling methods.

If your calorie intake has been in a deficit for a significant amount of time – two to three months – and your fat loss seems slower than it should be (on paper), you will continue applying progression in your training and tightening the belt anywhere you recognize your compliance has slipped. But you may also need to apply a new and different strategy. Your body is starting to adapt to the low calories and become more efficient at doing the workouts. Sometimes the best thing you can do is temporarily raise your calories in order to restimulate your fat-burning hormones.

That doesn't mean pig out or go off the nutrition programme. It's simply a way of giving your body a break from continuous deprivation. Eating more gives your metabolism a boost, resets regulatory hormones, and gives you a psychological break as well. For the most part, keep your food quality high and eat more of the same nutrient-dense foods. Here's how:

One or two days a week, raise your calories – especially the carbs – up to maintenance instead of staying on low calories every day.

This is known as the re-feeding or cycling method. I've mentioned it before and you'll learn more about the specifics in the final chapter, where I show you a complete cycling plan, including how much more to eat, when to eat, and what to eat to make it work the best. Yes, this is counterintuitive. Do it anyway. You'll thank me.

### 3. Late-stage plateau: Break it with rest and recovery.

Training more and dieting harder are not always the best strategies. Sometimes when you're stuck in the mud, pushing on the accelerator just spins your wheels and digs you into a deeper rut.

If you've been training hard, long, and often for months – three to four or more – your plateau could be related to overtraining or adaptation to high-volume exercise. Your body adapts to high-volume training in a similar way it does to calorie restriction: It becomes more efficient. If you suspect this is causing your stagnation, sometimes the best thing to do – at least temporarily – is cut back on your volume or go back to a minimalist routine. If you're seriously overtrained, you may need a short time off to let your body fully recover.

If you've been dieting hard for at least three to four months, you've leaned out quite a bit, but you're struggling with the last of the stubborn fat, you might want to consider taking a diet break. This is the most counterintuitive of all the plateau-breaking strategies because a diet break means that you'll eat more by returning your calories to maintenance level for at least one full week.

Although you might gain some weight, it's usually only a few pounds and it's mostly water and increased glycogen storage. You won't gain fat if you only return your calories to maintenance. The increase in calories shuts off the starvation alarm, stimulates your metabolism, and resets the fat-burning and starvation hormones. You also get a psychological break from the diet as well, which makes it easier to stick with the programme when you go back to it.

When you return to your calorie deficit after a break, or to your training programme after a rest, your body will respond again the way it did when you first started the programme. So don't worry about losing ground by taking time for recovery. When you need a rest, take a rest. You'll probably hold steady. But even if you do take a step back, look at your break as one step back to prepare for two steps forward. When you get back to work with a fully recovered body, you'll be amazed how easily you'll blast beyond your old plateau, capture new ground, and reach a new personal best.

## ADAPTATION AND THE ART OF COAXING PROGRESS

Your body will forever be adapting to everything you throw at it and you will always be working against your body's tendency to remain the same. Energy balance is dynamic; the amount of calories you need is constantly changing, and during weight loss and calorie restriction that amount is decreasing. To continue making progress and reduce the time spent on plateaus, the bottom line is that you must change your approach as your body changes.

If you have a week with no progress and you keep doing the same thing, you'll keep getting the same results. Part of the art in body transformation is knowing what variables to change and when to change them. The more options you have, the better your chances of success, so let me show you some of your basic options.

## PROGRESSION VARIABLES TO BREAK FAT-LOSS PLATEAUS AND KEEP MAKING PROGRESS

Here's the master checklist of the eight most important training and nutrition variables you can adjust each week to break plateaus and keep your progress coming.

### 1. Eat less.

The whole idea of *Burn the Fat, Feed the Muscle* is to eat more and burn more for a faster metabolism and better nutrition. Sometimes, however, there's no way around it: To break a fat-loss plateau, you must reduce your food intake. If you've stopped losing body fat, it means you're no longer in a calorie deficit.

Reducing food intake is the ideal choice for reestablishing the deficit if you've only recently started the programme or if you think you overestimated your initial calorie needs. However, if your calories are already low or you've already cut them to break previous plateaus, cutting calories more can backfire. So cut calories when you have breathing room to do so, but always remember that there are two sides to the equation: You can eat less, burn more, or use a combination of both.

## 2. Change your macronutrient ratios.

Decreasing your carbs (increasing your protein ratio) can often help break a plateau, especially when you're already lean and you want to get leaner. This change in macronutrient ratios may give a slight metabolic or hormonal advantage over a high-carb diet, especially for endomorphs or carb-intolerant types who have problems with blood sugar and appetite control. A small change in macronutrients won't make or break your success, but when you have to cut calories, it makes sense to cut the carb calories first while keeping your lean protein, fibrous carb, and healthy fat intake stable. You'll learn more about the specifics of macronutrient manipulation and lower-carb diets in the final chapter.

## 3. Improve your food quality.

Breaking a plateau is mainly an issue of calorie quantity and re-establishing an energy deficit. However, when fat loss slows down, I believe it pays to be stricter about the quality of your food choices. Eat fewer processed foods and more natural foods. It's always better for your health, and it may help you with your deficit. The trick there is to increase nutrient density while controlling the calorie density. This is much easier to do with natural foods like vegetables and fish compared to man-made foods like pastries or fast-food burgers. You could get away with eating low-quality, highly processed foods and still lose weight as long as you stayed in a calorie deficit, but when your calories are getting lower and lower, it only makes sense to get the highest nutrient density possible from every calorie you eat.

## 4. Increase the duration of your cardio.

On the *Burn the Fat, Feed the Muscle* programme, most people average about 30 minutes of cardio training per session for fat loss. If this doesn't produce the desired results, you can increase your calorie burn by extending your duration incrementally five to ten minutes at a time. Measure the results of each increase on a weekly basis until you find the level where you break the plateau and start dropping fat at the rate you want. For most people, 30 to 45 minutes per session gives excellent results. You can go longer, but after 45 to 60 minutes you usually get a diminished rate of return compared to using other plateau-breaking strategies.

## 5. Increase the frequency of your cardio.

If you're already doing long workouts, continuing to increase your duration can become impractical. At this point, one option is to increase your frequency. A realistic starting point is a minimum of three days per week of cardio training. To break a plateau or increase the rate of fat loss, incrementally add one day per week until you reach six or seven days per week. Don't try to keep up daily cardio for months on end or use it as a crutch for poor nutrition. But used as a way to break a fat-loss plateau and reach peak condition, daily cardio can work wonders to get you lean superfast. It's not a coincidence that so many bodybuilders and fitness models do cardio every day before they step onstage or in front of the camera.

Twice-a-day cardio is another advanced strategy some people might use for short periods to break a plateau or to get extremely lean. This is an extreme strategy that's neither mandatory nor practical for most people who aren't full-time athletes. But many bodybuilders and figure athletes use double cardio before competitions and swear it's the one thing that gets them through any plateau and, more importantly, sheds the last few pounds of stubborn fat. Two-a-day cardio is also a strategy you might use when there's a deadline and you need maximum fat loss in a short period of time.

High-volume cardio done for prolonged periods while in an aggressive calorie deficit can actually increase metabolic adaptation, so this strategy could backfire if you don't use it with caution. If you ever advance to double cardio, don't overdo the duration or intensity at every workout and don't continue with double cardio sessions for long. This is a peaking or plateau-breaking strategy, not something you do year-round.

## 6. Increase the intensity of your cardio.

The most time-efficient way to break a plateau is to increase the intensity of the cardio you're already doing. This simply means work harder! Push yourself to burn more calories in the same time you were already spending. Of course, you can increase intensity only so much because eventually you approach the anaerobic threshold. That's when you push harder and start to lose your breath and have to slow down or stop to recover the oxygen debt before you can continue. But most people who have been doing low- or moderate-intensity workouts have plenty of room to boost the intensity level. Many people forget that that intensity is not a switch with two settings, high or low; it's a dial with low, medium, high, and everything in between. Smart physique athletes turn up the dial on intensity as one of the progression variables to accelerate fat loss or break plateaus. This applies to both steady-state and interval training.

## 7. Add high-intensity interval training or sprint work into your cardio programme.

As you learned in chapter 15, interval training can give you a very high calorie burn in a short period of time. As little as 20 to 25 minutes of intervals (counting the warm-up and cooldown) can burn enough calories for some serious fat loss. Interval training also increases your metabolic rate so you keep burning calories after the workout is over. The higher the intensity, the higher the "afterburn" effect. Intense interval training is usually not recommended for beginners, but after several weeks of building up a fitness base, introducing more intense training is the next step. If you've hit a plateau, that's a perfect time to implement it.

## 8. Change the type of cardio.

If you have a favourite type of cardio you really enjoy, by all means, stay with it, and when you're getting good results, never change for the sake of change. When your progress is starting to flatline, however, a change alone can restimulate your progress and your motivation.

For example, if you've been walking, change the type of exercise to stair-climber, cross-trainer, or stationary bicycle. If you've been using the cross-trainer, try an intense kickboxing or boot camp class. Try anything your body isn't used to. Changing your workouts is also a great way to prevent boredom and recharge your enthusiasm while avoiding repetitive overuse injuries.

## FAT-LOSS PLATEAUS VERSUS MUSCLE-BUILDING PLATEAUS

Keep in mind that most of this information has been directed at breaking a fat-loss plateau. But as you learned in the section on weight training, your body adapts not only to diets but to all kinds of training as well. In a matter of weeks or months, your muscles will adapt to every resistance training programme you follow. Once your body has adapted, continuing with the same training programme doesn't always produce the same results. There's a popular saying among trainers and strength coaches: Everything works, but nothing works for long.

If your goals currently include gaining muscle or if they change to gaining muscle in the future, progress plateaus are going to happen during that endeavour as well. In some ways, continuing to gain lean muscle for months on end after the beginner gains have ended can be more challenging than keeping the fat loss coming.

It goes beyond the scope of this book to go into detail about breaking muscle-building plateaus, but in chapters 16 and 17 you already got the basic tools you need. All you have to do is follow the resistance-training success principles, especially progressive overload, variation, and periodization, and you'll continue making great progress in strength and lean muscle.

Keep in mind especially that beginners can make progress on the same routine longer. The more advanced you become, the more quickly your body adapts and the more often you should change. Changing programmes regularly not only outsmarts your body's adaptive mechanisms, it also beats boredom and keeps your enthusiasm high, and those factors alone can help you keep the results coming.

## THE FOOL-PROOF SECRET TO BREAKING ANY PLATEAU

Progress plateaus are rarely caused by some genetic anomaly or hormonal defect. The simplest explanation is almost always the correct one: If your fat loss has stopped, your body has adapted and you're no longer in a calorie deficit. The questions to ask are: What happened to your calorie deficit and what is the best strategy to use in your situation to get progress rolling again?

To stay motivated, it's important to keep reminding yourself that when you hit a plateau, it's not a bad thing; it's a normal thing. It's simply your body's signal that it has adapted to the stresses you've been imposing on it, and you need to do something different and more challenging for positive adaptations to continue. Now you have an entire arsenal of techniques you can use to push through to the next level of progress.

Combine the information in this chapter with what you learned in chapter 5 about using feedback loops and tracking progress, and you have a fool-proof success system to break any plateau. Measure everything you want to improve, use the progress chart, get into a weekly feedback loop, hold yourself accountable for results, and let your results dictate your next move. If you get stuck, choose a strategy to re-establish your deficit, restimulate your metabolism or restart your progress, go back to work for another seven days, and measure your results again. If it worked, keep it up. If it didn't work, repeat this process until you succeed.

Coming up next, you're going to read about a strategy that you can use not only to break tough plateaus: It's also a secret weapon to accelerate your fat loss. You can use it to reach the most challenging of goals, such as peaking for a competition, getting in photo-shoot shape, or getting lean enough to see six-pack abs. It's the technique that bodybuilders, figure athletes, and fitness models depend on more than any other, and you can use it to reach your goals too. Learn how in the final chapter.

# CHAPTER 19

# How to Accelerate Your Fat Loss

"Basically, I manipulate my carbohydrate intake to turn my body into a fat burning machine!"

– Chris Faildo, Mr. Universe natural bodybuilding champion

## THE *BURN THE FAT, FEED THE MUSCLE* APPROACH TO ULTIMATE LEANNESS

You've learned the fundamentals, you've put all the elements into action, and you're getting results. But what if you want results faster? What if you want to reach an extraordinary level of leanness? What if you want to break through a tough plateau, burn off the final 10 pounds (4.5 kg) of stubborn fat, uncover a set of six-pack abs, or get in peak condition for a contest or photo shoot? You'll learn how to do all these things in this final chapter.

These are the advanced techniques for getting ripped that physique athletes and fitness models use. They're also the same techniques I've used to hit low-single-digit body fat for more than two dozen bodybuilding competitions. These are the methods that unlock the final level of leanness. Think of them as your "sprint to the finish line." It all revolves around a few unique twists on the old low-carb diet.

Most low-carb diets are, by definition, dogmatic. Carbs are the bad foods, and you're only allowed to eat so many grams, full stop. Not so with this programme. This new approach is superior because it's carb customized for your goals and preferences. In *Burn the Fat, Feed the Muscle*, using carb restriction at all is optional. You may not want to or need to restrict carbs. However, to accelerate fat loss, the flexibility to easily apply these carb manipulation techniques is built right into the programme.

## WHEN TO USE A LOW-CARB DIET

Most people have no trouble getting results without resorting to major carb restriction. But there's always a subset of people who struggle more than others and are frustrated with their lack of results despite honest efforts. Broadly, we call them endomorphs. These people sometimes eat fewer carbs to begin with and cut them even more to really get fat loss cranking. Others get results steadily for weeks or even months while eating generous amounts of carbs, but then hit a plateau or find themselves falling behind schedule for an important deadline. A reduced-carb diet with more healthy fat and protein can be an important part of the solution.

*Burn the Fat, Feed the Muscle* is not, however, a low-carb diet by default. In fact, when I talk about the low-carb approach, I intentionally use the word "diet" because when carbs are cut substantially I consider it a short-term adjustment. I don't see very-low-carb eating as a lifestyle for most people. A more balanced macronutrient split that doesn't severely restrict food groups, combined with plenty of exercise, is the real ideal lifestyle plan.

Why and when would you reduce carbs? Here are three situations where low-carb dieting is most appropriate:

### 1. Accelerating fat loss

You're making progress, but it's too slow. Maybe your goal was 2 pounds (0.9 kg) of fat loss per week and you're losing only 1 pound (0.5 kg). Or perhaps you'd be satisfied with a pound a week, but it's more like a pound a month. You think to yourself, "I'm patient, but this is ridiculous. There has to be a way to get results faster without spending more hours in the gym."

### 2. Breaking a plateau

Even if you drop fat slowly and sensibly, it's natural for your fat loss to eventually slow down as you get leaner and leaner – that is, unless you have some plateau-breaking strategies in your fat-burning tool kit. Pulling back on the carbs while keeping the protein high is as close to a sure thing as you'll find. Using a cyclical low-carb diet (which you'll also learn about in this chapter) is even better because it can boost a sluggish metabolism or help prevent plateaus before they happen.

### 3. Peaking for bodybuilding, physique, fitness, figure, or transformation contests

Reduced-carb diets are controversial in some corners of the fitness world, but most physique athletes use them. Some restrict aggressively, others only moderately, but when it comes time to get ultra-lean for a competition or photo shoot, almost all of them follow a high-protein diet with at least some degree of carb restriction. I find this commonality striking, and since bodybuilders are the leanest muscular athletes in the world, you might want to take notice too.

## HOW DOES REDUCING CARBS INCREASE FAT LOSS?

Any diet that puts you in a deficit can cause weight loss, so you could cut calories across the board and you'll lose weight. But there are several reasons why cutting carb calories specifically can help with advanced fat-loss goals. If you jump into a low-carb diet without understanding why you're doing it and how it works, you're likely to fall down a rabbit hole of carbophobia and unnecessary food avoidance. A unique trait of physique athletes is that they're not afraid of carbs; they learn how to manipulate carbs, eating more at times and less at other times. Here are the reasons why they (and you) might reduce them:

### 1. Low-carb, high-protein diets are highly thermic.

Protein has the highest thermic effect of any food, up to 30 per cent. For example, if you eat 100 calories of chicken breast, 30 of those calories are burned off just to digest and utilize it. The net calorie value is only 70 calories. Ironically, it's high protein that gives you the metabolic advantage, not the low carbs, so it may be more accurate to say that high-protein, low-carb diets help accelerate fat loss rather than credit the low carbs alone. Because of the high thermic effect, protein is less likely to be converted to fat than any other macronutrient.

### 2. Low-carb diets help control calories, reduce hunger, and increase satiety.

Protein is the most satiating of all the macronutrients. Dietary fat makes food taste richer, so it has a psychologically satisfying effect, but it doesn't physiologically quell hunger the way protein does. Protein makes you feel fuller and decreases hunger hormonally. High-protein meals increase glucagon-like peptide (GLP-1), a hormone that makes you feel fuller, and the hormone peptide YY (PYY), which reduces appetite.

### 3. Low-carb diets help control insulin.

When you reduce carbs, you reduce insulin output. Since high insulin levels prevent stored fat from being released, controlling insulin with carb restriction may help assist fat loss, especially the last few pounds of stubborn fat. Certain types of stubborn fat deposits are highly sensitive to the effects of insulin and more resistant to releasing stored fatty acids. When insulin is lower, stubborn fat is more easily released into circulation and then burned for energy.

### 4. Low-carb, high-protein diets help reduce water retention.

A high-protein, low-carb diet tends to decrease water retention. This gives a more defined look to your muscles. Bloating and puffiness from water retention is only temporary and shouldn't be confused with real changes in body composition. However, improved muscle definition is one more reason physique athletes say they prefer this type of diet for their final peaking phase.

## DISADVANTAGES OF THE LOW-CARB DIET

Before you consider cutting carbs or trying a competition diet, it's important to understand the downsides and why we don't consider it a lifestyle but a short-term strategy to reach a specific goal. This section lists eight of them, which can help you make an informed decision about whether carb restriction is right for you.

### 1. Low-carb diets are more difficult to stay on.

Low-carb diets are more restrictive and harder to follow. On the most extreme type of low-carb diet, you're only allowed to eat protein (or protein and fat) with limited amounts of leafy greens and nonstarchy vegetables. I'm sure almost anyone can grin and bear that for a while, but it requires tremendous restraint and may set you up for cravings and binges.

### 2. Low-carb diets have a high relapse rate.

If you lose weight quickly on a strict low-carb diet, the odds of relapse and weight regain are usually higher. It doesn't just happen to weight-loss dieters. I've seen seasoned bodybuilders gain 20 pounds (9 kg) the week after a contest because they went on a sugar binge after a four-month diet of protein, salad, and veggies. Transitioning off a low-carb diet must be planned carefully and executed gradually, preferably reintroducing the carbs a little at a time with each passing week. It takes self-control and discipline to pull it off.

### 3. Low-carb diets may be unbalanced and lack essential nutrients.

A balanced nutrition programme, by definition, has a nice mix between proteins, carbs, and fats and includes a wide variety of foods. Any diet that requires you to eat mostly one food or to remove or severely restrict an entire food group is not balanced. That makes it more likely to be missing important nutrients. Some low-carb diets are so strict that fruit is off-limits and even vegetables are kept to a minimum. This can leave you short on fibre and important vitamins and minerals.

### 4. Low-carb diets may be unhealthy.

Low-carb diets that are mostly protein almost guarantee rapid weight loss, but without adequate fibre and micronutrient intake, a low-carb diet can be unhealthy, especially if you follow it for a long time. Some low-carb diets (ketogenic) are actually high in fat, not high in protein. This could also be unhealthy if the types of fat aren't well balanced or if the fat is so high it pushes out other nutrients. It's also never smart to eat large amounts of processed low-carb foods.

### 5. Low-carb diets can kill your energy levels.

A complaint from many low-carb dieters is the drop in energy and training performance. That's why most athletes eat more carbs. Many low-carb dieters notice there's an adaptation phase where they admit the initial weeks on the diet are miserable, but they say it gets easier as the body gets used to it. However, most people who are serious about their training agree that maintaining energy and workout intensity on low carbs is an ongoing challenge.

### 6. Low-carb diets can produce deceiving weight-loss results.

Much of the weight loss in the initial phase of a low-carb diet comes from water and glycogen depletion. It's not uncommon to see 4 to 8 pounds (1.8 to 3.6 kg) a week drop off in the first two weeks in people who start out heavy. But when you judge your results by body composition instead of body weight, you'll see the results are deceiving. For example, if 1 pound (0.5 kg) is fat, 1 pound (0.5 kg) is muscle, and 3 pounds (1 kg) are water, a 5-pound (2-kg) weight loss isn't so impressive any more.

### 7. Low-carb diets affect your mental state.

Low-carb diets are known for producing "brain fog." When you deprive yourself of carbs, it's not uncommon to become moody, irritable, and an all-around grouchy S.O.B. Ask anyone who has ever done a strict low-carb diet (or anyone who has lived with a low-carb dieter), and they'll tell you. The stories (and jokes) about grumpy low-carb dieters and the Jekyll and Hyde personality change are numerous – even legendary!

### 8. Low-carb diets may increase the risk of muscle loss.

Preventing muscle loss is a challenge on any calorie-restricted diet, but when you restrict carbs, your body can easily use protein for energy through a process called gluconeogenesis. More often than not, I've seen all kinds of low-carb diets increase the risk of muscle loss, especially if protein isn't high enough, if calories are too low, and if the dieter isn't weight training.

## THE FOUR SECRETS OF MAKING LOW-CARB DIETS MORE EFFECTIVE AND EASIER TO FOLLOW

Reading the list of potential drawbacks is enough to make some people steer clear of low-carb diets and stick with their baseline nutrition plans. But there are ways to get the benefits of low carbing without all the side effects. These include:

1. **Progressive carb reductions.** Decrease your carbs slowly, only if you need to, based on your weekly results.

2. **Moderate carb restriction.** Cut some carbs but don't remove them completely.

3. **Carb targeting.** Eat carbs in the pre- and post-workout meals on training days.

4. **Carb cycling.** Cycle the carbs instead of staying on low carbs all the time.

For people who are training, these methods are vastly superior to the old style of low-carb diets found in most popular diet programmes. When you put them together, you can achieve incredibly low body-fat levels, develop super muscle definition, and maintain all your hard-earned muscle without making your life miserable.

## PROGRESSIVE REDUCTION OF CARBS

Most popular weight-loss programmes start you with the strictest version of their diet right from day one. Typically this means severe restrictions on carbohydrates. A 30- to 70-gram-per-day limit is common. After you've lost the weight, you're allowed to gradually "loosen it up," putting some carbs back in. Some of these programmes call the initial phase "induction," while others call it a "quick start."

The quick loss of scale weight can be motivating and makes the programme appear more effective, but essentially they've put you on a crash diet. *Burn the Fat, Feed the Muscle* does it the other way around. We emulate the bodybuilder's method, in which you start with a normal (higher) carb intake (similar to a bodybuilder's off-season eating plan) and gradually "tighten it up" by reducing calories and carbs as your weekly results dictate and you get closer to peak condition (similar to a bodybuilder's pre-contest diet).

Why should you gradually reduce carbs and calories? One reason is because *Burn the Fat, Feed the Muscle* is an athlete's style of eating, so it's a foregone conclusion that you'll be training hard. This alone calls for a higher carb intake than a sedentary person. The sudden removal of carbs that you're accustomed to using for fuel can wreak havoc on your training intensity.

The second reason is because if you play all your cards on day one and you hit a plateau later, what then? There's nowhere to go: Your carbs and calories are already slashed to a minimum. The smarter approach is to keep an ace in the hole. Why not eat the most carbs you can while still losing body fat?

The third reason to gradually reduce carbs is: Why suffer unnecessarily? The last few pounds are always hardest to get rid of because of how your body adapts as you lose weight. Your initial weight loss should always be the easiest, so making the diet too strict from day one doesn't make sense. I know people who made one or two changes – little things like cutting out fizzy drinks and reducing visits to fast-food restaurants – and followed a simple workout programme. These changes got them 80 per cent of the way to their goal. No major carb cutting, no forbidden foods, nothing crazy at all – just training, a calorie deficit, and healthier choices. Only later, for the final push toward six-pack abs, did they get stricter.

If you're having a hard time losing even the first few pounds, there's something seriously wrong with your nutrition strategy. Crash diets are the last thing you need;

you must focus on fundamentals. It's the final phases of fat loss – achieving goals like single-digit body fat or six-pack abs – that takes serious tightening of the diet belt. If you must cut more calories somewhere, cutting carbs is one of the best ways to tighten up.

## MODERATE CARB RESTRICTION: THE ACCELERATED FAT-LOSS DIET

Some studies have shown that replacing just one serving of carbs with one serving of lean protein per day is enough to make a difference. A moderate 10 per cent to 15 per cent reduction in carbs with a corresponding increase in protein (and/or good fats) can sometimes work wonders, especially for endomorphs. After this initial drop in carbs, the shift in macronutrient ratios might look something like this:

### THE MODERATE-CARB, HIGH-PROTEIN ACCELERATED-FAT-LOSS DIET:
**40 per cent carbohydrates**
**40 per cent protein**
**20 per cent fat**

Forty per cent carbs is not a low-carb diet by many people's standards; it's considered moderate carb. But it's lower in carbs than the baseline and higher in protein. This usually works out to about 140 to 180 grams of carbs per day for women and 200 to 250 grams per day for men, although the grams of each may vary based on a person's size and activity.

In some cases, people with serious fat-loss goals, such as competing or doing photo shoots, might consider advancing to yet another level and decreasing carbs to as low as 25 per cent to 30 per cent of total calories. For the average male, a competition diet is usually about 150 to 200 grams of carbs per day. For the average female, carb intake is usually around 100 to 130 grams per day.

Here the diet is tightened up to the strictest level. This is the final progression, because in *Burn the Fat, Feed the Muscle* we never cut carbs completely.

### THE LOW-CARB, VERY HIGH-PROTEIN "COMPETITION DIET":
**25 per cent to 30 per cent carbohydrates**
**45 per cent to 50 per cent protein**
**20 per cent to 25 per cent fat**

It's not mandatory to progress to this final phase. This is a very strict diet consisting mostly of lean protein and fibrous vegetables with only limited starchy carbs. It's not for everyone and it's not a prescription. It's simply the way many physique champions prep for fitness or bodybuilding contests, which is why it's called a competition or peaking diet.

Peaking diets, because they're restrictive, aren't used longer than the contest or photo-shoot prep period, which typically lasts about 12 weeks. The actual duration of a contest prep phase depends on an athlete's starting body fat level. If you're already lean, it might take you only 6 to 8 weeks to peak. If your body fat is high, it might take you 14 to 16 weeks to peak. Afterward, athletes gradually shift back to a more balanced nutrition plan with more carbs and less protein for the maintenance or muscle-building phase.

## Your Daily Carb Intake: How Low Is Too Low?

Some low-carb diet advocates argue that we don't need carbs at all. Technically speaking, they're right. The textbook definition of "essential" refers to whether your body can manufacture a nutrient on its own or must obtain it from food. There are essential amino acids, essential fatty acids, essential vitamins, and essential minerals, but there are no essential carbs.

If you have all the essentials, plus adequate energy, you could survive and even stay healthy on protein and fat with near-zero carbs. The question is: Do you merely want to "survive?" You can survive for weeks without food, but that doesn't mean it's a good idea to eat nothing for weeks on end. You can lose weight on a 100 per cent Twinkie (Mini Roll) diet, provided your calories are in a deficit every day. That doesn't mean it's a good idea to eat nothing but Twinkie (Mini Rolls).

Just because you can survive on protein and fat doesn't mean that's the best way to do it, especially if you're athletic. If you want peak performance, a muscular body, and a lifestyle you can enjoy, without long lists of forbidden foods, then you need carbs. It's simply a matter of finding the right amount for you.

When it comes to cutting carbs, there's a point of diminishing returns. This point is not the same for everyone, and it takes some experimenting to find yours. When you're testing different carb levels, pay attention to how you feel physically and mentally, in and out of the gym; your experiments can help you fine-tune your intake. You'll know it when you reach your "critical level," because once you've dropped your carbs too much, the side effects I mentioned earlier begin to rear their ugly heads.

Extreme carb cuts may also have downsides that don't occur with moderate carb cuts. For example, cutting carbs too low can reduce thyroid levels. One study found that active thyroid levels fall when carbs drop below 120 grams per day. Studies also show that the anti-starvation hormone leptin falls with both reduced calories and reduced body fat levels. It's an increase in carbs that restores leptin to normal levels and helps reduce symptoms of the starvation response.

Coincidentally, the dietary reference intake (DRI) for carbs is 130 grams per day. All this data gives us some pretty good reasons to suggest approximately 120 to 130 grams per day as a sensible low end for carb intake for anyone active and in training. This corresponds closely to our recommendation of no less than 25 per cent to 30 per cent of total calories from carbs.

Your personal response may vary. Some people tolerate low carbs better than others. Women, who have lower energy needs, can often go a little lower (100 grams or so) on the stricter competition diets. But most athletes will tell you that very low-carb diets are a real drag on their energy, performance, and mood.

## CARB TARGETING: THE NUTRIENT TIMING TECHNIQUE FOR BETTER BODY COMPOSITION AND PEAK PERFORMANCE

In the past, a big deal was made out of the time of day you eat, especially carbs. I've known thousands of people over the years who said they got leaner by eating fewer starchy carbs at night (carb tapering). However, advancing research on nutrient timing suggests putting more attention on when you eat relative to when you train. I've almost always trained in the morning or early afternoon, which is probably why I thrived on more food early in the day and less food later.

There's no shortage of theories or opinions about the best time of day to work out or eat your meals. But the primary objective of nutrient timing that most experts agree on is to provide more fuel and nutrients when you need them the most. Earmarking some of your daily carb calories for around your workouts when you need them for energy, recovery, and growth is known as carb targeting.

One of the best places for a high-carb-plus-protein meal is right after intense weight training. If you have enough carbs to work with, you can use the bracketing method and put carbs in your pre-workout meal as well. This helps provide fuel and nutrients to improve your performance during your workout and recovery after. It can help improve body composition as well, as nutrients are partitioned into muscle for growth and glycogen repletion instead of into fat stores.

# OUTSMART YOUR METABOLISM WITH CYCLICAL DIETING

Here's the great catch-22 of all diets: If you want to burn fat, you must reduce your calories. But dropping your calories, especially your carb calories, can decrease your metabolism, increase your appetite, and trigger all kinds of adaptations that make it harder to keep getting leaner. It's also tough to follow restrictive diets. The good news is there's a solution. By adding one simple twist to the old low-carb diet, you can get all the low-carb benefits while minimizing the side effects.

Typical diets have you cut calories and keep them at the same low level. But what if you didn't stay on low calories all the time? What if you dropped your calories for a short while, then increased them again at regular intervals? Every time you take a higher-calorie day, you boost your metabolism, satisfy your hunger, and help avoid the starvation response. This is cyclical dieting, also known as nonlinear dieting or zigzag dieting. It's an incredibly effective way to improve your body composition, increase compliance, avoid diet monotony, and break plateaus – or even avoid them completely.

Many dieters have been advised to apply this concept by having a "cheat day." Once a week they eat anything and everything for a full day – cheesecake, pizza, doughnuts, anything goes – hoping to get the benefits I just mentioned. Although the full cheat day works for some people after an entire week of depletion, I've seen it fail more often than not. The reason it backfires is because "free-for-all" cheat days too often turn into uncontrolled binge days that erase the hard work you did the week before. There's a better way.

## CARB CYCLING: SECRET WEAPON OF
## THE LEANEST PEOPLE IN THE WORLD

The most effective way to do a cyclical diet is with a special variation on low carbing known as carb cycling. Carb cycling involves rotating lower-carb days and higher-carb days instead of keeping carbs low all the time.

On the low days, follow your high-protein, low-carb ratios with a moderate or aggressive calorie deficit. You'll eat mostly lean protein and fibrous carbs with only small amounts of starchy carbs. Think of these as maximum fat-burning days. On the high days, you'll add calories, mostly from starchy carbs, until you hit maintenance level or slightly higher. High days are also known as "re-feeds." Think of these as anabolic rebuilding and replenishing days.

The benefits are numerous. More than any other macronutrient, carbs restimulate your metabolism-regulating hormones. Your depleted glycogen levels are restored, your muscles fill out, your skin gets tighter, you feel a surge of energy, and you get a good pump in the gym again. The influx of carbs even has an anabolic effect that helps you retain lean body mass far better than a linear low-carb diet. On top of all this, you don't need to fear the carbs being stored as fat because carb-depleted muscles soak up carbs into glycogen like a dry sponge.

The re-feed day is also a psychological trick that makes your plan easier to stick with. On the lower-calorie, lower-carb days, you might be hungry and craving carbs, but if you're carb cycling, you can say to yourself, "I can wait. There's another high carb day coming soon." (Compare this to "I can never eat pasta again.")

### When to Use Carb Cycling

Carb cycling is usually considered an advanced technique. It's the ace you pull out of your sleeve in the later phases. If you're a beginner, establish your basic healthy eating habits first. If you want to try carb cycling in the early phase of a fat-loss programme, you can, but your body won't need the high days as often. The re-feeds are more important when your body is dieted down.

Your starting body fat level is also a factor. The higher your body fat, the less necessary it is to re-feed. When your body fat is high, you have less risk of muscle loss or metabolic slowdown. When you're leaner and have less energy in body fat storage (toward the end of a diet phase), the risk is higher. Re-feed days help prevent these problems.

There are no hard-and-fast rules on re-feeding frequency except that for fat loss there must be more deficit days than re-feed days or you won't establish enough of a weekly deficit. A full re-feed day is also essential because, while a single high-carb meal may be psychologically satisfying, it's not enough to trigger all the physiological benefits.

My suggestions: If you're a beginner or your body fat is on the high side (men 20 per cent and up; women 25 per cent and up), a re-feed is optional, or take one re-feed day every 7 to 14 days as you see fit to give you a break from continuous calorie restriction and to restore some physical and mental energy.

For anyone in the lean or better category (men under 12 per cent; women under 18 per cent), re-feed at least once per week. Twice a week is probably ideal for contest prep or the lean (dieted-down) physique athlete. Among *Burn the Fat, Feed the Muscle* followers, the most popular carb cycling method for getting super-lean is three days low followed by one day high (3:1 carb cycling).

## What Kind of Carbs to Eat When Carb Cycling

You eat mostly the same types of carbs on your high-carb days as you normally would on this programme; you simply eat more of them. Low-carb days emphasize fibrous carbs like nonstarchy vegetables, salads, and leafy greens. Because the amount of calories you need to add can be significant, the high-carb days emphasize starchy carbs like oats, potatoes, yams, and brown rice.

On high-carb days, you can also be more liberal with starchy carbs like pastas, cereals, and breads, preferably the whole grain varieties. These are the slightly processed starches so they may have more calorie density and less nutrient density than the natural carbs, but a re-feed day is an ideal day to include them if you choose.

For some dieters, knowing they can have a carb-rich meal like a plate of pasta once or twice a week makes sticking to the programme infinitely easier. Just remember that this is a "controlled re-feed," not an all-you-can-eat cheat day.

## How Many Carbs to Eat When Carb Cycling

It's not possible to give one carb cycling schedule with calorie and carb amounts that apply to everyone. You have to customize. But let me show you a typical example for an average man with a 2,800-calorie-per-day maintenance level and an average woman with a 2,100-calorie-per-day maintenance level.

On low days, most people drop their carbs all the way down to the low-carb, very high-protein ratios. Calories are set at an aggressive deficit, around 30 per cent below maintenance; that's around 1,500 for women and 2,000 for men, on average. On the high days, you increase your calories all the way back up to maintenance, which is about 2,100 for women and 2,800 for men. The easiest way to set up a carb cycling diet is to simply add more carbs on the high day and change nothing else.

Don't worry too much about the percentages; the main thing to remember is this: On high days, "just add carbs." But for all my number-crunching readers, it looks like this: For women, it usually works out to about 100 to 130 grams of carbs on low days and about 200 to 275 grams of carbs on high days. For men, it's typically 150 to 200 grams of carbs on low days and 300 to 400 grams on high days.

| CARB CYCLING SCHEDULE FOR AN AVERAGE MALE | | | |
|---|---|---|---|
| **Low-Carb Day (2,000 calories)** | | **High-Carb Day (2,800 calories)** | |
| Protein | 250 g | Protein | 245 g |
| Carbs | 150 g | Carbs | 350 g |
| Fat | 44 g | Fat | 47 g |

| CARB CYCLING SCHEDULE FOR AN AVERAGE FEMALE | | | |
| --- | --- | --- | --- |
| Low-Carb Day (1,500 calories) | | High-Carb Day (2,100 calories) | |
| Protein | 169 g | Protein | 153 g |
| Carbs | 112 g | Carbs | 263 g |
| Fat | 42 g | Fat | 47 g |

### What's the Most Effective Way to Carb Cycle?

The carb cycling theory is based on sound psychology and physiology. However, there are no studies directly confirming what kind of carb cycling schedule is best. Almost all the information we have on carb cycling is based on personal experience from the bodybuilding, physique athlete, and fitness model community. I've seen all kinds of complicated carb cycling schemes, including diets with low, medium, and high days, with carb amounts based on training volume and with lists of specific carbs that must be eaten at specific times on particular days. A popular method is to synchronize your high-carb day with your days of most intense weight training. There's probably merit to all these strategies, especially the last one, but I've always found that the more complex you make it, the more confused you get. Simpler is better.

Here's the big idea to let sink in: On your low-carb days, follow a strict calorie deficit, high protein, and low carbs (mostly fibrous carbs like salad leaves and fibrous vegetables), plus the healthy fats. On your high-carb days, eat more by adding mostly starchy carbs like rice, oats, yams, and potatoes until you hit maintenance calories.

You don't need to make it more complicated than that. In fact, enjoy the process! Everyone loves high-carb day. It's a welcome relief from the traditional low-carbs-all-the-time diets, so it's not only more effective, it's easier. Some even say it's fun!

### *BURN THE FAT, FEED THE MUSCLE* ACCELERATED-FAT-LOSS TEMPLATES

The two core ingredients of the accelerated-fat-loss meal are a lean protein and fibrous carb. The biggest difference between this and the baseline plan is that you'll be eating fewer starchy carbs. As your progress dictates, in some meals, you might remove the starchy carbs completely.

If you ate nothing but lean protein and fibrous carbs at all of your meals, you'd see the fat fall off, even if you didn't count calories or macros, because it's almost impossible to overeat lean proteins and fibrous carbs. Don't drop all your starchy carbs, though, because you need some to support your training energy and recovery. In fact, even when you drop your starches to a moderate level, you may need to increase the lean protein and healthy fat portions to prevent your calories from dropping too low.

Here's what the meal template looks like:

**STEP 1:** Choose a lean protein for every meal.
**STEP 2:** Choose a fibrous carb for every meal.
**STEP 3:** Add in a small portion of starchy carbs or remove completely.
**STEP 4:** Add healthy fats as needed to reach your daily macronutrient goal.

A typical daily mean plan template looks like this:

| | |
|---|---|
| **Meal 1**<br>**Time:** | Lean protein<br>Fibrous carb (or fruit)<br>Starchy carb (full serving) |
| **Meal 2**<br>**Time:** | Lean protein<br>Fibrous carb<br>Starchy carb (full serving) |
| **Meal 3**<br>**Time:** | Lean protein<br>Fibrous carb<br>Starchy carb (small serving or none) |
| **Meal 4**<br>**Time:** | Lean protein<br>Fibrous carb |
| **Meal 5:**<br>**Time:** | Lean protein<br>Fibrous carb |

Here's an example of an accelerated-fat-loss daily meal plan for men, based on the previous template:

| | | Qty. |
|---|---|---|
| **Meal 1** | Scrambled eggs/omelette (2 whole, 3 whites) | 5 |
| | Old-fashioned rolled oats | 65 g (2¼ oz) |
| | Spinach | 30 g (1 oz) |
| | Mushrooms | 90 g (3¼ oz) |
| **Meal 2** | Vanilla whey protein | 2 scoops |
| | Old-fashioned rolled oats | 65 g (2¼ oz) |
| | Grapefruit | 1 large |

| Meal 3 | Chicken breast | 175 g (6 oz) |
|---|---|---|
| | Baked potato | 225 g (8 oz) |
| | Green salad with cucumber and tomato | 135 g (4¾ oz) |
| | Olive oil and balsamic dressing | 2 tbsp |
| Meal 4 | Salmon | 175 g (6 oz) |
| | Asparagus | 225 g (8 oz) |
| Meal 5 | Lean beef, topside | 175 g (6 oz) |
| | Broccoli | 140 g (5 oz) |

Total: 2,100 calories; 218 grams protein, 197 grams carbs, 52 grams fat

Here's an example of an accelerated-fat-loss daily meal plan for women:

| | | Qty. |
|---|---|---|
| Meal 1 | Scrambled eggs/omelette (1 whole, 3 whites) | 4 |
| | Old fashioned rolled oats | 55 g (2 oz) |
| | Spinach | 30 g (1 oz) |
| | Mushrooms | 90 g (3¼ oz) |
| Meal 2 | Whey protein, vanilla | 1½ scoops |
| | Old-fashioned rolled oats | 55 g (2 oz) |
| Meal 3 | Chicken breast | 115 g (4 oz) |
| | Baked potato | 175 g (6 oz) |
| | Green salad with cucumber and tomato | 135 g (4¾ oz) |
| | Olive oil and balsamic dressing | 2 tbsp |
| Meal 4 | Salmon | 150 g (5 oz) |
| | Asparagus | 150 g (5 oz) |
| Meal 5 | Lean beef, topside | 115 g (4 oz) |
| | Broccoli | 100 g (3½ oz) |

Total: 1,569 calories; 158 grams protein, 138 grams carbs, 41 grams fat

## TIPS FOR ACCELERATING FAT LOSS WITH REDUCED-CARB MEAL PLANS

1. **Eliminate refined carbs.** Reduce starchy carbs and grains. Eat more fibrous carbs and leafy greens.

2. **You may use fat-free and low-fat dairy products, but emphasize lean meats, fish, eggs, and fibrous carbs first.** Many physique athletes prefer to remove dairy products on competition diets.

3.  **Initially set macronutrient ratios at approximately 40 per cent carbs, 40 per cent protein, and 20 per cent fat, give or take 5 per cent.** If you reach a fat-loss plateau or want to accelerate fat loss, you can reduce starchy carb calories more (to about 25 per cent to 30 per cent of total calories). That leaves mostly fibrous carbs and lean proteins with small amounts of healthy fats. Starchy carbs will be very low, but not removed completely.

4.  **Use the nutrient timing method on weight training days, saving most of your carbs for around your workouts.** If you train early in the day, front-load your carbs early. If you train later in the day, save most of your starchy carbs for your evening post-workout meal. On nontraining days, place your starchy carbs wherever you want them. I prefer having them for breakfast and then eating fibrous carbs and protein the rest of the day (carb tapering).

5.  **Always include at least one or two servings per day of healthy fats.** When you cut your carbs significantly, some people feel fuller and more energetic by compensating with a slight increase in fat. If calories get too low, you can increase healthy fats (along with increased protein).

6.  **Use this plan for maximum fat loss or contest dieting, not long-term maintenance.** After you reach your goal, gradually reintroduce more calories from starchy carbs and shift back to baseline carb levels. Introduce 100 to 200 more carb calories per week and measure results before increasing again.

## CONCLUSION

That's it! You've just learned some of the most powerful fat-loss techniques in existence. But remember: Any diet taken to an extreme can do more harm than good, and that includes the low-carb diet. In *Burn the Fat, Feed the Muscle*, there are progressive phases with increasing reductions in carbs and corresponding increases in protein, but nowhere do I recommend the complete removal of carbs. Nowhere do I say carbs are evil or completely off-limits. Sensible and strategic carb manipulation with increased protein to accelerate the fat-loss process? Absolutely! Zero or close to zero carb diets? No, thanks!

**APPENDIX**

# EXTRA TOOLS

## BURN THE FAT, FEED THE MUSCLE PROGRESS CHART *

| Week | Date | Sum of Skinfolds (mm)† | Body fat percentage | Body Weight | Pounds of Body Fat | Pounds of Lean Body Mass (LBM) | Weekly LBM change | Weekly Body Fat Change | Weekly Weight Change | Total Weight Change To Date |
|---|---|---|---|---|---|---|---|---|---|---|
| Start (Baseline) | | | | | | | | | | |
| Week 1 | | | | | | | | | | |
| Week 2 | | | | | | | | | | |
| Week 3 | | | | | | | | | | |
| Week 4 | | | | | | | | | | |
| Week 5 | | | | | | | | | | |
| Week 6 | | | | | | | | | | |
| Week 7 | | | | | | | | | | |
| Week 8 | | | | | | | | | | |
| Week 9 | | | | | | | | | | |
| Week 10 | | | | | | | | | | |
| Week 11 | | | | | | | | | | |
| Week 12 | | | | | | | | | | |

\* Download free interactive Excel spreadsheet versions of this progress chart at www.BurnTheFatFeedTheMuscle.com.

† If you use an accu-Measure, there is only one skinfold, the iliac crest (hip bone) site. If you use a multi-site test, add up the total of each skinfold and log the sum in your chart. If you don't use skinfolds as your body fat-testing method, you can leave the skinfold column blank.

## *BURN THE FAT, FEED THE MUSCLE*
## GOAL-SETTING WORKSHEET

**Your long-term ideal body goal.** What does your ultimate ideal body look like? Don't hold back: Think big. You may want to use another person's physique for inspiration. If so, who is your role model?

_____

_____

_____

**Your one-year goals.** What is your body weight and body composition goal for 12 months from now? What are some fitness, strength, performance, and lifestyle change goals you want to achieve during that year?

_____

_____

_____

**Your three-month goal.** What is your body weight and body composition goal for three months from now? (This is your "focus-priority" goal and the one you'll also put on a goal card and carry with you at all times, reading it as often as possible.)

_____

_____

_____

**Your one-month goals.** What is your schedule for the next 28-day training block? What are your cardio and resistance training goals for this 4-week period?

_____

_____

_____

**Weekly goals.** What is your weekly body weight and body composition goal? What will be your official weigh-in and body-fat-testing day every week? How will you measure?

_____

_____

_____

**Daily goals.** What are the most important behaviours you must develop into habits and repeat every day to reach all your fitness and body composition goals?

_____

_____

_____

**Personal record (PR) goals.** What lifetime personal best records for performance, fitness, and physical condition do you want to achieve?

_____

_____

_____

## THE GOAL-ACHIEVING FORMULA CHECKLIST

[ ] Are your goals specific?

[ ] Are your goals measureable?

[ ] Have you set your goals big enough? (You're not selling yourself short, are you?)

[ ] Have you set realistic deadlines for all your goals?

[ ] Have you written your goals in the form of present-tense, personal, positive affirmations?

[ ] Have you prioritized your most important goal and made sure it doesn't conflict with other goals?

[ ] Do you have a goal card with your number one goal written on it?

[ ] Do you know the emotional reasons why you want to achieve your goals?

[ ] Are you visualizing your goals as already achieved?

[ ] Are you writing, reading, and visualizing your goals with faith and belief?

[ ] Do you reward yourself when you achieve big goals?

[ ] Do you update and rewrite your goals constantly?

[ ] Are you keeping a list of achieved goals to revisit past successes for motivation?

To download printable copies of this goal-setting worksheet, visit www.BurnTheFatFeedTheMuscle.com.

## CALORIE WORKSHEET

### The Averages Method

Use this method if want a ballpark estimate and you don't want to do any maths. Use the lower end of the ranges if you are small-framed and/or inactive. Use the high end of the ranges if you are large-framed and/or active. (These numbers are based on the average man or woman. If your body size or activity levels are much higher than average, use one of the other methods).

| AVERAGE CALORIE INTAKES DAILY FOR FAT LOSS | |
| --- | --- |
| Men | 2,100–2500 calories |
| Women | 1,400–1,800 calories |

| AVERAGE CALORIE INTAKES DAILY FOR MAINTENANCE | |
| --- | --- |
| Men | 2,700–2,900 calories |
| Women | 2,000–2,200 calories |

## YOUR CUSTOMIZED DAILY CALORIE GOAL

| Fat Loss | |
| --- | --- |
| Maintenance | |

## The Quick Method

Use this method if you want a customized estimate with one quick calculation (current body weight times a multiplyer between 11 and 20). Use the lower number if you're lightly active, the middle number for moderately active, and the higher number for very active. The formula is based on body weight, so it's the same for men and women.

### DAILY CALORIE INTAKE FOR FAT LOSS

| Fat Loss | 11–13 calories per pound of body weight |
| --- | --- |
| Maintenance | 14–16 calories per pound of body weight |
| Weight gain | 18–20 calories per pound of body weight |

### YOUR CUSTOMIZED DAILY CALORIE GOAL

| Fat Loss | |
| --- | --- |
| Maintenance | |

## The Harris–Benedict and Katch–McArdle Formulas

Use this four-step method if you want the most accurate estimate of your ideal calorie needs based on body size and activity level and you don't mind crunching a few numbers. If you don't know your lean body mass, use the Harris–Benedict equation to calculate your BMR.

---

### STEP 1: CALCULATE YOUR BASAL METABOLIC RATE (BMR)

#### OPTION (A): HARRIS–BENEDICT EQUATION

| Men | BMR = 66 + (13.7 × weight in kg) + (5 × height in cm) – (6.8 × age) |

| Women | BMR = 655 + (9.6 × weight in kg) + (1.8 × height in cm) - (4.7 × age) |

Your Basal Metabolic Rate
(BMR)

---

#### OPTION (B): KATCH–MCARDLE EQUATION

| Men and Women | BMR = 370 + (21.6 × lean mass in kg) |

Your Basal Metabolic Rate
(BMR)

---

### STEP 2: CHOOSE YOUR ACTIVITY LEVEL (MULTIPLIER)

| Activity Level | Multiplier | Description |
| --- | --- | --- |
| Sedentary | BMR × 1.2 | Little or no exercise, desk job |
| Lightly active | BMR ×1.375 | Light exercise or sports, 3–5 days/week |
| Moderately active | BMR × 1.55 | Moderate exercise or sports, 3–5 days/week |
| Very active | BMR × 1.725 | Hard exercise or sports, 6–7 days/week |
| Extremely active | BMR × 1.9 | Hard daily exercise or sports and physical labour job or twice-a-day training (football camp, etc.) |

Your Activity
Multiplier:

---

### STEP 3: CALCULATE YOUR MAINTENANCE LEVEL (TDEE)

BMR        × your activity multiplier        = TDEE (maintenance level)

---

### STEP 4: CHOOSE A CALORIE DEFICIT AND CALCULATE YOUR IDEAL CALORIE INTAKE FOR FAT LOSS

| Your Maintenance Level (TDEE) | Very Conservative Deficit (TDEE 15%) | Conservative Deficit (TDEE 20%) | Moderate Deficit (TDEE 25%) | Very Aggressive Aeficit (TDEE 30%) | Other Deficit _____ % |
| --- | --- | --- | --- | --- | --- |

To download free printable copies of this worksheet, visit www.BurnTheFatFeedTheMuscle.com.

# GRAMS OF FAT DAILY FOR
## 15% TO 30% MACRONUTRIENT RATIOS

| Calories | 15% Fat | 20% Fat | 25% Fat | 30% Fat |
|----------|---------|---------|---------|---------|
| 1,200 | 20.0 | 26.7 | 33.3 | 40.0 |
| 1,300 | 21.7 | 28.9 | 36.1 | 43.3 |
| 1,400 | 23.3 | 31.1 | 38.9 | 46.7 |
| 1,500 | 25.0 | 33.3 | 41.7 | 50.0 |
| 1,600 | 26.7 | 35.6 | 44.4 | 53.3 |
| 1,700 | 28.3 | 37.8 | 47.2 | 56.7 |
| 1,800 | 30.0 | 40.0 | 50.0 | 60.0 |
| 1,900 | 31.7 | 42.2 | 52.8 | 63.3 |
| 2,000 | 33.3 | 44.4 | 55.6 | 66.7 |
| 2,100 | 35.0 | 46.7 | 58.3 | 70.0 |
| 2,200 | 36.7 | 48.9 | 61.1 | 73.3 |
| 2,300 | 38.3 | 51.1 | 63.9 | 76.7 |
| 2,400 | 40.0 | 53.3 | 66.7 | 80.0 |
| 2,500 | 41.7 | 55.6 | 69.4 | 83.3 |
| 2,600 | 43.3 | 57.8 | 72.2 | 86.7 |
| 2,700 | 45.0 | 60.0 | 75.0 | 90.0 |
| 2,800 | 46.7 | 62.2 | 77.8 | 93.3 |
| 2,900 | 48.3 | 64.4 | 80.6 | 96.7 |
| 3,000 | 50.0 | 66.7 | 83.3 | 100.0 |
| 3,100 | 51.7 | 68.9 | 86.1 | 103.3 |
| 3,200 | 53.3 | 71.1 | 88.9 | 106.7 |
| 3,300 | 55.0 | 73.3 | 91.7 | 110.0 |
| 3,400 | 56.7 | 75.6 | 94.4 | 113.3 |
| 3,500 | 58.3 | 77.8 | 97.2 | 116.7 |
| 3,600 | 60.0 | 80.0 | 100.0 | 120.0 |
| 3,700 | 61.7 | 82.2 | 102.8 | 123.3 |
| 3,800 | 63.3 | 84.4 | 105.6 | 126.7 |
| 3,900 | 65.0 | 86.7 | 108.3 | 130.0 |
| 4,000 | 66.7 | 88.9 | 111.1 | 133.3 |
| 4,100 | 68.3 | 91.1 | 113.9 | 136.7 |
| 4,200 | 70.0 | 93.3 | 116.7 | 140.0 |
| 4,300 | 71.7 | 95.6 | 119.4 | 143.3 |
| 4,400 | 73.3 | 97.8 | 122.2 | 146.7 |
| 4,500 | 75.0 | 100.0 | 125.0 | 150.0 |

## GRAMS OF PROTEIN DAILY FOR
## 30% TO 45% MACRONUTRIENT RATIOS

| Calories | 30% Protein | 35% Protein | 40% Protein | 45% Protein |
|---|---|---|---|---|
| 1,200 | 90.0 | 105.0 | 120.0 | 135.0 |
| 1,300 | 97.5 | 113.8 | 130.0 | 146.3 |
| 1,400 | 105.0 | 122.5 | 140.0 | 157.5 |
| 1,500 | 112.5 | 131.3 | 150.0 | 168.8 |
| 1,600 | 120.0 | 140.0 | 160.0 | 180.0 |
| 1,700 | 127.5 | 148.8 | 170.0 | 191.3 |
| 1,800 | 135.0 | 157.5 | 180.0 | 202.5 |
| 1,900 | 142.5 | 166.3 | 190.0 | 213.8 |
| 2,000 | 150.0 | 175.0 | 200.0 | 225.0 |
| 2,100 | 157.5 | 183.8 | 210.0 | 236.3 |
| 2,200 | 165.0 | 192.5 | 220.0 | 247.5 |
| 2,300 | 172.5 | 201.3 | 230.0 | 258.8 |
| 2,400 | 180.0 | 210.0 | 240.0 | 270.0 |
| 2,500 | 187.5 | 218.8 | 250.0 | 281.3 |
| 2,600 | 195.0 | 227.5 | 260.0 | 292.5 |
| 2,700 | 202.5 | 236.3 | 270.0 | 303.8 |
| 2,800 | 210.0 | 245.0 | 280.0 | 315.0 |
| 2,900 | 217.5 | 253.8 | 290.0 | 326.3 |
| 3,000 | 225.0 | 262.5 | 300.0 | 337.5 |
| 3,100 | 232.5 | 271.3 | 310.0 | 348.8 |
| 3,200 | 240.0 | 280.0 | 320.0 | 360.0 |
| 3,300 | 247.5 | 288.8 | 330.0 | 371.3 |
| 3,400 | 255.0 | 297.5 | 340.0 | 382.5 |
| 3,500 | 262.5 | 306.3 | 350.0 | 393.8 |
| 3,600 | 270.0 | 315.0 | 360.0 | 405.0 |
| 3,700 | 277.5 | 323.8 | 370.0 | 416.3 |
| 3,800 | 285.0 | 332.5 | 380.0 | 427.5 |
| 3,900 | 292.5 | 341.3 | 390.0 | 438.8 |
| 4,000 | 300.0 | 350.0 | 400.0 | 450.0 |
| 4,100 | 307.5 | 358.8 | 410.0 | 461.3 |
| 4,200 | 315.0 | 367.5 | 420.0 | 472.5 |
| 4,300 | 322.5 | 376.3 | 430.0 | 483.8 |
| 4,400 | 330.0 | 385.0 | 440.0 | 495.0 |
| 4,500 | 337.5 | 393.8 | 450.0 | 506.3 |

# GRAMS OF CARBS DAILY FOR
## 25% TO 50% MACRONUTRIENT RATIOS

| Calories | 25% Carbs | 30% Carbs | 35% Carbs | 40% Carbs | 45% Carbs | 50% Carbs |
|---|---|---|---|---|---|---|
| 1,200 | 75.0 | 90.0 | 105.0 | 120.0 | 135.0 | 150.0 |
| 1,300 | 81.3 | 97.5 | 113.8 | 130.0 | 146.3 | 162.5 |
| 1,400 | 87.5 | 105.0 | 122.5 | 140.0 | 157.5 | 175.0 |
| 1,500 | 93.8 | 112.5 | 131.3 | 150.0 | 168.8 | 187.5 |
| 1,600 | 100.0 | 120.0 | 140.0 | 160.0 | 180.0 | 200.0 |
| 1,700 | 106.3 | 127.5 | 148.8 | 170.0 | 191.3 | 212.5 |
| 1,800 | 112.5 | 135.0 | 157.5 | 180.0 | 202.5 | 225.0 |
| 1,900 | 118.8 | 142.5 | 166.3 | 190.0 | 213.8 | 237.5 |
| 2,000 | 125.0 | 150.0 | 175.0 | 200.0 | 225.0 | 250.0 |
| 2,100 | 131.3 | 157.5 | 183.8 | 210.0 | 236.3 | 262.5 |
| 2,200 | 137.5 | 165.0 | 192.5 | 220.0 | 247.5 | 275.0 |
| 2,300 | 143.8 | 172.5 | 201.3 | 230.0 | 258.8 | 287.5 |
| 2,400 | 150.0 | 180.0 | 210.0 | 240.0 | 270.0 | 300.0 |
| 2,500 | 156.3 | 187.5 | 218.8 | 250.0 | 281.3 | 312.5 |
| 2,600 | 162.5 | 195.0 | 227.5 | 260.0 | 292.5 | 325.0 |
| 2,700 | 168.8 | 202.5 | 236.3 | 270.0 | 303.8 | 337.5 |
| 2,800 | 175.0 | 210.0 | 245.0 | 280.0 | 315.0 | 350.0 |
| 2,900 | 181.3 | 217.5 | 253.8 | 290.0 | 326.3 | 362.5 |
| 3,000 | 187.5 | 225.0 | 262.5 | 300.0 | 337.5 | 375.0 |
| 3,100 | 193.8 | 232.5 | 271.3 | 310.0 | 348.8 | 387.5 |
| 3,200 | 200.0 | 240.0 | 280.0 | 320.0 | 360.0 | 400.0 |
| 3,300 | 206.3 | 247.5 | 288.8 | 330.0 | 371.3 | 412.5 |
| 3,400 | 212.5 | 255.0 | 297.5 | 340.0 | 382.5 | 425.0 |
| 3,500 | 218.8 | 262.5 | 306.3 | 350.0 | 393.8 | 437.5 |
| 3,600 | 225.0 | 270.0 | 315.0 | 360.0 | 405.0 | 450.0 |
| 3,700 | 231.3 | 277.5 | 323.8 | 370.0 | 416.3 | 462.5 |
| 3,800 | 237.5 | 285.0 | 332.5 | 380.0 | 427.5 | 475.0 |
| 3,900 | 243.8 | 292.5 | 341.3 | 390.0 | 438.8 | 487.5 |
| 4,000 | 250.0 | 300.0 | 350.0 | 400.0 | 450.0 | 500.0 |
| 4,100 | 256.3 | 307.5 | 358.8 | 410.0 | 461.3 | 512.5 |
| 4,200 | 262.5 | 315.0 | 367.5 | 420.0 | 472.5 | 525.0 |
| 4,300 | 268.8 | 322.5 | 376.3 | 430.0 | 483.8 | 537.5 |
| 4,400 | 275.0 | 330.0 | 385.0 | 440.0 | 495.0 | 550.0 |
| 4,500 | 281.3 | 337.5 | 393.8 | 450.0 | 506.3 | 562.5 |

# CALORIE AND MACRONUTRIENT QUICK REFERENCE CHART

## LEAN PROTEINS

| Food Item | Qty | Calories | Protein (g) | Carbs (g) | Fat (g) |
|---|---|---|---|---|---|
| Beef, mince, 90% lean | 110 g (4 oz), raw | 199 | 22.7 | 0 | 11.3 |
| Beef, top sirloin, lean | 110 g (4 oz), raw | 144 | 34.4 | 0 | 9.1 |
| Beef, top round | 110 g (4 oz), raw | 146 | 26.1 | 0 | 3.8 |
| Chicken breast, skinless, 99% fat free | 110 g (4 oz), raw | 120 | 26 | 0 | 1.0 |
| Egg, whole | 1 large | 70 | 6.3 | 0.4 | 4.0 |
| Egg, white | 1 large | 17 | 3.6 | 0.2 | 0.0 |
| Fish, tuna, chunk light in water | 110 g (4 oz) | 120 | 26 | 0 | 1.0 |
| Fish, Salmon, Atlantic | 110 g (4 oz), raw | 206 | 28.8 | 0 | 9.2 |
| Fish, Sardines (Herring) | 85 g (3 oz) | 150 | 19 | 0 | 8.0 |
| Fish, Cod | 110 g (4 oz), raw | 88 | 20.2 | 0 | 0.8 |
| Fish, Tilapia | 110 g (4 oz), raw | 110 | 23 | 0 | 2.0 |
| Lobster | 110 g (4 oz), raw | 102 | 21.3 | 0.6 | 1.0 |
| Protein powder, whey | 1 scoop (30 g/1 oz) | 110 | 24 | 2 | 1.0 |
| Turkey, ground 99% lean | 110 g (4 oz), raw | 120 | 0 | 0 | 1.0 |
| Turkey Breast, skinless | 110 g (4 oz), raw | 178 | 33.9 | 0 | 3.7 |
| Shrimp | 110 g (4 oz) | 120 | 23 | 1 | 2.0 |

## COMPLEX CARBS (STARCHY)

| Food Item | Qty | Calories | Protein (g) | Carbs (g) | Fat (g) |
|---|---|---|---|---|---|
| Beans, black | 125 g (4½ oz) | 100 | 7 | 20 | 0.5 |
| Beans, chickpeas | 125 g (4½ oz) | 110 | 7 | 19 | 1.5 |
| Black eye peas | 125 g (4½ oz) | 90 | 6 | 16 | 1 |
| Bread, whole wheat | 1 slice (30 g/1 oz) | 100 | 5 | 20 | 1.5 |
| Bread, sprouted (Ezekiel) | 1 slice (30 g/1 oz) | 80 | 4 | 14 | 0.5 |
| Corn | 155 g (5½ oz) | 90 | 2 | 18 | 1 |
| Lentils | 50 g (2 oz) | 150 | 10 | 27 | 1 |
| Oats, rolled, old-fashioned | 40 g (1½ oz) | 150 | 5 | 27 | 3 |
| Oats, steel-cut | 40 g (1½ oz) | 150 | 5 | 27 | 2.5 |
| Peas | 85 g (3 oz) | 60 | 4 | 11 | 0 |
| Potato, sweet | 170 g (6 oz) | 136 | 2.1 | 31.6 | 0.4 |
| Potato, white | 225 g (8oz) | 210 | 4.4 | 49 | 0.2 |
| Pumpkin | 425 g (15 oz) | 175 | 3.5 | 35 | 0 |
| Pita, whole wheat | 55 g (2 oz) | 145 | 6 | 27 | 1.5 |
| Pasta, whole grain spelt | 55 g (2 oz) | 190 | 8 | 40 | 1.5 |
| Pasta, whole wheat | 30 g (1 oz) | 105 | 4.5 | 20 | 1 |

| | | | | | |
|---|---|---|---|---|---|
| Rice, long grain brown | 200 g (7 oz) | 216 | 5 | 44.8 | 1.8 |
| Shredded Wheat | 55 g (2 oz) | 170 | 6 | 40 | 1 |
| Quinoa | 170 g (6 oz) | 156 | 6 | 27.3 | 2.6 |
| Yam | 140 g (5 oz) | 167 | 2.2 | 39.5 | 0.2 |

## DAIRY PRODUCTS

| Food Item | Qty | Calories | Protein (g) | Carbs (g) | Fat (g) |
|---|---|---|---|---|---|
| Milk, skim | 240 ml (8 fl oz) | 90 | 8 | 12 | 0 |
| Milk, 1% lowfat | 240 ml (8 fl oz) | 100 | 8 | 11 | 2 |
| Cheese, fat-free | 2 slices (55 g/2 oz) | 60 | 10 | 4 | 0 |
| Cheese, feta, lowfat | 55 g (2 oz) | 120 | 12 | 0 | 8 |
| Cottage cheese, 1% lowfat | 110 g (4 oz) | 100 | 17.5 | 5 | 1.3 |
| Cottage cheese, nonfat | 110 g (4 oz) | 100 | 16.2 | 7.5 | 0 |
| Cream cheese, nonfat | 2 tbsp (85 g/3 oz) | 30 | 16 | 4 | 2 |
| Sour cream, non fat | 2 tbsp (30 g/1 oz) | 25 | 2 | 4 | 0 |
| Yogurt, fruit, 1% lowfat | 225 g (8 oz) | 250 | 9 | 50 | 2 |
| Yogurt, nonfat | 225 g (8 oz) | 100 | 8 | 17 | 0 |
| Yogrut, Greek fruit | 225 g (8 oz) | 160 | 19 | 14 | 3 |
| Yogurt, Greek, plain | 170 g (6 oz) | 120 | 18 | 7 | 0 |
| Yogurt, Greek, vanilla | 170 g (6 oz) | 120 | 16 | 13 | 0 |

## FRUIT

| Food Item | Qty | Calories | Protein (g) | Carbs (g) | Fat (g) |
|---|---|---|---|---|---|
| Apple | 1 med (155 g/5½ oz) | 80 | 0.0 | 21 | 0 |
| Applesauce, natural | 240 g (8½ oz) | 100 | 0.0 | 26 | 0 |
| Banana | 1 med (130 g/4½ oz) | 110 | 1.0 | 29 | 0 |
| Blueberries | 240 g (5 oz) | 82 | 1.0 | 20.4 | 0.6 |
| Cantaloupe | ½ med (270 g/9½ oz) | 94 | 2.3 | 22.3 | 0.7 |
| Grapefruit | 240 g (5 oz) | 53 | 1.1 | 13.4 | 0.2 |
| Grapes (seedless) | 100 g (3½ oz) | 72 | 0.6 | 17.8 | 0.2 |
| Nectarine | 1 med (240 g/5 oz) | 67 | 1.3 | 16 | 0 |
| Orange | 1 med (240 g/5 oz) | 65 | 1.0 | 16.3 | 0.3 |
| Peach | 1 med (240 g/5 oz) | 59 | 1.0 | 15 | 0 |
| Pear | 1 med (170 g/6 oz) | 100 | 1.0 | 26 | 1 |
| Plum | 1 med (55 g/2 oz) | 30 | 0.0 | 8 | 0 |
| Pineapple | 170 g (6 oz) | 82 | 1 | 22 | 0 |
| Raspberries | 110 g (4 oz) | 60 | 1.0 | 15 | 1 |
| Strawberries | 155 g (5 oz) | 46 | 1.0 | 10.6 | 0 |
| Watermelon (diced) | 155 g (5 oz) | 50 | 1.0 | 11.4 | 0.6 |

## COMPLEX CARBS (FIBROUS)

| Food Item | Qty | Calories | Protein (g) | Carbs (g) | Fat (g) |
|---|---|---|---|---|---|
| Asparagus | 10 spears (185 g/6½ oz) | 40 | 4 | 8 | 0 |
| Broccoli | 85 g (3 oz) | 30 | 2 | 4 | 0 |
| Brussel sprouts | 85 g (3 oz) | 38 | 3 | 7.3 | 0.1 |
| Cabbage | 85 g (3 oz) | 21 | 1 | 5 | 0 |
| Carrots | 1 large (85 g/3 oz) | 31 | 0.7 | 7.3 | 0.1 |
| Cauliflower | 100 g (3½ oz) | 25 | 2 | 5 | 0 |
| Celery | 100 g (3½ oz) | 6 | 0.3 | 1.5 | 0.1 |
| Spring greens | 85 g (3 oz) | 22 | 2.1 | 4.3 | 0 |
| Cucumber | 1 small (170 g/6 oz) | 20 | 2 | 4 | 0 |
| Aubergine | 85 g (3 oz) | 22 | 0.8 | 5 | 0.2 |
| Green beans | 110 g (4 oz) | 33 | 2.6 | 8 | 0 |
| Kale | 70 g (2½ oz) | 34 | 2.2 | 6.8 | 1.4 |
| Lettuce, Romaine | 170 g (6 oz) | 30 | 2 | 6 | 0 |
| Mushrooms | 70 g (2½ oz) | 18 | 2 | 2 | 0.4 |
| Onion | 70 g (2½ oz) | 30 | 0.9 | 6.9 | 0.1 |
| Salsa | 4 tbsp (110 g/4 oz) | 20 | 0 | 5 | 0 |
| Spinach | 85 g (3 oz) | 20 | 2 | 3 | 0 |
| Pepper, green or red | 110 g (4 oz) | 20 | 0.7 | 4.8 | 0.1 |
| Tomato | 1 med (155 g/5 oz) | 25 | 1 | 6 | 0 |
| Courgette | 85 g (3 oz) | 16 | 1.4 | 3.2 | 0.2 |

## FATS

| Food Item | Qty | Calories | Protein (g) | Carbs (g) | Fat (g) |
|---|---|---|---|---|---|
| Almonds | 30 g (1 oz) | 160 | 7 | 6 | 14 |
| Avocado | 100 g (3½ oz) | 161 | 2 | 8.5 | 14.5 |
| Coconut (shredded) | 40 g (1½ oz) | 141 | 1.3 | 6.1 | 13.4 |
| Coconut oil | 1 tbsp | 120 | 0 | 0 | 14 |
| Fish oil (supplement) | 5 softgels (5 g) | 50 | 0 | 0 | 5 |
| Flaxseed Oil (supplement) | 1 tbsp | 130 | 0 | 0 | 13.3 |
| Olives, black, pitted | 10 medium (30 g/1 oz) | 50 | 0 | 2 | 4 |
| Olive oil, extra virgin | 1 tbsp | 120 | 0 | 0 | 13.6 |
| Peanut Butter, natural | 1 tbsp | 95 | 4 | 3 | 8.5 |
| Salad dress, olive oil vinegar | 1 tbsp | 75 | 0 | 0.5 | 8 |
| Salad dress, light balsamic | 2 tbsp | 45 | 0 | 2 | 4 |
| Udo's essential oil blend | 1 tbsp | 134 | 0 | 0 | 14.2 |
| Walnuts | 30 g (1 oz) | 190 | 7 | 3 | 18 |

* All food items are weighed raw or dry (uncooked) unless indicated otherwise

## ACKNOWLEDGEMENTS

*Burn the Fat, Feed the Muscle* has been through many evolutions, and putting this book into a brand-new print edition was a huge team effort. I'd like to express my gratitude to everyone who helped. First, I'd like to thank, once again, Stephen Barbara of Foundry Literary media. Without your support, encouragement, and persistence over a long period of time, this book would not be in our hands in hardcover. Endless thanks to Yfat Reiss-Gendell, also of Foundry Literary. I'm glad you are on our team. And thanks to everyone else at Foundry.

I'm thrilled to have the honour of being published by Random House/Harmony. I'd like to thank everyone who has been involved in every way from start to finish. In particular, I want to thank editor Mary Choteborsky for the amount of time, effort, and creativity put into this project. The improvements in this new version of the book are fantastic, and the new content, improved format, increased user-friendliness, and a lot more can be in large part credited to you.

To Lee Allen Howard: Thank you for your editorial help, not just in this new edition, but through two iterations of the book. Your feedback has helped in many ways, especially in helping make *Burn the Fat, Feed the Muscle* as streamlined as a "bible" of fat loss can be.

Special thanks to: Dr. Chris Mohr, R.D., our go-to guy for registered dietician advice and the nicest guy in the business. Will Brink: the first person to ever promote the early editions of *Burn the Fat, Feed the Muscle* online – your support has always been remembered and appreciated. Christian Finn: Thank you for your outstanding contributions to our field and for supporting *Burn the Fat, Feed the Muscle* all these years. Brad Schoenfeld: I appreciate your work and you generously giving me your time to chat about the science of muscle. I hope this book finally achieves that perfect balance between the science and the art. Alan Aragon: Thanks for your feedback and all the great work in evidence-based fitness. Shawn Phillips: Thanks for keeping us strong and always making us think. Kostas Marangopoulos: Thanks for everything, including being the number one advocate and supporter of *Burn the Fat, Feed the Muscle* and everything it stands for since day one. John Sifferman, Lee Wennerberg, Leigh Peele, and Scott Tousignant: Thanks for your feedback on the new material at various stages of rewriting.

Thank you to the whole *Burn the Fat* online team: webmasters, blogmasters, site managers, admins, assistants, programmers, contributors, guest writers, and challenge judges. Big thanks to Matt Dietz, webmaster extraordinaire: We wouldn't have been online for so many years, without you. Kyle Battis and Dominick Iosca: Thank you for all your support and behind the scenes work. Without you guys, the *Burn the Fat* Challenge would not keep happening. Simon Harrison, blogmaster and jack of all other Internet trades: Thanks for your help so far, and for what is yet to come.

I'm grateful to all our members at the *Burn the Fat* Inner Circle. We have the best, most unique support group in the world; it's like family. I'd like to thank all our *Burn the Fat* challenge winners and hall-of-famers for your participation and congratulate you for your achievements in our *Burn the Fat* events. To our star members: Some of you shine super-bright and burn ultra-hot; you know who you are and you have lit the way for many others. To all of our *Burn the Fat* fans and followers who have shared your transformation success stories: Thank you. You've not only transformed yourselves but also inspired thousands of others through your examples, and you are more influential than you think.

To all our hundreds of thousands of original *Burn the Fat, Feed the Muscle* readers and *Burn the Fat* newsletter subscribers: I thank all of you for your support. I appreciate everyone who posted comments and sent me encouraging e-mails; above all else, your personal messages are what kept me going all these years.

To every affiliate and partner who supported *Burn the Fat* online: Thank you. The next chapter is just beginning and I look forward to continuing to work with you.

To my family: Thank you for supporting all the work I do and how I do it.

And to every new reader of this book who is on the path of lifelong self-improvement: I applaud your commitment and thank you for putting your faith in this programme and in me.

Train hard and expect success,

Tom Venuto

Get all the free tools, exercise demos, worksheets, and downloads for *Burn the Fat, Feed the Muscle* at: http://www.BurnTheFatFeedTheMuscle.com

Join our private (subscription/members-only) community at: http://www.BurnTheFatInnerCircle.com

Join our public *Burn the Fat, Feed the Muscle* fans group on Facebook at: http://www.Facebook.com/burnthefat

Follow *Burn the Fat, Feed the Muscle* author Tom Venuto on Twitter at: http://twitter.com/tomvenuto

Subscribe to and bookmark the official *Burn the Fat* Blog at: http://www.BurnTheFatBlog.com